Guidelines for Pediatric Home Health Care

Section on Home Health Care
American Academy of Pediatrics

Mark S. McConnell, MD, FAAP
Editor

Sonia O. Imaizumi, MD, FAAP
Associate Editor

Section Editors
Allen I. Goldberg, MD, FAAP
Burton Grebin, MD, FAAP
Ronald M. Perkin, MD, FAAP
Arnold Schussheim, MD, FAAP

American Academy of Pediatrics
141 Northwest Point Blvd
Elk Grove Village, IL 60009-0927

Dedication

"Home care will be the next frontier of pediatric practice." This prophetic statement was made by the late Frank Oski, MD, FAAP, who inspired this volume. As a legendary leader of pediatrics in America, Dr Oski encouraged us to pursue our passion for home care and to help others understand the importance of home care.

AAP Department of Marketing and Publications

Maureen DeRosa, Director, Department of Marketing and Publications
Mark Grimes, Director, Division of Product Development
Diane Beausoleil, Senior Product Development Editor
Sandi King, Director, Division of Publishing and Production Services
Jill Rubino, Manager, Editorial Services
Jason Crase, Editorial Specialist
Leesa Levin-Doroba, Manager, Print Production Services
Linda Diamond, Manager, Graphic Design
Peg Mulcahy, Graphic Designer
Jill Ferguson, Director, Division of Marketing and Sales
Linda Smessaert, Manager, Publication and Program Marketing
Natalie Arndt, Department Coordinator

Photo credits:

Figure 18-1 used with permission from American Academy of Pediatrics. *Textbook of Pediatric Education for Prehospital Professionals.* Sudbury, MA: Jones & Bartlett Publishers; 2000

Figures 21-1, 21-2, and 21-3 courtesy of Rani Kathirithamby, MD

Library of Congress Control Number: 2001132027

ISBN: 1-58110-073-6

MA0169

The recommendations in this publication do not indicate an exclusive course of treatment or serve as a standard of medical care. Variations, taking into account individual circumstances, may be appropriate.

Contributors

Marvin E. Ament, MD
Stephen Arpadi, MD
Jean B. Belasco, MD
Judy Bernbaum, MD
Vinod Bhutani, MD
Peter Boling, MD
Sharyn Boyle-King, RNC, BSN, CCM
Danuta Buzdygan, MD
Denise Callarman
Deborah Calvert, MSW, LSW
Constance Cleary, RN
JoAnn D'Agostino, RN, MSN, CPNP
Dennis Deleon, MD
Margaret C. Fisher, MD
Donald E. George, MD
Marsha Gerdes, PhD
Allen I. Goldberg, MD
Bruce P. Himelstein, MD
Nancy Host, MBA
Sonia O. Imaizumi, MD
Beverley H. Johnson
Lois H. Johnson, MD
Rani C. Kathirithamby, MD
Thomas Keens, MD
John Kerner, Jr, MD
Edward Korycka, RN, CRNI, OCN
Lourdes R. Laraya-Cuasay, MD
Linda Larson, MS, RN
Rosemary De Marco Laudani, BSN
Leann Lazzari
Beth Leonberg, MS, RD, CSP
Russell Libby, MD
Karen Ann Lichtenstein, MA

Rachel K. Lockwood, RNC, NNP
Mhairi MacDonald, MBChB, FRCPE, DCH
Carol Marsiglia, RN, BSN, CCM
Mark S. McConnell, MD
Barbara McCord, MS
David Nash, MD, MBA
Fred Y. Nishioka, PharmD
Mark O'Gwynn, RRT, MPH
Alexander Okun, MD
Robert Orr, MD
Howard Panitch, MD
Francine Pasek, RN
Gilbert O. Pereira, MD
Ronald M. Perkin, MD
Robert L. Poole, PharmD
Catherine Prophet, RN, BSN
Denise E. Ramsden, RN
Laurie Reyen
Daniel Robertson, RRT, MBA
Robert J. Rose, MD
Jennifer Rosen, JD, MSW
Tove Rosen, MD
Elizabeth Ruppert, MD
Richard Rutstein, MD
Juliette Schlucter
Ann Schwoebel, MSN, CRNP
Alan Spitzer, MD
Stephanie Storgion, MD
Marion Townsend, RN
Sally L. Davidson Ward, MD
William Wenner, MD
Pamela Wood, MD
Hanna Zafar, MHS, MSII

Foreword

Home care represents one of the traditions of medical practice; sending a patient home has healing results. I frequently tell pediatric residents that the physician can learn more during one house call than from 10 visits to the office. A visit in person provides essential insights into psychosocial, cultural, social, economic, and environmental factors that affect global health of the patient and family.

I have always been a strong believer in and advocate for pediatric home health. As surgeon-in-chief at the Children's Hospital of Philadelphia, I encouraged pioneering work during the 1970s that led to the modern era of home care for infants and children. Home care benefited my patients who were dependent on technology and their families after pediatric surgery in those situations that still required prolonged life-sustaining technology for optimal health, growth, and development. As US surgeon general during the 1980s, I made efforts to increase public awareness and promote public policies to support the development of home care for all children with special needs. As surgeon general, I convened a National Surgeon General's Workshop on the home care of children dependent on a ventilator, believing that if we could master that challenge, other less complicated and risky applications of home care would be less risky and more easily accomplished. More recently, I have given thought to the potential of telemedicine at home and have personally experienced the benefits of home care. I know firsthand that, whenever possible, the home is where patients and their families want to be.

In recent years, there has been major development in and improvement of home care. As the need has grown, so has a home care industry to serve this market. Consequently, home care expenditures have increased and public policies have responded. At the same time, the body of knowledge of home care has grown. Nevertheless, physicians have not been adequately involved and there has been little to encourage them to do so. No curriculum has been formally adopted in medical schools and residency programs to prepare physicians-in-training for their essential roles and responsibilities in home care. Nor have they been adequately taught the need to recognize the risk of home care enterprises moving into the market of pediatric home care without comprehension of the unique problems of child growth and development in home care. The American Academy of Pediatrics (AAP) should be congratulated on its efforts to enhance the practicing physician's awareness of and knowledge about home care by support of the activities of the Section on Home Health. Its initiatives have provided pediatricians ways to learn about the realities of home care to help them integrate it into their practices. The depth and breadth of the guidelines herein developed fill an enormous pediatric need.

The growth of home care continues to present challenges for new opportunities along with additional risks. Home care requires a knowledge of what is medically necessary, an understanding of the unique situations facing children with special needs, and an adequate commitment of resources. In addition, there is need for promotion of physician involvement. This will only happen with physician education. The AAP *Guidelines for Pediatric Home Health Care* will be a major step in this direction. Readers have an opportunity to develop the insight and knowledge to ensure that children will receive proper care in the home and that payers recognize that home care services are an essential component of the continuum of care. Hopefully, more pediatricians will get involved with the delivery of home care services to their young patients and experience the joy of this tradition of medicine.

C. Everett Koop, MD, ScD

Preface

Pediatric home health care began in the 1970s when children dependent on technology were sent home from intensive care units where they had no option but to "live" for months or even years. In 1982, home care became a possible alternative to long-term hospitalization for all children with chronic disabilities as a result of the 1982 Surgeon General's Workshop convened by C. Everett Koop, MD, ScD, FAAP, in collaboration with Merle McPherson, MD, FAAP, and the late Vince Hutchins, MD, FAAP, US Public Health Service, Division of Maternal and Child Health.

In a landmark 1993 conference, "Home-Based Care for a New Century," then-administrator of the Health Care Financing Administration (HCFA) (now Centers for Medicare and Medicaid Services [CMS]), Bruce Vladeck, PhD, stated that home care has been the fastest growing public expenditure of health care in America. He further stated that pediatrics was its fastest growing segment. This growth was attributed to earlier patient discharges because of lower prospective reimbursement for hospitalized patients and managed care pressures, increased survival of infants at high risk and other children dependent on technology, and improved quality of life of children with special needs because of chronic illness or disability. As a consequence, increasingly complex patients were being discharged sooner from the hospital to home. The home now represents an accepted alternative site to hospital care and an extension of office-based practice.

At the same 1993 keynote address, Dr Vladeck expressed concern that home care requires direct physician involvement, yet, at that time, physicians were not educated or trained to provide pediatric home health care. The American Academy of Pediatrics (AAP) Section on Home Health was formed to bring together a diverse group of pediatricians and other health care professionals whose goals are to increase the knowledge base of pediatric home care, improve the quality of care for children in the home, and promote the use of home care among pediatricians. Since its inception, the Section on Home Health has undertaken a variety of projects to meet these goals, such as regularly inviting experts to conduct educational programs at national AAP meetings and developing a resident training curriculum (see Appendices). However, the section soon realized that to further promote the understanding and appropriate use of home care, developing guidelines for practicing pediatricians had to become a priority. The section then sought AAP support and obtained approval for its educational endeavor.

The AAP Section on Home Health proudly presents to interested health care professionals these guidelines for pediatric home health care. The Section on Home Health was formed in 1994 to serve the AAP as a resource for its members and others who seek information about caring for patients at home. The authors of this manual, who were invited by the editors and the Executive Committee of the Section on Home Health to contribute, will guide your understanding of pediatric home care based on their years of extensive experience.

These guidelines focus sharply on a future vision. We share a core value that the optimal health of children and families improves when physicians provide care in the home setting. Our authors have had first-hand experience providing or facilitating pediatric home care. They realize that home care will play a major role in the future of pediatric practice and that no standards exist to guide all interested parties in understanding or establishing safe, medically necessary, family-centered home care for pediatric patients.

Guidelines for Pediatric Home Health Care addresses most of the issues physicians and other caregivers face in managing the care of children in the home. The principles and practices promoted in these guidelines will be helpful to the physician establishing a medical home for children with a variety of special needs. No matter what your role in caring for children in the home, you will benefit from these guidelines. This manual was written to help you integrate home care into your practice; to assist your involvement as a leader or participant in home care activities such as academic programs, organization, delivery, finance, or public policy; and simply to educate you on what home health care is all about. Because home health care is a team effort of diverse professionals, with parents as partners, the authors represent a broad spectrum of viewpoints.

Although very little had been written about pediatric home care in the past, the editors were delighted to find that pediatric nurses and other health care professionals were pursing similar projects independently. The section was fortunate that these professionals were willing to contribute their work, knowledge, and resources to this manual from the AAP. Such collaboration has given these guidelines a broader, more realistic, and practical focus that will undoubtedly appeal to those in many health care disciplines and other interested readers.

Because little evidence-based research exists in the growing field of pediatric home care, addressing issues with an entirely evidence-based approach, in its strictest sense, was not feasible in this manual. As a result, the editors compiled a series of best-practice guidelines written by experts in the pediatric home health field. Whenever possible, each author has annotated his or her chapter with relevant medical literature, which is listed in the bibliography of each chapter.

This manual is organized into five parts. Part One, Organization of Pediatric Home Health Care, provides an overview of pediatric home care and discusses the past, present, and future of pediatric home health. Also covered are home care delivery models, technology, funding, and family-centered and family-directed models of pediatric home care. Part Two, Guidelines for Pediatric Home Health Care Programs, establishes guidelines for a variety of home care treatment programs, including infusion, parenteral and enteral feeding, chemotherapy, antibiotic therapy, pain management, and durable medical equipment including phototherapy. Also addressed are the uses of assistive technology in home care, transporting children who are medically fragile, and acquiring durable medical equipment. Part Three, Disease-Management Programs, applies the guidelines set forth in the previous part as they relate to specific pediatric medical conditions, eg, using enteral feedings in short-bowel syndrome, caring for children who require mechanical ventilation, and caring for children with human immunodeficiency virus infection. Case management and home care programs for infants who are socially at risk are also covered in Part Three. Part Four, Other Considerations for Pediatric Home Health Care, deals with universal home health care issues such as ethics, quality assurance, infection control, out-of-home child care and medical day treatment programs, and home visits by physicians. Part Five contains Appendices that include helpful tools to promote effective pediatric home care, including the Home Health Care Curriculum for Residents in Pediatrics, the Emergency Information Form for Children With Special Needs, and a self-assessment inventory on family-centered care for home care agencies.

The manual is designed to be a practical reference for use by health care professionals from many disciplines who have an interest in pediatric home care. We hope that this manual will serve as a catalyst for the design of outcome-focused research studies to improve the quality of care and services provided to children who are cared for in the home.

In closing, we must credit the leadership of the Executive Committee of the AAP Section on Home Health, our manual section editors, and our authors for sharing our vision to develop a vitally needed resource like this. We would also like to thank the AAP Board of Directors and its support staff, including Diane Beausoleil, Teri Salus, Maureen DeRosa, and others, for their diligent work in making this project a reality. We would especially like to recognize the important efforts of Susan Aronson, MD, FAAP; F. Lane France, MD, FAAP; and Gilbert Buchanan, MD, FAAP, for their extensive review of the entire manuscript. We sincerely hope that this manual will improve the knowledge and quality of health care for all children at home with their families where they belong.

Mark S. McConnell, MD, FAAP, Editor
Sonia O. Imaizumi, MD, FAAP, Associate Editor

Bibliography

Oski F. No place like home. *Contemp Pediatr.* September 1992:7

Vladeck BC. Keynote address. In: *Home-Based Care for a New Century.* Harriman, NY: Arden House; 1993

Table of Contents

Chapter 30

**Guidelines for Home Management and
Phototherapy for Neonatal Hyperbilirubinemia**

Chapter 31

Apnea and Home Cardiorespiratory Monitoring

Chapter 35

Quality Improvement in Pediatric Home Care 463

PART ONE

Organization of Pediatric Home Health Care

Chapter 1

History of Pediatric Home Health Care

Allen Goldberg, MD

Prehospital Era: From Colonial Times to the 21st Century

Physician involvement in pediatric home care has strong traditional roots in the United States. In the earliest years, the customary site for providing child care for acute illness or chronic disability was the home. Only those without the economic means required institutions. Middle- and upper-class families converted bedrooms into sick rooms, babies were delivered at home, and relatively uncomplicated surgery was conducted at home.

Even families living in poverty had options other than an institution. Indigent families could access home care services organized by religious orders and secular groups. The Boston, MA, home nursing service was established in 1796. By the end of the 19th century, visiting nurse associations (VNAs) supported by philanthropy provided most home care in the United States.

Early Hospital Era

The modern hospital era began with late 19th- and early 20th-century advances of asepsis, anesthesia, surgery, and medical technology responsive to wartime needs. Such advances allowed safe and efficient diagnosis and treatment not possible at home. Facilities were designed according to modern industrial processes and organizational principles, making it feasible to justify their capital and operational expenses. Hospitals could afford to buy and use expensive medical technologies and doctors sought hospitals that gave access to these technologies. It became easier for pediatricians to see and manage patients in the hospital than at home.

Although the hospital became the site for treating serious illness, most families preferred care at home with self- or family-provided care supplemented by privately funded VNAs. World War II stimulated more demand for community-based care, and physicians were actively making house calls in the 1950s.

Precritical Care Era: Post-Polio Experience

▸ The First Generation of Children Dependent on Technology

The polio epidemic stimulated the organization of special respiratory care units (the precursor of intensive care units [ICUs]) and the development of long-term mechanical ventilation by negative pressure (eg, tank/iron lung, cuirass). High mortality from bulbar polio with negative-pressure ventilation encouraged development of modern upper airway management by tracheostomy and positive-pressure mechanical ventilation. Patient care was provided by an interdisciplinary team of physicians, nurses, and therapists (the precursor of the modern critical care team).

Many infants' and children's lives were extended by these new methods of organizing the care team and new life-saving technologies. However, a small number of children became dependent on technology to sustain their lives. Some of the families of these patients, working with their health team, participated in the first home mechanical ventilation procedure. Care was arranged to be provided at home by family members, along with professionals, personal care attendants, and equipment/supplies under the funding and service auspices of the National Foundation for Infantile Paralysis (later called the March of Dimes).

The Critical Care Era

▸ The Second Generation of Children Dependent on Technology

Origin and Design of High-Technology Home Care

In the United States, successful research to prevent polio resulted in mass immunization and the near total eradication of the disease. With a few exceptions in public hospitals, the polio special respiratory care centers were discontinued and professionals with expertise evolved the practices of rehabilitation, neonatology, and pediatric critical care medicine. The few polio patients dependent on ventilators at home were unknown to younger physicians-in-training.

Neonatologists and pediatric intensivists soon faced a second generation of children assisted by ventilators. These few patients survived acute illness because of modern advances in pediatric medicine, surgery, and anesthesia, but required prolonged use of life-sustaining technologies. Such children were living in ICUs without institutional or community-based alternatives. Their presence critically limited regional ICU capacity designed for more acute life-threatening conditions. Bed shortages resulted in the turning away of life-threatening emergencies and cancellation of life-saving surgeries.

The Katie Beckett Story: Origin of the Medicaid Waiver

The critical care era led to the development of an ICU-based interdisciplinary team approach to home mechanical ventilation and the coordination of a discharge process involving ICU and community providers, payers, and parents. This management approach later evolved further after an Iowa family with a child dependent on medical ventilation was visiting Children's Memorial Hospital in Chicago, IL, during the initial home care discharge of a similar child in Illinois. The Cedar Rapids family and the pediatrician attempted to bring about a similar discharge at home without success because of restrictive Iowa Medicaid policy. The resourceful mother, Julie Beckett, contacted key local political leaders with access to the White House. At the time, President Ronald Reagan sought examples of how government bureaucracy intruded into and limited family life. Vice President George Bush gave him an excellent example, which the president made public with his mandate to send Katie Beckett home. Katie did go home by Christmas 1981, as an exception to (waiver from) Medicaid regulations.

Public Policy Formulation: From the Surgeon General's Workshop to the Department of Health and Human Services (HHS)/Office of Technology Assessment (OTA) Task Force

The president of the United States creates a crisis by making a public example of a situation like that facing the Beckett family and mandating an action by presidential decree. Public programs must respond for future public policy formulation. The Waxman Committee (Health and Environment Subcommittee of the House Commerce Committee) had to determine subsequent congressional action. Department of Health and Human Services (HHS) Secretary Schweiker appointed the Katie Beckett Ad Hoc Task Force with a similar charge for the administration. They both were concerned with the potential for unlimited financial exposure for the government because of the unmet needs of similar children with special needs that could benefit from home care. They considered this catastrophic cost to the government because these cases would "come out of the woodwork" (the "woodwork effect").

The final proposal authorized finite numbers of community-based waivers from Medicaid policy by a process of individual state application and with approval by the Health Care Financing Administration. In October 1982, C. Everett Koop, MD, FAAP, convened a Surgeon General's Workshop ("Children with Handicaps and Their Families — Case Example: The Ventilator-Dependent Child") in an effort to bring together all sectors and represent all essential stakeholders in developing programs and formulating public policy for children dependent on technology *and* children with special needs. This was the beginning of several public policy initiatives that focused on the needs of the large population of children with chronic disease or disability who required community-based services. Included were studies by the US Congress, Office of Technology Assessment (OTA) ("Technology-Dependent Children: Hospital vs Home Care") and the HHS Secretary's Ad Hoc Task Force on Technology-Dependent Children ("Fostering Home and Community-Based Care for Technology-Dependent Children").

The Managed Care Era

▶ The Initial Phase: Negotiation With Commercial Insurance and Initial Case Management

In early pediatric home care experience, catastrophic-cost home care had no precedent or policy. Thus, every case required individualized, coordinated financial planning with negotiation with public and/or private funding sources. When confronted with huge financial liability for institutional care, private insurance companies saw an advantage of using funds *that were already committed by contract* to be applied to well-designed home care on an individual case-by-case basis. Private insurers responded to cost shifting (increasing private insurance claims made to offset public funding inadequacies during the era of cost-plus reimbursement) by establishing catastrophic long-term care case management. These case managers and their medical directors usually were approachable and amenable to well-conceived and designed home care plans. During this early period, there was no public policy (prior to Katie Beckett). However, public authorities were payers of institutional care after private insurance ran out. Thus, it was possible for pediatricians to work with Title V (Crippled Children's Services [CCS]) and Title XIX (Medicaid) medical directors and initiate innovative home care programs to offset institutional care that was or would become obliged under Medicaid.

▶ Current Situation: Case Management, Cost Containment, and Quality Management

As managed care organizations have increased their market penetration, more high-technology home care has required managed care negotiations. As most contracts are determined by employer preferences, parents working with employers and physicians working with managed care medical directors have negotiated home care arrangements. Such arrangements have required catastrophic cost management with attention to cost containment and quality management. Collaborative arrangement with family involvement has led to innovative home care programs with enormous cost savings for managed care organizations. However, most recent public funding and managed care policies have been restrictive, leading to enormous payment denials and delays discouraging pediatric home care service delivery.

Current Realities and Future Expectations

Current and future organization of pediatric home care must reflect several trends in global health care delivery. Pediatric home care must be considered one component of integrated health care delivery systems and community health networks. It must be reimbursed as one system cost in a more global contractual relationship with public and private payers sharing the financial risk.

Services must be managed with computerized information systems that integrate physician, clinical, and administrative functions and permit coordination of services across the care continuum (acute, subacute, long-term).

Services must be managed with computerized information systems that integrate physician, clinical, and administrative functions and permit coordination of services across the care continuum (acute, subacute, long-term). Physicians must embrace interactive communication technologies that enable them to make diagnoses and therapeutic decisions with devices designed for home use. Physicians must have access to information networks and share management decisions with families at home. This is what informed families will expect and demand.

Bibliography

Aday LA, Aitken MJ, Wegener DH. *Pediatric Home Care: Results of a National Evaluation of Programs for Ventilator Assisted Children.* Chicago, IL: Pluribus Press; 1988

Engström CG. Treatment of severe cases of respiratory paralysis by the Engström universal respirator. *Brit M J.* 1954;2:666-669

Fostering Home and Community-based Care for Technology-Dependent Children: Report to Congress and the Secretary by the Task Force on Technology-Dependent Children. Baltimore, MD: US Dept of Health and Human Services, Health Care Financing Administration; 1988. Publication HCFA 88-02171

Ginsberg E, Balinsky W, Ostow M. What the literature reveals. In: *Home Care: Its Role in the Changing Health Services Market.* Totowa, NJ: Rowman and Allanheld; 1984:6-41

Goldberg AI. Home care for a better life for ventilator-dependent people. *Chest.* 1983;84:365-366

Goldberg AI. Outcomes of home care for life-supported persons: long-term oxygen and prolonged mechanical ventilation [comment]. *Chest.* 1996;109:741-749

Goldberg AI. Pediatric high-technology homecare. In: Rothkopf MM, Askanazi J, eds. *Intensive Homecare.* Baltimore, MD: William & Wilkins; 1992:199-213

Goldberg AI. The regional approach to home care for life-supported persons. *Chest.* 1984;86:345-346

Goldberg AI, Faure E, Vaughn C, Snarksi R, Seleny F. Home care for life-supported persons — an approach to program development. *J Pediatr.* 1984;104:785-795

Goldberg AI, Kettrick R, Buzdygan D, Lis E, Schraeder B, Vaughn C. Home ventilation program for infants and children [abstract]. *Crit Care Med.* 1980;8:238

Goldberg AI, Noah Z, Fleming M, et al. Quality of care for life-supported children who require prolonged mechanical ventilation at home. *QRB Qual Rev Bull.* 1987;13:81-88

Goldberg AI, Trubitt MJ. An integrated approach to home health care. *Physician Exec.* 1994;20:45-46

Keenan JM, Boling PE, Schwartzberg JG, et al. A national survey of home visiting practice and attitudes of family physicians and internists. *Arch Intern Med.* 1992;152:2025-2032

Koop CE. *Report on the Surgeon General's Workshop on Children With Handicaps and Their Families. Case-Example: the Ventilator-Dependent Child.* Washington, DC: US Maternal and Child Health; 1983. Publication PHS 83-50194

Kristensen HS, Neukirch F. Very long-term artificial ventilation (28 years). In: Rattenborg CC, Via Reque E, eds. *Clinical Use of Mechanical Ventilation.* Chicago, IL: Yearbook; 1981:209-221

Lis EF, Goldberg AI, Monahan CA, Murphy KE, and the Children's Home Health Network of Illinois (CHHNI). *Pediatric Home Ventilation: a Model of Discharge and Home Planning.* Rockville, MD: US Dept of Health and Human Services, Public Health Service, Maternal and Child Health; 1987. Publication MC5172262

Make BJ, Hill NS, Goldberg AI, et al. Mechanical ventilation beyond the intensive care unit. Report of a consensus conference of the American College of Chest Physicians [comment]. *Chest.* 1998;114:1794-1795; May 113 (5 Suppl):289S-344S

Rehabilitation Institute of Chicago. *What Ever Happened to the Polio Patients?: Proceedings of an International Symposium.* Chicago, IL: Rehabilitation Institute of Chicago; 1982

US Congress, Office of Technology Assessment. *Technology-Dependent Children: Hospital vs Home Care — a Technical Memorandum.* Washington, DC: US Government Printing Office; 1987

Chapter 2

Present and Future of Pediatric Home Health Care

Hanna Zafar, MHS, MSII; David Nash, MD, MBA

Introduction

More than 40 years ago, when authorities caught up with the million-dollar bank robber Willy Sutton and asked why he robbed banks, he replied, "Because that's where the money is." Today, the same logic is applied to answer, "Why bring pediatric health care into the home?" — because that is where the children are. Home health care was the fastest-growing division of personal health care spending in the United States in the early 1990s. While much of this growth was because of the increased use of home care services among the elderly, the former Health Care Financing Administration (HCFA) (now the Centers for Medicare and Medicaid Services [CMS]) Administrator Bruce Vladeck designated pediatrics as the fastest growing segment within home health care.

Recent medical advances not only have saved and extended the lives of infants and children, but also have made the home a viable site for delivery of care to medically fragile and chronically ill children who are often dependent on technology.

This chapter describes the three major players in the current model of pediatric home care — patients, providers, and payers — and closes with a summary of the key issues facing pediatric home health care in the future.

Patients: Who Are These Children?

▶ Diagnoses

Current home care services span the spectrum of health care services from outreach and education programs to infusion therapy and technology-dependent life support. One way to define home care is to use three dimensions: time (acute, intermediate, long-term); need for support (none, intermittent, continuous); and technology (none, low, high). A sampling of home care services includes the following: intravenously administered medication; parenteral nutrition; nasogastric or enterostomy feedings; peritoneal dialysis; oxygen administration; ventilator support; physiologic monitoring; bilirubin therapy; and physical, occupational, and speech therapies for developmental needs.

The wide range of therapies administered in the home is reflective of the broad array of primary diagnoses under which children are admitted to home care. A recent study analyzing data from the 1994 National Home and Hospice Care Survey found that the three most common diagnoses of children receiving home care were cerebral palsy, lack of expected physiologic development, and preterm births. However, when combined, these diagnoses accounted for only 15% of the pediatric home care population; and, although many home care recipients remain dependent on technology, closer analysis shows that the majority of pediatric home care patients are chronically ill but not dependent on technology (eg, cerebral palsy and Down syndrome). Accordingly, intermittent care, consisting of one or more visits per week, accounts for more than 90% of home care visits versus continuous care consisting of 8- to 12-hour shift care.

While such statistics illustrate the diversity of severity, complications, and diseases these children present to the home care provider, the underlying diagnosis for the majority of the children is preterm birth and its associated sequelae (respiratory, cardiac, and feeding problems). Among infants receiving home care, the 1994 National Home and Hospice Care Survey data show that two of the three most common diagnoses are related to perinatal conditions. This age group characteristically uses a larger volume of home health services because of the high costs associated with care (the average cost of caring for a low-birth-weight infant in a neonatal intensive care unit [NICU] is $72,000). Estimated savings of $20,000 per case after transitioning these children from the NICU into the home make home health an attractive option to payers. Even among older pediatric age groups, chronic and developmental conditions, including cerebral palsy and mental retardation, likely are associated with preterm birth.

Examination of the epidemiology surrounding preterm birth reveals a clustering of social risk factors, namely low socioeconomic status and single marital status, as well as decreased education levels and poor compliance. Such issues pose additional challenges to delivering home health care to this population beyond operational hurdles.

▶ Access

Addressing social barriers is a top priority to the home health care provider who must work with families to effectively care for the patient. Agencies may have to arrange for escorts to accompany nurses into neighborhoods, communicate with families that have no phone, or treat a child in a home that has no hot running water. Access into the home is an invaluable tool for identifying root causes of poor compliance that may not be apparent during an office visit. A visit to a child who fails to thrive may reveal a lack of formula in the home or an overwhelmed mother. For the home health nurse, the goal is not simply to treat an illness but to treat the physical and emotional needs of the child and the family. Agencies should be able to educate parents on what public assistance programs are available to their children and how to better care for themselves, in addition to training parents on how to care for the child.

Many children with a chronic illness are not physically able to get to the doctor's office because of transportation or other logistical reasons. Children whose parents are not able to go to a physician's office cannot receive health care. At St Mary's Hospital for Children in Bayside, NY, home health nurses drive out to visit children through a Vehicular Access to Neighborhoods program. "We can reach kids who can't otherwise receive services…[at a] less expensive cost and using a more appropriate venue," said Bert Grebin, MD, president and chief executive officer of St Mary's Hospital for Children, which receives 65% of its revenue from home care and community outreach programs. Through philanthropic support, the program employs four vans with drivers to escort providers into unsafe areas and stay with the vans while services are delivered.

Children in rural areas face additional barriers because of their geographic distribution and presentation of rare, complex diagnoses to home health providers. Many patients are discharged from urban tertiary care centers into the charge of local physicians and nurses. As such, children may be located in counties without access to appropriately trained pediatric home health providers. Even in those areas where acute care pediatric nurses are available, the scattered location of children across a county may allow a nurse to travel to only a few patients each day. The distance between children in rural areas and appropriately trained providers in large tertiary care centers demands that local physicians and home health nurses be educated on treatment plans and therapies for every child.

To ensure continuity of care, rural home health nurses may travel to a hospital and train for specific cases involving new surgical procedures and uncommon diseases. While inefficient, this is the best model of care to fit the needs of these children today. Future models of care for isolated children will be improved further through the increased use of telemedicine. Telemedicine may save money and increase safety for families between physician visits through immediate physician and nurse contact. While technology does not replace hands-on care, it may expedite physician decision making.

▶ Funding

Navigation of existing services and funding undoubtedly is one of the toughest challenges in caring for the multiple clinical, social, and educational needs of this pediatric population. Difficulties exist in coordinating pediatric home care for all socioeconomic groups. However, recent unbundling of services among public assistance programs has increased problems with access to available services, such as home care, among poor populations. The removal of ties between programs like Medicaid and Aid to Families with Dependent Children (AFDC) likely will deny insurance to eligible children with special needs for available services, including home care and medical day care (*see* Chapter 37).

▶ Ethical Issues

Increasingly, the home has become an accepted environment to care for children with illnesses that previously required hospitalization. The success of technology in saving and extending the lives of these children has surpassed the expectation of health care professionals, families, and payers. As these children progress, their diagnoses and capabilities change. According to a recent study supported by the Agency for Healthcare Research and Quality (AHRQ), more than 40% of extremely small (with birth weights of 800 g or less) and premature newborns (born at 26 weeks of gestation or earlier) are expected to survive. However, approximately one in every five of these infants has a major neuro-developmental disorder such as cerebral palsy, mental retardation, blindness, or deafness.

Given the chronic needs of many of these children, the cost benefit of home health care depends greatly on whose perspective is adopted. This population consumes a high portion of resources in proportion to its numbers. Payers may see the increased savings that can be achieved through home care and want to discharge more children into this setting. A payer's economic motivation may not result in the best clinical outcome for these children. Cost-effective discharge of patients into the home essentially may be a cost shifting of the burden of care to the family.

Although home care will not always be the most cost-effective care option, it is desirable from the patient perspective. Home care may provide minimally lower rehospitalization rates, and improve social and cognitive development and the quality of life for patients. Given the societal preference to treat children in the home environment, there would seem to be a call for further research into such questions as when it is appropriate to treat these children at home and when other environments, such as pediatric long-term care facilities, are more suitable.

▶ Respite Care

Respite care programs allow parents and caregivers to take a weekend or week-long break from caring for children who are chronically ill. The number of existing programs and the variability in payer coverage for this service, contrasted with the number of children admitted to home care, calls into question the capability of existing systems to address the comprehensive needs of caregivers. In the long-term, there is a need to develop extended services and ensure quality of life for the expanding population of children who are chronically ill and their families. Such services include medical day care, respite facilities, long-term pediatric facilities, day schools for children with special needs, school-based health centers, bereavement camps, and domestic abuse prevention programs for siblings, and hospice and palliative care facilities.

▶ Family Issues

Expanded programs become necessary as families attempt to handle the burden of care that is shifted from the well-staffed and resource-rich hospital to the home. Earlier discharge of perinatal and neonatal children increases family stress and expenses. The primary goal of home care is to discharge the child from the agency with sufficient patient/family knowledge for early detection of problems and appropriate follow-up. However, little research has been done on what level of training should be acquired by caregivers before discharging children home. More important questions are: (1) how much burden can be shifted onto these families? and (2) how realistic is it to expect families to become medical providers? If both parents need to work outside the home to support the cost of their child, who will provide the care inside the home to meet the needs of the child? Given the social burden many of these families face, every child may not have a caregiver capable of assuming responsibility for home care.

▶ Patient Population

Currently there are no available national statistics addressing growth among the pediatric population with special needs over the next 5 to 10 years. Predictions on home care demand are confounded further by uncertainty about the exact number of children using services and children eligible for

...increasing numbers of referrals into home care lead experts to believe there will be overall growth in the pediatric home care population.

services. Recent statistics reflecting increasing numbers of premature births point to increasing numbers of children eligible for home care. Despite these unknowns, most agencies are preparing to increase services across the board, citing two underlying trends. First, as mentioned previously, advances in technology not only have saved and extended lives that previously would have been lost, but also have made home care a practical option. Second, cost-conscious payers now are transitioning children out of the decreasing numbers of hospital beds and into step-down units or the home setting more frequently. Retention of the existing patients as well as increasing numbers of referrals into home care lead experts to believe there will be overall growth in the pediatric home care population.

Institutions: Who Is Providing Care?

While some agencies, such as those affiliated with children's hospitals, specialize in pediatric home care, some other large agencies have a pediatric specialty division in addition to adult home care services. Smaller agencies employ a more generalized model where staff serve pediatric and adult patients. Depending on the specialization of agency staff, different levels of service are offered. Agencies may focus on intermittent or visit-based care, including nursing and custodial home health aide, in addition to therapy (physical, occupational, and speech) and medical social work. During these visits, nurses focus on assessment, intervention, and patient/family teaching. Alternatively, the agency also may provide continuous or private duty nursing, which offers 8- to 12-hour shift care for the entire day or while caregivers work or sleep. Additional services, which are often subcontracted by smaller agencies, include pharmacy infusion services and respiratory/durable medical equipment (DME). Enteral and parenteral infusion therapy include a pharmacist and dietician, in addition to the nurses who provide patient care and caregiver teaching. The DME services, including oxygen, nebulizers, apnea monitors, beds, commodes, and wheelchairs, require a respiratory therapist to assist with equipment setup and maintenance.

▶ Staffing

Typically, agencies will have registered nurses (RNs), licensed practical nurses (LPNs), home health aides (HHAs), therapists (physical, occupational, and speech), medical social workers, psychologists, and dieticians on staff or accessible through subcontracts. Diminished availability of trained home health nurses has become one of the greatest hurdles agencies must contend with in delivering care. The average age of all RNs in 1996 was 44.3 years. Given declining enrollment in nursing schools, this points to a significant decrease in nursing staff as a large number of RNs retire over the next 15 years. Such decreases are not unique to RNs; they also have been seen in LPNs and HHAs. At the same time, the Bureau of Labor Statistics has predicted that the percentage of home health RNs will rise from 5.95% in 1994 to 10.8% in 2005.

In the face of these statistics, agencies have begun to assume some responsibility for training staff in pediatric care. The investment in completely training a nurse in pediatric home care may not be effective, however. In the home health care environment, many field nurses work on a per diem basis, contracting with several agencies and receiving work as needed. Training becomes a misuse of time and resources for agencies because of the unpredictable volume of cases. Once a nurse is trained, he or she already may be employed by another agency.

Perhaps the greatest advantage a hospital system-based home care agency has is the use of hospital nurses in home care services. Hospital nurses offer a flexible workforce that potentially is the greatest asset an agency can possess in this dynamic field. Subcontracting for hospital-employed pediatric nurses who already receive benefits through the hospital can lower agency costs. More importantly, physicians feel comfortable making referrals for home care because they are comfortable with the competency level of the nurses they work with.

▶ Admission to Home Care

Referrals for home care mainly come from local hospitals and payers but also may come from community physicians and families themselves. Case management of children usually falls to a designated agency home care nurse after physician referral is made and approval of services is received from the child's payer. Prior to discharge, the case manager or primary care nurse will review the plan of treatment with the discharging physician and perform predischarge teaching with the family. Part of this teaching involves an initial home visit to check logistical details, such as rewiring for medical equipment, as well as identification of a secure caregiver.

Two of the greatest challenges in pediatric home health are caregiver training and coordination between service agencies and providers. On the operations side, case managers will coordinate agency services (therapy and social work), subcontracted services (pharmacy infusion or DME), as well as child life specialists. On the clinical side, communication between different home care providers also is coordinated through the case manager. Progress reports on visits made to the child (respiratory therapist or RN) are given to the primary care nurse, who is responsible for calling the physician as needed. In an effort to ensure quality of care, children's charts are reviewed approximately every month during weekly case manager meetings — although this is not an industry standard.

▶ Physician Involvement

The role of physicians in home care has not been well defined to date. Although pediatricians are responsible for initiating, supervising, and terminating home care for these children, their level of involvement ranges across the board. It is thought that the marginal role of most physicians in pediatric home care is because of lack of guidelines on home care, poor reimbursement, and inadequate education on what home care entails.

At present, there is a dearth of organized research on both established selection criteria for home care patients and clinical home care guidelines linked to positive outcomes. Although there have been some studies that have linked home care criteria with outcomes, physicians are asked to discharge children into the home with little or no information about specific outcomes research. The litigious environment of health care leaves physicians caught between clinical care and financial realities.

Reimbursement

Reimbursement also remains an obstacle to physician participation as part of the multidisciplinary team caring for home care children. Although *Current Procedural Terminology (CPT)* codes are available for home care services, they are not commensurate with the time and effort that physicians put into managing these children. So while many of these children, particularly those who are chronically ill and dependent on technology, would benefit from collaborative management of the primary care pediatrician, they are not receiving such attention uniformly.

Education

In addition to operational and financial disincentives to entering home care, education is another barrier from the physician's perspective. There is no standardized home health exposure during clerkship and residency training. Practicing physicians may not be aware of available home care techniques and therapies. Home care involvement ranges from discharge planning to case management via interactive telecommunications. Usually, home care does not require direct delivery of care but supervision of other care providers. However, a home visit is important when you have a complex patient who is dependent on technology with high resource needs at home.

Given appropriate education on, and input in, operational design, home care could represent a growth segment for some pediatricians. The home care nurse needs access to physicians who are able to deal with issues like disease management, payment, coordination of DME, and educating families. Physician involvement will have to increase to effectively advocate to payers that skilled nursing services are necessary for certain children. The door is open for collaborative research between community physicians, faculty at academic medical centers, home health agencies, and payers into the development of cost-effective and health-promoting criteria for home care of children with special needs.

▶ Continuity of Care

Continuity of care for home health patients across multiple services and providers remains a challenge. Providers face a number of logistical barriers to obtaining information once children are released into the home environment. While agencies scramble to coordinate services across multiple settings, the nursing shortage has created additional barriers to home care. First, the seasonal nature of home care nursing does not always permit the same one, or even two, nurses to care for a single child. Therefore, care of children frequently is fragmented with reeducation of nurses about a specific case occurring often. Second, nurses hired by many agencies do not always have adequate pediatric acute care experience to be knowledgeable about when to call in a physician and how to communicate effectively with other ancillary staff. These issues create more disincentives for physicians to discharge children home.

Information Technology

Some issues can be addressed through improved information systems. Most field nurses use cellular phones or fax machines to communicate with agency case managers or physicians. While timely, these techniques do not document clinical data or communicate information across the home, laboratory, and physician's office in an organized, easily accessible manner. Information systems offer additional solutions to case managers charged with communicating children's progress to payers. Often, as children progress during home care visitation, their needs and capabilities change accordingly. Active involvement is required of the agency case manager to monitor patient progress and document the need for skilled nursing services to payers versus less costly custodial care. As technology advances and field staff are able to capture clinical data at the bedside, outcomes tracking will be facilitated greatly among the home care population.

This level of sophisticated technology comes at a cost for most agencies. The lack of standardized data collection requirements for accreditation can be discussed only after the development of pediatric-specific software combining financial and clinical data. Currently, most agencies track financial data by comparing charges to collection by individual payer and breaking out costs among treatment categories. A few agencies have invested in customized software with the capability to break down costs by patient and diagnosis, but such detailed analysis remains the exception. Others agencies rely on individual piecemeal systems to address pharmacy or finance reports, leaving clinical data still very much paper based.

▶ Clinical Protocols and Outcomes

Home health agencies are attempting to improve information flow across multiple providers, and clinical protocols and outcomes tracking lend themselves well to this effort. The variety of diagnoses among the pediatric home care population has led many agencies to shy away from developing clinical protocols, excluding large, well-researched populations, such as patients with asthma. However, the repetitive nature of continuous care and larger clusters of diagnostic groupings merit guideline development when appropriate.

The smaller margin of error when treating children necessitates the use of protocols in the home, debatably more than in the hospital. The need for protocols is magnified further in the home environment where home care providers work relatively unsupervised. In the hospital environment, mistakes may be seen by another provider and corrected in a timely manner. In the home, protocols can help compensate for this lost quality control. Written guidelines not only help nurses by outlining their responsibilities, but assist families by clarifying what to expect from home visits.

Evaluating Outcomes

With regard to outcomes, most agencies still are tracking crude indicators such as hospital readmission, discharge, length of stay, and death. Other agencies have invested in customized software or borrowed hospital software that tracks costs of service, percentage of goals achieved, and patient satisfaction. As home care continues to develop, there will be an emergence of children who are chronically ill for whom the treatment goal is stabilization rather than cure. Positive indicators for a patient receiving nasogastric feedings may be days transitioning to oral feeding, whereas appropriate measures for a child dependent on mechanical ventilation may be days free from infection. The severity and number of diagnoses require clinical personnel to develop appropriate outcome measures.

Another consideration for agencies seeking to track outcomes is the education of field staff. Many nurses are trained to think in terms of delivering services and leaving the home, rather than working on a timeline toward measurable goals and documenting progress. As accreditation moves toward outcomes collection, the emphasis of caring for these children may shift when total costs, rather than initial costs, are examined. It seems likely that further research into outcomes will reveal the hidden costs of using non-specialized home care agencies, such as increased rates of rehospitalization and delayed discharge from acute care units. When payers are provided with conclusive data demonstrating that skilled pediatric care providers and agencies provide the best value for their home care dollar, over time they are more likely to invest in skilled providers.

Future outcomes work is needed to answer the following questions:

- What type of provider is best suited to deliver services?
- What level of competency is required by caregivers prior to patient discharge into the home?
- How can services be streamlined without affecting quality?
- What is the number and length of home visits dictated by patient need to achieve optimal patient outcomes?
- How can financial and nonfinancial barriers to care be reduced?
- How can agencies best address the psychosocial needs of patients through teaching and outreach to prevent hospital readmittance and increased acute care visits among early discharges?

Before home care can be accepted fully as a safe and effective model of care delivery, outcomes research must address these areas.

▶ Quality

Increasingly, accreditation for adult home care is moving toward outcome measures; pediatric home care accreditation likely will do the same over the next 5 to 10 years. Currently, most agencies measure quality through patient satisfaction surveys and mock reviews. As the pediatric home care population increases, parents and payers are sure to demand cogent, reliable standardized data sets comparing quality of care for children with chronic conditions across multiple settings.

Accreditation

Because pediatric home care providers essentially are islands unto themselves, isolated agencies may develop protocols internally but have no neutral forum for benchmarking data and comparing methodologies with other like-minded providers. Current attempts by established accrediting bodies to create a uniform national outcome data set for home health agencies have focused on the elderly population. Both the Joint Commission on Accreditation of Healthcare Organizations' ORYX tool and the CMS' Outcome and Assessment Information Set (OASIS) tool are hailed as the home health industry standard for accreditation. Typical activities of daily living as measured by these instruments are geared toward adults and include the ability to answer the phone and bathe independently. While such measures are not relevant to children, payers still require accreditation approval with these tools for agencies to receive reimbursement.

The low prevalence of any one diagnosis in the pediatric home care population makes it difficult to capture data through a disease-specific checklist approach. Currently there are two useful measurement instruments for this population that focus on gauging consumer experience of general satisfaction levels for children who are chronically ill or disabled. First is the Consumer Assessment Health Plan tool developed by AHRQ, which offers the additional advantage of separating children who are chronically ill in private insurance from those in Medicaid. Second is the Living With Illness Screening and Supplemental Survey Module, which was developed by the Foundation for Accountability and created for children with terminal illness. This tool uses a non-categorical case-finding approach to highlight areas such as provision of patient education and provider communication that are common to all children with special needs.

Payers: Who Is Financing This Care?

Although society has cared for children in the home since the practice of medicine began, the recent demand for pediatric home care is being driven in part by the payer community. Payment for pediatric home care is fragmented and coverage of services varies widely by plan for private insurance and by state for public insurance. Typically, family health insurance is the primary payer, either public or private, although additional sources of payment include Medicaid waiver programs, designated state funds, and philanthropic sources.

The two largest payers for pediatric home care services are commercial managed care companies and Medicaid. These include traditional fee-for-service (FFS) Medicaid, Medicaid managed care, and Medicaid waiver programs for special groups, such as children who are dependent on technology or people with acquired immunodeficiency syndrome (AIDS).

▶ Medicaid

Medicaid is a joint federal/state program whose largest beneficiaries are parents and children participating in the AFDC program. This program provides health care coverage to families that fall below a state-designated income maximum (also known as the state poverty level). Therefore, families and children lose and regain eligibility as their income and assets fluctuate. States may customize benefits among eligible groups beyond the requirements for clinical and dental services and prescription drugs (*see* Chapter 3).

▶ Types of Reimbursement Contracts

Reimbursement for care varies based on the case. Intermittent care cases are negotiated at a per-visit rate, such as postpartum visits, which are relatively standardized across agencies at one visit. Continuous care cases usually are contracted at a per-hour rate, including children who are dependent on a ventilator where nursing may be needed around the clock or while parents sleep and work, for as long as 4 to 6 years. Other highly prevalent and well-researched diagnoses may be reimbursed on a per-case or per-episode basis in which, for example, an agency accepts a flat rate for management of patients with asthma within which they must manage patient costs of hospitalization, care, education, and drugs. Such risk arrangements are not the norm. Usually agency and payer case managers negotiate the length and number of visits allowed on a case-by-case basis.

▶ Managed Care

In Medicaid as well as private insurance, the dominant form of insurance for children remains managed care. From the perspective of agencies, managed care has affected the level and speed of payment. Caring for children usually costs more, but agencies are being reimbursed at the same level as adults. In addition, it is not unusual for agencies to receive payment 3 months or more after delivering a service. Although there are data supporting improved coverage for preventive services under managed care, there are no data to date indicating how this transition will affect pediatric home health. For both adults and the elderly, better outcomes were achieved under FFS, but at the price of higher volume of services and higher costs. It is not unreasonable to assume that this effect holds true for pediatric patients.

Given the larger social issues that cluster with treating children who are chronically ill and medically fragile, managed care organizations (MCOs) are spending large amounts of money to effectively manage this population. At the same time, the pool of money that states draw on to treat children is diminishing because of competition from other beneficiaries. The Balanced Budget Act of 1997 led to a high initial influx of adult home care recipients into nursing homes because of reduced funding available for home care visits. As a result, funding for Medicaid, which covers long-term care, was diminished for other beneficiaries, including pediatric home care patients. Underfunding and high demand for services across all age groups have left many Medicaid MCOs on unstable footing and led to decreased length and number of authorized visits. Maintaining agency solvency while providing needed home care to patients without financial resources is a major ethical problem in home care. The lack of organized data collection and analysis in this area underscores the need for research to delineate how such reimbursement measures will impact patients.

▶ Changing Market of Health Care Finance

Home care has gained momentum over the past decade, in large part because the current cost-conscious climate views home care as a less expensive option than inpatient care. To better understand the economic drivers that have made home health care popular, it is important to understand how the financing of health care itself has changed over the past 2 decades.

Cost-based Reimbursement

Until the mid-1980s, pediatric home care was paid for by cost-based reimbursement, also known as FFS. In this model home care agencies would provide bills to payers and receive retroactive reimbursement for each service provided. Usually Medicaid paid less per visit than Medicare, but, under FFS, agencies were motivated to perform more services to generate higher

payment. The FFS medicine held the federal government at financial risk
and placed little effort on containing costs aside from compliance with
federal reimbursement regulations. The home health agency was responsible
for coordinating home care services (eg, therapy, DME, and pharmacy) as
well as serving as the patient advocate.

Medicaid costs escalated throughout the 1980s under cost-based reimbursement, due in large part to the long-term care component of the
program. Although the concept of managed care has existed since the early
1900s, concern over the dramatic rise in health care costs led to rapid adop-
tion of managed care cost-containment principles by the private sector
during the late 1980s. Essentially, managed care is a system that integrates
the clinical and financial sides of health care, and as such puts the provider
of services at financial risk for managing a population of patients. Under this
payment mechanism, health care services, which traditionally generated revenue, now become costs, shifting the incentives for authorization and delivery of care. Not long after the success of managed care in the private sector,
this concept was embraced by the public sector in the early 1990s using state
managed care demonstration waiver programs. By 1997, managed care plans
constituted 74% of US health care enrollees, compared with 52% in 1992
and 29% in 1988. Although MCOs share many of the same guiding principles, different techniques are used to obtain common goals.

Indemnity

Traditional indemnity is similar to FFS in that providers are reimbursed for
all or part of covered expenses after a service is provided by submitting an
insurance form. Enrollees may select a provider of choice for services for
which they typically pay an annual deductible. Under this plan, the payer
assumes financial risk for overuse of services as well as some responsibility
for cost-containment efforts. Medical and financial authorization for services
remain with the physician. Coordination of services and the role of patient
advocate remain with the home care agency.

Preferred Provider Organizations

Preferred provider organizations (PPOs) are organized around a purchaser
(an insurance company, employer, or employee union) who selects a limited
number of providers to contract with (hospitals, physicians, home care agen-

cies, etc). In return for access to this patient population, providers, who may belong to several PPOs, receive discounted FFS reimbursement for all services to plan members. Enrollees have the option of self-referring to a provider not included on the panel, also known as out-of-network providers, but pay higher fees to exercise this choice. In this model, financial risk still remains with the payer, and providers still are incentivized, as under FFS, to benefit from high use of services. To control use of services and costs, payers usually require pre-authorization prior to providing home care. Coordination of services and the role of patient advocates again rest on the home care agency.

Health Maintenance Organizations

A health maintenance organization (HMO) operates by providing a purchaser (usually an employer or insurance company) with coverage of specific health care services to a select panel of physicians, hospitals, or home health agencies for a fixed prepaid premium. This fee is paid regardless of the amount and type of services provided to enrollees. Providers are then at risk for offering agreed-upon services to each enrollee within the budget provided by the HMO.

A withhold, in which part of a provider's fixed payment is retained every month and can be earned back during the year upon successful group or panel financial performance, may be included by an HMO. Alternatively, if a provider does not meet the financial target, all or part of the withhold may be kept by the HMO. Numerous risk pools are created in this arrangement so that if one provider exceeds its rate limit other providers will not be penalized. Often, low-volume service providers, such as pediatric home care, are paid at a negotiated FFS basis. A home care agency's risk typically is limited to the performance of ancillary service providers. Under this model, financial risk is shared by both the payer and the provider. While the segregation of risk pools seeks to minimize risk for home health agencies, reimbursement still may be affected adversely by an unusually high number of catastrophic cases requiring costly DME. Such an event then would result in a negative effect for all other providers in the payment pool. Similar to the PPO arrangement, medical authorization remains with the physician and financial authorization remains with the payer. Payers may shoulder the burden of case management through implementing use management and quality control. In this scenario, the agency and the payer share coordination of services, with the role of patient advocate remaining with the home care agency.

Alternatively, HMOs may be fully capitated, meaning all providers receive a negotiated portion of the per-member, per-month payment from each enrollee. This arrangement would make the pediatric home care agency responsible for providing contractually negotiated services to all children under the plan regardless of the cost of those services. The HMO identifies patients in need of home health services and both financial and medical authorization for home care services now come under the jurisdiction of the physician. Cost containment becomes the responsibility of the home care agency, which must ensure that services do not exceed the originally assigned predetermined sum. While the home health agency is responsible for coordination of services, the HMO and the agency share the role of patient advocate. Table 2-1 compares certain home care responsibilities based on the type of payer.

▶ Cost Tracking

In managed care, children eligible for home health care must compete with the needs of a plan's entire population to determine how to allocate resources accordingly. This explains why, despite a projected increase in the volume of children referred to home health, payers are pushing to decrease the number of authorized visits per child, leaving the net number of visits performed by agencies relatively unchanged. Because 5% to 7% of a payer's population is typically pediatric, coverage of these services remains low on the list of priorities for health plans.

Risk Reimbursement

Despite the low number of children eligible for pediatric home care, the high costs of this population already have led the payer community to approach agencies about assuming risk for some patients. Adult home care already has begun to adopt risk-sharing reimbursement. Individually, agencies have rolled out capitation products for adult enrollees. Nationally, prospective payment rates for the Medicare program were implemented on October 1, 2000. Other pediatric subacute providers, such as home rehabilitation programs, have begun to develop levels of care, or pathways, linked to clinical protocols, including fixed hours of therapy, skilled nursing, and physician consultation.

TABLE 2-1. Comparison of Responsibilities in Pediatric Home Health Across Insurance Types

			Insurance Type		
	Fee for Service (FFS)	Traditional Indemnity	Preferred Provider Organization (PPO)	Health Maintenance Organization (HMO) With Withhold	HMO Capitated
Finance					
What is the unit of payment to pediatric home health agencies?	Per-visit/per-hour	Per-visit/per-hour	Per-visit/per-hour	Per-episode	Capitation
Who bears financial risk?	Payer	Payer	Payer	Payer/home health agency	Home health agency
What is the financial risk to the agency?	None	None	None	Work more without additional payment	Lose money working more without additional payment
Case Management					
Who is responsible for medical/financial authorization of home care services?	Physician	Physician	Physician	Physician/payer	Physician/home health agency
What is the incentive to agency staff about providing services?	Deliver more services	Deliver more services	Deliver more services	Deliver services in the most cost-efficient way	Deliver fewer services in the most cost-efficient way
Who coordinates home care and support services?	Home health agency	Home health agency	Payer/home health agency	Payer/Home health agency	Home health agency
Who is the patient advocate?	Home health agency	Home health agency	Home health agency	Home health agency	Shared

Levels are assigned by diagnosis upon admission to a program and evaluated periodically for appropriateness relative to actual patient costs.

Although other home health and pediatric providers have begun to offer risk reimbursement, pediatric home health agencies are only dabbling in this arena with flat rate, per-episode reimbursement for selected groups such as pediatric patients with asthma. Poor data collection and tracking of cost by diagnosis and child have led a number of agencies to stay away from risk assumption until the exact cost of caring for children, including equipment and nursing costs, can be measured. However, it is recognized among these providers that they must begin to track costs, develop guidelines, and chart outcomes to prepare for the future of risk assumption. Risk reimbursement requires knowledge of historical use of services by patients. While the variety and severity of diagnoses among pediatric home health recipients have been cited by agencies as incompatible with risk arrangements, others disagree.

Ultimately, thorough documentation over time is the only way to understand the total cost of care associated with these children. Developing an acceptable reimbursement scheme for pediatric home care can only be addressed through further research into the long-term costs and outcomes associated with caring for children at home. Until then, it is difficult for agencies to enter into risk agreements and demand adequate reimbursement.

Summary

Several themes explored in this chapter were brought up during discussions with pediatric home health providers and experts. Below is a list of the top eight issues, as flagged by home care providers in the field, that must be addressed over the next 5 to 10 years for home health to remain viable.

1. Staffing
   - Nurses constitute the largest providers of pediatric home health care, and the current nursing shortage will continue to remain a top issue for pediatric providers well into the future. As the demand for qualified home health nurses rises over the next 10 years, agencies will be forced to address training and retention of field staff in what has been a "seasonal business" to date. Already, many agencies have loosened hiring requirements. This is a troubling trend in light of the smaller margin of error for this population and the decreased safety net in

the home. Alternative care providers should be explored at this time to prevent staffing difficulties in the future.

- Training of home health nurses is a concern because they are relatively isolated from experimental technology and surgery procedures to which hospital nurses are routinely exposed. Often, they may not be familiar with procedures that patients have undergone. As more home health nurses without pediatric-specific experience enter this field, it may be better to require case-specific training for home health providers prior to hospital discharge.

- Smaller pediatric home health agencies will continue to compete with hospitals and large institutions offering benefit packages and other conveniences for the select pool of nurses with pediatric acute care experience. It is likely that systems-based agencies will emerge on top because of flexibility of staffing with affiliated acute care providers and security of referring physicians with competency in home health staff.

2. Reimbursement

- Agencies repeatedly have voiced concern about low reimbursement rates for home health visits. The survival of pediatric home health care, according to many agencies, does not boil down to a data or accreditation issue but a financial issue. Negotiating and collecting appropriate reimbursement for the level of service provided is an ongoing challenge for agencies. Medicaid continues to reimburse at levels that are below cost for a population that requires increased spending because of underlying social issues.

- Speed of payment is a handicap for smaller agencies that must contend with the delay between delivery of services and collection of payments. Reimbursement remains unpredictable and varies greatly on a state-to-state basis because of geographical differences in standards of living and instability among Medicaid MCOs. The challenge for agencies is how to try and prepare for local and global changes in payment, given this unpredictability. As payers move toward risk arrangement contracts, such issues will become increasingly important. Cash flow shortages have been the death knell for many smaller pediatric home care agencies nationwide.

3. Outcomes Data
   - There remains an overall lack of organized research delineating selection criteria and specific guidelines for pediatric home care tied to improved outcomes measures. Although there have been studies examining how children progress at home, the information remains sparse in relation to the number of diagnoses and children who are discharged.
   - Present research in adult home care is examining issues of provider competency in terms of outcomes of patients and education of families. To date, this area of pediatric care has not been studied well. Although payers increasingly are moving toward less expensive providers (eg, LPNs versus RNs), this decision comes at the cost of knowledge about when to communicate with physicians and how to prevent acute care situations. Agencies are more likely to sway payers to pay for more costly skilled nursing care with data demonstrating clearly improved outcomes and cost savings.

4. Information Systems
   - At present there are no pediatric-specific information systems available that combine clinical and financial data. Most agencies continue to track patient progress manually on the clinical side, and only are able to compare payer collections versus charges on the financial side. As accrediting agencies continue to ramp up outcomes data requirements, smaller agencies will be forced to invest in costly software, while contending with issues of reimbursement collection.
   - Information systems also will be a boon to coordinating care across multiple providers for this population in real time. Such services would assist physicians and agencies in providing and justifying care through rapid correspondence and documentation.

5. Expansion of Services
   - As life expectancy increases among this population of children, demand is created for services beyond the home, including respite care, pediatric long-term care, medical day care, and school-based programs. Existing school-based services are not prepared to address and grow with the medical and educational needs of these children. Although programs exist for nurses to accompany children into schools, these services are costly for the agency and the payer. More medical day care programs and day schools may be needed to develop age- and

diagnosis-appropriate goals and curricula for such children. Collaboration between hospitals, agencies, payers, and public schools is needed to address this area.

6. Access
   - Barriers to public assistance will leave numerous eligible children without home care services and invalidate estimations on the real demand for pediatric home health care. There is no information available on the need for these services or the benefit.
   - In rural areas and homes where parents are left to care for children dependent on technology, telemedicine increasingly will play a large role in delivering care. Technology must be appropriately designed so it is adaptable to the home environment.
   - In addition, home health agencies need to explore programs that address the barrier of transportation for children who otherwise may not be able to access physician services.

7. Family Involvement
   - As critical members of the health care team, families and child care providers spend the majority of the day with children and know best what they as caregivers can and cannot do. Yet they often are not included in the design of home care treatment. Given that the goal of health care is to discharge children into the care of competent and knowledgeable caregivers, families need to be more involved with the planning and implementation of treatment for children.
   - As technology improves and more children with chronic illnesses and disabilities are kept alive, family support and involvement in treatment must be addressed. The ethical issue of how to best care and maintain quality of life for children that were not expected to survive long-term is present. There is an investment required from payers in ongoing treatment and services that has not been well described to date.

8. Physician Involvement
   - Physicians will have to become active participants in the home care design process. The clinical expertise of physicians is a valuable resource in organizing future research on pediatric home care. Partnerships between agencies, payers, and physicians could be fruitful in describing selection criteria and developing appropriate protocols and outcomes for treatment.

- To encourage physicians to become more involved in home care, reimbursement levels will have to match the time and effort required.
- Home health should be integrated actively into medical education. Only then will physicians begin to understand how to case-manage patients in the home and appreciate the social barriers that many patients face in that environment.

Acknowledgments

The authors would like to thank the following individuals who gave their time to contribute to the chapter: Elizabeth Madigan, PhD, RN; Sharon Johnson, MSN, RNC, CNA; Richard Chesney, MBA; Lynn Rinke, RN, MS; Susan Chatman, RN, BSN, MAHCA; Veronica Schuck, RN, BSN, MHA; Janet Prozzillo, RN, BSN; Bonnie MacNew, RN, MSN; Christina Smith, BSN, RN; Mike McBride, RN, BSN; Susan Walsh, RN; Tara Haupt, MA; Deeley Middleton; Janet Serwint, MD; June Chan, RN, MSN, MSA; Allison Filippone; Joe Sansone, MBA; Ellen Parker; William Wenner, MD; Allen Goldberg, MD; Lisa Remington; Bert Grebin, MD; Catherine Prophet, RN, BSN, PhN; Lorry Frankel, MD; Rick Millard, PhD, MBA; Donna Grimm, RN; and Doug Henderlight, MS, RN, CHCE.

Bibliography

Arnold L, Gennaro S, Kirby A, Atendido M, Laverty M, Brooten D. The perinatal evaluation center: a nurse practitioner service delivery model. *J Perinat Neonatal Nurs.* 1995;9:45-51

Berkowitz GS, Papiernik E. Epidemiology of preterm birth. *Epidemiol Rev.* 1993;15:414-443

Brooten D, Knapp H, Borucki L, et al. Early discharge and home care after unplanned cesarean birth: nursing care time. *J Obstet Gynecol Neonatal Nurs.* 1996;25:595-600

Brooten D. Perinatal care across the continuum: early discharge and nursing home follow-up. *J Perinat Neonatal Nurs.* 1995;9:38-44

Brooten D, Naylor M, Brown L, et al. Profile of postdischarge rehospitalizations and acute care visits for seven patient groups. *Public Health Nurs.* 1996;13:128-134

Brown LP, Gennaro S, York R, Swinkles K, Brooten D. VLBW infants: association between visiting and telephoning and maternal and infant outcome measures. *J Perinat Neonatal Nurs.* 1991;4:39-46

Congressional Budget Office. *Baseline: Medicare Staff Memorandum.* Washington, DC: Congressional Budget Office; 1997

Goldberg AI, Gardner HG, Gibson LE. Home care: the next frontier of pediatric practice. *J Pediatr.* 1994;125:686-690

Lorenz JM, Wooliever DE, Jetton JR, Paneth N. A quantitative review of mortality and developmental disability in extremely premature newborns. *Arch Pediatr Adolesc Med.* 1998;152:425-435

Madigan EA. An introduction to pediatric home health care. *J Soc Pediatr Nurs.* 1997;2:172-178

Madigan EA, Youngblut J, Haruzivishe C. Pediatric home healthcare: patients and providers. *Home Healthc Nurse.* 1999;17:699-705

McConnell M. Pediatrics: providers partnering with case manager. *Remington Report.* 1995;14-17

Nash DB. *The Managed Care Manual.* Boston, MA: Total Learning Concepts; 1997

Chapter 3

Pediatric Home Health Care: Public Funding

Danuta Buzdygan, MD

Introduction

The extent to which home care is delivered today would not be possible without public financing. Private insurance plans vary considerably in the type and amount of coverage they provide. A common feature among them is maximum liability. Once the benefits are exhausted, an individual or the family must seek other resources. The uninsured must rely on publicly funded programs or charity from the start.

Recent decades have brought a significant expansion of public funding for home care for the aged, blind, and disabled. Children, in particular, have benefited from the new programs and expansions of Medicaid eligibility, as well as the array of services available through its Early and Periodic Screening, Diagnosis, and Treatment (EPSDT) program. New federal programs have expanded eligibility of families in state-administered public insurance programs with the goal of providing medical insurance for most children.

Early Funding

Enacted in 1935 as Part 2 of Title V of the Social Security Act, the Services for Crippled Children program provided funds that enabled states to pay for medical, surgical, corrective, and other services and care for "children who are crippled or who are suffering from conditions which may lead to crippling." For 30 years, or until the enactment of Title XIX of the Social Security Act in 1965, Title V remained the main source of public funding for pediatric home care. This program financed nursing visits and rehabilitation therapies, but there were no provisions for long-term care. Children who were more severely handicapped were likely to receive services in an institutional setting, such as a chronic disease hospital or a hospital school. Most children who were severely disabled were institutionalized or, if cared for at home, totally dependent on their families for care.

Medicaid

Title XIX of the Social Security Act is known as Medicaid. Eligibility for Medicaid is determined by family income. Although the standard, defined as the eligibility for Aid to

Families with Dependent Children (AFDC), varies from state to state, in most instances it hovered around 50% of the federal poverty line (FPL). A series of Medicaid expansions raised the income eligibility levels for the defined population groups starting with the Omnibus Budget Reconciliation Act of 1987, which permitted states to grant Medicaid eligibility to pregnant women and children up to 1 year of age whose family income was at or below 185% of FPL. Currently, children up to the age of 6 years may qualify for Medicaid when the family income is below 133% of FPL, and children who were born after September 30, 1983, qualify if their family income is at or below 100% of FPL.

Welfare reform of 1996, which replaced AFDC with the Temporary Assistance for Needy Families (TANF) program, de-linked cash assistance from the medical assistance (Medicaid), meaning that a cash grant does not automatically carry eligibility for Medicaid and, conversely, one may be eligible for medical assistance in the absence of a cash grant. However, the old AFDC standard continues to define Medicaid eligibility. It is important to understand that Medicaid eligibility varies from state to state and pediatric practitioners must become familiar with the eligibility guidelines in their own states.

Supplemental Security Income

Another means of gaining Medicaid eligibility is as an adjunct to eligibility for Supplemental Security Income (SSI), a cash benefit program for people with disabilities administered by the Social Security Administration. The determination of eligibility for SSI takes into account financial and disability criteria, including the family's financial status as well as the degree of disability measured in terms of the individual's ability to engage in gainful employment. The disability criteria for the child is based on the child's ability to engage in age-appropriate activities such as school attendance.

▶ Mandatory Services Covered by Medicaid

Medicaid benefits are defined in the state's plan approved by the Centers for Medicare and Medicaid Services (CMS) (formerly the Health Care Financing Administration [HCFA]). Home care is one of the mandatory services covered by Medicaid. It provides for skilled nursing visits; physical, occupational, and speech therapies; nutritional and social work consultations; as well as durable medical equipment and supplies. It should be noted that private duty nursing is not subsumed under the category of home care but is considered a separate, optional Medicaid service. This means that a state may choose to include it in its state plan but is not obligated to do so.

▶ Early and Periodic Screening, Diagnosis, and Treatment Program

The EPSDT program is another mandated Medicaid service. Limited to Medicaid recipients under 18 and, optionally, up to 21 years of age, the EPSDT program ensures comprehensive child health services. It emphasizes preventive care (ie, periodic screenings) aimed at early detection and correction or amelioration of any health problem. It requires all diagnostic and treatment services to be available when needed by an EPSDT program recipient. By waiving certain federal requirements, the EPSDT program allows states to offer child beneficiaries services not available to the rest of the eligible population. This is particularly significant in states with a limited array of services. Under the EPSDT program requirement, all optional and mandatory Medicaid services, even those not included in the given state's Medicaid plan, must be made available to EPSDT program beneficiaries. Generally, the EPSDT program is an important but underused Medicaid benefit because of poor understanding of the program and state bureaucratic barriers.

By waiving certain federal requirements, the EPSDT program allows states to offer child beneficiaries services not available to the rest of the eligible population.

Disabled Children's Program

Historically, much credit for the expansion of home care for children dependent on technology belongs to the short-lived SSI Disabled Children's Program enacted in 1976. Through its special funding, the program sought to improve services for children with disabilities by filling the gaps left by Medicaid. The new funds enabled states to try innovative services such as case management and a wider scope of home care services. With the assistance of this program, several eligible children dependent on ventilators were discharged from the hospital to home care. In 1980, the SSI Disabled Children's Program was incorporated in the Title V Maternal and Child

Health Block Grant, but the success of the precedent it established paved
the way for other community-based programs.

In 1981, through an executive order from President Ronald Reagan,
certain Medicaid eligibility requirements were waived to enable a child
dependent on a ventilator to return home from the hospital. This became
known as the "Katie Beckett waiver." Soon, other home- and community-
based services waivers followed. All of these waivers had the same basic
premise that it is more beneficial and cost effective to support services in
the community than to maintain individuals confined to hospitals or other
institutions. To expand community-based services, states had to be allowed
to waive a rule of eligibility, a rule of service, or both. Some state waiver
programs targeted individuals with a specific disease or disability, such as
acquired immunodeficiency syndrome (AIDS), or traumatic brain injury.
Others, by allowing coverage for nontypical Medicaid services such as
private duty nursing or respite care, aimed at redirecting individuals at risk for
institutional long-term care from the nursing home to the community.

Medicaid Managed Care Organizations

In recent years, many states opted to implement the concept of managed
care for Medicaid beneficiaries. To do so required another type of federal
waiver that permitted the state to limit the beneficiary's choice of provider.
States must demonstrate the benefit of using a managed care model. The
benefit often is improved access to services because the managed care
organizations (MCOs) that seek a Medicaid contract must demonstrate
an adequate provider network as one condition of participation. Improved
access may be a problem when states accept an MCO's list of providers, who
may accept only a limited number of Medicaid patients in their practices.

When a Medicaid agency contracts with an MCO, the MCO becomes
the Medicaid provider and the individual practitioners are reimbursed for
their services by the MCO. Medicaid beneficiaries who are not enrolled
in Medicaid MCOs continue to receive services in the traditional way,
through fee-for-service participating providers. The system of managed
care is based on primary care providers who coordinate and direct care for
patients in their panels. Thus, each managed care beneficiary must have a
medical home. When a home care referral becomes necessary, it must be
to a home care provider within the MCO's network. Federal data show

that children in fee-for-service Medicaid arrangements received more preventive care than those enrolled in a Medicaid MCO. Both the physician and the patient must be aware of constraints and disincentives before joining a Medicaid MCO.

State Children's Health Insurance Program

The State Children's Health Insurance Program (SCHIP) is the most recent addition to the array of publicly funded programs for children. Enacted as the Title XXI of the Social Security Act in 1997, it is an example of a federal/state partnership. Under this program, states are allowed to expand their Medicaid program, set up a new program, or use both in combination. All Medicaid regulations pertain to the Medicaid expansion. However, a new program, as a subsidized insurance program, is not bound by these regulations. Beneficiaries can be expected to pay coinsurance and contribute to the cost of services. Because states are free to determine what services will be covered under this insurance, it can be expected that the availability and extent of home care benefit will vary from state to state.

Summary

- Pediatricians contemplating home care for pediatric patients who are not insured, or whose benefits do not cover home care or already have been exhausted, need to understand the various public funding options described in this chapter.
- Medicaid EPSDT benefit provides access to all optional and mandatory Medicaid services for qualified beneficiaries.
- When this is not feasible, a Medicaid home and community services waiver may be an option.
- In some states, Title V services for children with special needs may continue to offer direct services for children not eligible for other programs.

Bibliography

American Academy of Pediatrics. *A Pediatrician's Guide to Managed Care.* Nelson RP, Minon ME, eds. 2nd ed. Elk Grove Village, IL: American Academy of Pediatrics; 2001

Chapter 4

Pediatric Home Health Care Providers

Rosemary De Marco Laudani, BSN

Introduction

Pediatric home care involves the delivery of medical care in the home to children who are ill, recovering, or disabled. It can be as simple as dressing changes or as complex as providing mechanical ventilation. The benefits of home care for children are many, including having the child cared for in the familiar surroundings of a home environment, continued access to social support such as friends and siblings, better growth and development, and less cost compared with continued hospitalization. Home care also may decrease the cost of health care by preventing or decreasing hospitalization stays.

Successful pediatric home care requires a commitment of resources and personnel to meet the unique needs of the pediatric population. Not every home care agency or organization can care for children.

Modern home care programs were developed primarily to serve the elderly population. Through Medicare, federal funding for home care programs began in earnest as a means to decrease the nation's increasing health care budget. Home care was viewed as a preferable alternative to continued hospitalization because of the salutary benefits to the patient and the considerable cost savings. As a result, the recent growth in home care was fueled by Medicare dollars that focused almost exclusively on the elderly patient population.

When competition for Medicare dollars increased, home care agencies looked to other markets to expand their services and, as a result, pediatric home care became one of the fastest-growing segments of the industry. Prior to this, pediatric home care was relegated mainly to children dependent on technology (ie, home mechanical ventilation). Competitive pressures also led to technological advances and innovative therapies in pediatric home care, making care more safe and reliable.

Unfortunately, the federal regulations that governed the industry did not change to accommodate this new population of home care patients. The Medicare conditions of participation for home care providers focused almost exclusively on the elderly population and were, at times, inappropriate for children. Pediatric home care providers were required to meet these regulations, however, if they wanted to receive reimbursement from Medicaid or Medicare. This situation remains today.

Many home care providers do an excellent job of caring for children despite these federal regulatory burdens, but some agencies remain focused on the elderly population and serve the pediatric population as an afterthought. These elderly focused agencies may not have the personnel or resources necessary to care adequately for children. This chapter describes the various types of home care organizations, as well as the personnel necessary to care for children

...some agencies remain focused on the elderly population and serve the pediatric population as an afterthought.

in the home. It is important to understand the different types of home care providers and personnel to make an educated referral of a pediatric patient to home care.

The Business of Pediatric Home Care

There are various business models used to deliver pediatric home care. These models include the not-for-profit agency, for-profit agency, Visiting Nurse Association (VNA), and hospital-affiliated agency.

▶ Not-for-profit Agency

Not-for-profit agencies do not have shareholders or stockholders. Usually, a board of directors of the agency exercises oversight of the business and clinical aspects of care. These agencies can be private or governmental. An example of a private not-for-profit agency is a VNA. Local municipal health departments may also provide home care services for children. These services vary by municipality and may include standard home care services or intermittent visits by public health nurses.

▶ For-profit Agency

For-profit agencies can be privately owned or publicly traded companies. For-profit agencies use a business model to deliver home care services. Any profits generated through the agency will be shared with the owners or stockholders. The efficiency of the care provided may have more importance to a for-profit agency, especially if the agency enters into risk-sharing contracts with insurers and other payers. In reality, given current market dynamics in the home care industry, both not-for-profit and for-profit agencies work to provide the most efficient care possible to optimize agency income.

▶ Visiting Nurse Association

The VNAs are an association of community-based not-for-profit home health agencies found in 40 states from coast to coast. The earliest community home care agencies began more than 100 years ago and were called visiting nurse agencies. In 1983, many not-for-profit agencies united to form an association to provide better advocacy and marketing for these community-based agencies. Although many agencies use the term *visiting nurse agency*, not all of these agencies are associated with the Visiting Nurse Association of America.

▶ Hospital-Affiliated Agency

Hospital-affiliated agencies are home care companies owned or operated by a hospital. This helps the hospital better manage patients along a continuum of care. Recent federal regulations require hospitals to offer patients a choice of home care providers on discharge and not solely refer to their own home care agency. These new regulations have decreased the number of hospital-affiliated home care agencies nationwide.

Organizational Structure of Home Care Companies

The organizational structure of home care companies generally can be separated into administrative and clinical functions. A home care agency's organization can be complex depending on the size and type of services the agency offers. The administrative functions include financial planning, billing, payroll, human resources, marketing, and materials management. The clinical functions include nursing administration, clinical policies and procedures, equipment delivery, and patient care. The clinical team includes the home care nurse, intake supervisors, area supervisors, a nurse educator, therapy personnel, and clinical specialties such as intravenous (IV) and terminal care teams.

Types of Home Care Providers

Pediatric home care agencies specialize in providing medical care to children in the home. The scope of services offered vary by agency and include intermittent nursing, shift nursing, respite care, home health aids, nutrition therapy, physical therapy, occupational therapy, speech therapy, respiratory therapy, social work, infusion therapy (pharmacy), and medical equipment.

▶ Home Nursing Agencies

Pediatric nursing agencies provide nurses to administer care in the home. The range of skills offered varies depending on the agency. Some agencies offer registered nurses (RNs) and licensed practical/vocational nurses, while some provide home health aids. The type of nurse needed will depend on the physician's request and the skilled needs of the patient. Often, nursing agencies will also provide therapy services including physical therapy, occupational therapy, and speech therapy. Nursing agencies usually do not provide infusion services or medical equipment, but some nursing agencies contract with home infusion agencies to supply nurses to administer medications.

▶ Durable Medical Equipment Providers

Durable medical equipment (DME) agencies provide medical equipment and supplies such as wheelchairs, dressing supplies, and respiratory equipment. The DME agencies should have appropriate-sized pediatric equipment and pediatric-specific policies and procedures. They also should have staff who are knowledgeable about the pediatric population and who are available 24 hours per day.

▶ Home Infusion Agencies

Home infusion agencies provide pharmaceuticals and supplies such as antibiotics, chemotherapy, nutritional therapy, enteral therapy, and infusion pumps. They may have their own nurses or subcontract for services with a home nursing agency. They should have an experienced pediatric pharmacist available. Pharmacy personnel should be available 24 hours per day.

▶ Infusion Centers

Infusion centers are specialized centers where patients can receive medication infusions such as chemotherapy and antibiotics. Infusion centers may be associated with a clinic. They are used when a medication infusion cannot be given safely in the home and the patient does not necessarily require hospital admission.

▶ Integrated Home Care Providers

Integrated home care providers may be the best choice for pediatric patients with complex medical conditions if they meet all the needs of the patient. Integrated providers can offer all pediatric home care services directly or through subcontractor arrangements. These agencies usually provide nursing care, home infusion pharmacy, medical equipment, therapy services, and social work. By offering all services under one agency, there is usually less fragmentation of care and better coordination of services. Additionally, families need to remember one phone number to call, instead of calling separate agencies if problems occur. This is a good choice for families with a child who has multidisciplinary needs.

▶ Respite Providers

Respite providers supply personnel who can care for a child who is medically fragile — to temporarily relieve the family from health care responsibilities. Respite personnel include lay volunteers or paid nursing staff. Respite care can be provided in the home or at a location outside the home such as medical day care (*see* Chapter 37) or a respite home. Hospitals should be considered a respite option only in an emergency situation.

▶ Hospice Providers

Hospice care is provided in the home for the patient who is terminally ill. This includes palliative and comfort care. Pediatric hospice programs can be difficult to find. Care plans for adult hospice patients should not be used for children. For example, needs such as tube feedings may be considered comforting for a child but not to an adult. Some pediatric home care agencies provide hospice services or use pediatric nurses who are competent and comfortable working with children who are terminally ill.

Licensure, Certification, and Accreditation

The terms licensure, certification, and accreditation often are confused when used in the home care field. Most, but not all, states require that a home care agency obtain a license to operate within the state. Licensure implies that the agency has met certain state regulations. The state department of health then exercises some amount of oversight of the home care company.

Certification implies that the home care agency has met certain federal requirements for patient care and management to participate in Medicare or Medicaid programs. An agency must be certified to provide care to Medicare and Medicaid patients. The federal government requires that home care companies participating in federal insurance programs rigidly adhere to the guidelines no matter in which state an agency is located. Many private insurers require home care agencies to achieve Medicare certification prior to contracting.

A pediatric home care agency also may receive voluntary accreditation, which means they are recognized by a professional organization that sets national standards of care. The major accrediting organizations for home care include the Joint Commission on Accreditation of Healthcare Organizations and the Community Health Accreditation Program. The accreditation process involves an intensive on-site review of the clinical program, including patient visits. Accreditation often is granted for 3 years before reaccreditation is necessary. Although accreditation does not guarantee good patient care, an agency with such accreditation usually will have systems, policies, and procedures in place to deliver patient care that meets national standards of care.

Home Care Personnel

▶ Administrator and Director of Nursing

The administrator is responsible for overall agency management. The administrator usually has a business background but also can be a clinical person like the director of nursing. The administrator's role includes budgeting, financial planning, human resource management, and ensuring appropriate clinical management. The director of nursing directs the clinical program and often has a master's degree in nursing. The director should have management skills to operate the agency safely and efficiently. The director of nursing is responsible for all of the clinical aspects of the home care agency.

▶ Case Manager

The case manager coordinates and administers the care of patients in the home, especially those with complex medical needs, to ensure the most efficient delivery of care. The case manager serves as the family's point of contact for the home care agency and frequently will be responsible for scheduling nursing visits and equipment delivery. The case manager may be the home care nurse. As a family becomes more comfortable providing care, the role of the case manager can change. The family may assume the role of case manager, as in the family-directed model of home care (*see* Chapter 6).

▶ Home Care and Private Duty Nurses

The home care nurse usually is an RN who provides skilled services in the home such as physical assessments, administering injections, or changing dressings. The home care nurse usually only provides intermittent visits and does not stay for an extended length of time. A private duty nurse, however, is a nurse who stays for an extended length of time to care for a patient with continuous need for skilled services. Depending on the skills needed, the private duty nurse can be an RN or licensed practical nurse. Private duty nursing typically is used for children who require mechanical ventilation in the home. Private duty nurses tend to work in shifts of 8 to 12 hours, whereas home care nurses provide intermittent visits lasting from 1 to 4 hours.

▶ Home Health Aids

A home health aid (HHA) assists patients with activities of daily living (ADLs) such as feeding and bathing. An HHA may be a licensed caregiver but does not have the same expertise or training for performing skilled tasks as a nurse. The role of HHAs is regulated by federal Medicare guidelines. These caregivers are used infrequently in pediatric home care because insurers will not pay for the services, since parents usually can assist their child with ADLs.

▶ Trained Caregiver

A trained caregiver is trained to perform the duties necessary to care for the child. This person often is a parent, relative, volunteer, or foster parent who is not licensed but is approved by the parent or caregiver to perform the same services as the primary caregiver. Because children with complex medical needs should have backup caregivers identified prior to discharge, a trained caregiver may be incorporated into the child's backup plan by the case manager.

▶ Physical Therapist

A physical therapist assists with muscle strengthening, positioning and handling, and range of motion to promote healing and relieve pain. Physical therapy interventions are taught to the parent or nurse so that they are performed throughout the day. A physical therapist may order and fit specialized equipment such as a walker or wheelchair. The therapist also should set up a written plan in the home, and include pictures to illustrate the plan.

▶ Occupational Therapist

A home care occupational therapist provides home visits to improve fine motor development and may assist with feeding techniques for pediatric patients. The role of the occupational therapist may overlap with that of the physical therapist or speech therapist. Occupational therapists also may assist in ordering equipment such as hand splints. Like the physical therapist, the occupational therapist should set up a written plan in the home, and include pictures to illustrate the plan.

▶ Speech Therapist

A home care speech therapist evaluates the speech development of a child and may assist in feeding techniques and oral and cognitive stimulation. The speech therapist should set up a written plan in the home, and include pictures to illustrate the plan, just like the other therapists. The physical therapist, occupational therapist, and speech therapist should work together to optimize the child's development and create realistic goals.

▶ Respiratory Therapist

A home care respiratory therapist assists with management of respiratory care of children with chronic pulmonary problems. The respiratory therapist evaluates and assists in oxygen therapy, airway management, postural drainage, and ventilator management. A respiratory therapist helps train family members in proper care and management of these therapies. A respiratory therapist also assists in ordering appropriate equipment and supplies needed to care for the child's respiratory needs. Typically, respiratory therapists are used to set up a home mechanical ventilation plan for a child requiring this support.

▶ Social Worker

The social worker assesses the psychological and social needs of the patient and family and identifies resources to meet their needs. The social worker identifies financial and emotional supports for the patient and family in addition to making appropriate referrals to supportive agencies within the community. Unfortunately many insurers will not pay for social work services in the home. However, the unique insights that social workers provide by evaluating a patient in the home may allow for earlier interventions that promote the home care plan and avoid costly hospitalizations or fragmentations in care. If a child is enrolled in a government-sponsored early intervention program, social worker services often are available.

▶ Delivery Personnel

Delivery personnel are trained to deliver medical equipment and supplies. They are knowledgeable about handling equipment, such as oxygen, safely and setting up equipment appropriately. Complex medical equipment, such as a ventilator, should be assembled and tested by a nurse or respiratory therapist prior to use.

Summary

- Business models for pediatric home care include not-for-profit agencies, for-profit agencies, VNAs, and hospital-affiliated agencies.
- The organizational structure of home care companies includes administrative and clinical functions.
- Home care personnel deliver a variety of services, including intermittent nursing, nutrition services, physical therapy, occupational therapy, speech therapy, respiratory therapy, social work, infusion therapy, and medical equipment delivery and setup.
- Most states require home care agencies to be licensed.
- Home care agencies must be certified to participate in Medicare or Medicaid programs.
- A home care agency may undergo voluntary accreditation to determine whether it meets national standards of care.

Chapter 5

Technology and Home Health Care

Daniel Robertson, RRT, MBA; Mark McConnell, MD

Introduction

Pediatric health care professionals practicing outside the walls of the hospital in home care face a significantly different set of demands than their predecessors did 20 or 30 years ago. Health care professionals are more likely to be part of a network of providers striving to deliver timely, efficient, and effective care to patients outside of the hospital. This care is provided in an increasingly regulated environment requiring more documentation for quality and reimbursement purposes.

Information and other technologies have been developed to help meet the increasing documentation needs and to provide efficiency in caring for the patient at home. These technologies fall into four main categories: clinical information and reporting systems, administrative billing and decision support systems, enterprise systems, and patient monitoring systems. The upside of the availability of this range of technology is better and more efficient home care and patient monitoring.

Unfortunately, most smaller home care providers cannot afford to purchase sophisticated information technology systems in the current home care reimbursement environment. However, some government and private payers are now allowing reimbursement for some of these technologies.

Clinical Information and Reporting Systems

Many clinical information systems allow home care providers to capture patient clinical information in the home and transmit data to the main office. This information then can be stored as part of the patient's medical record. Such systems make it easier for clinical supervising personnel to monitor the provider's care and the patient's outcomes. Electronic clinical information can be analyzed to find trends in care to intervene earlier, prevent adverse patient events, or implement more effective practice models. This type of information gathering is required by the Centers for Medicare and Medicaid Services (CMS) (formerly the Health Care Financing Administration [HCFA]) for Medicare home care providers under its Outcome Assessment and Information Set (OASIS) project, and by the Joint Commission on Accreditation of Healthcare Organizations under its ORYX project.

The patient's clinical information can be input in the home by a parent or provider on a laptop or handheld computing device. This information is then downloaded over telephone lines or wirelessly to the main clinical database in the provider's office. These devices may reduce the time that nurses and other providers spend doing documentation, allowing more time to be spent caring for the patient.

▸ Monitoring Devices

Newer patient monitoring equipment allows direct capture of patient information from devices such as apnea monitors, blood pressure monitors, cardiac monitors, or peak flow monitors. This information is downloaded to a monitoring station or directly to the physician's or provider's office, where it is analyzed and alterations in the patient's plan of care are implemented more quickly than by sending a nurse or other provider into the home. These types of monitoring devices are sure to become more commonplace as technology advances and the cost of the devices decreases.

▸ Confidentiality and Security

Because clinical monitoring and information systems necessarily require the transmission of confidential patient information, it is important for home care providers to have policies and procedures that address patient confidentiality and delineate which employees have access to confidential medical information. In addition, such clinical information systems should have significant security systems with firewalls and passwords to prevent inadvertent and malicious access to stored information by someone outside of the home care organization.

Administrative Billing and Decision Support Systems

The other types of information systems commonly found in home care organizations are billing and decision support systems. These systems are important to ensure the financial viability of the organization. Billing systems should allow for accurate coding and billing for procedures done in the home. Errors in billing, even if unintentional, may subject providers to fraud and abuse charges by government investigators, leading to large fines and possible loss of licensure. It is important that physicians work closely and carefully with the home care provider to ensure that orders are signed in a timely manner and that home care and equipment certifications are accurate and returned promptly. A robust administrative information system can track completed procedures on a daily basis, ensure that the procedures done were consistent with physician orders, and generate an accurate bill.

An administrative decision support system allows the home care provider to track the expenses and reimbursement related to each patient or procedure. Such financial tracking, known as activity-based costing, allows the home care organization to track business more closely, on a patient-by-patient basis, to ensure its future financial viability. By using these decision support systems, home care providers can work more carefully under prospective payment systems and add or remove programs that may positively or negatively influence the organization's financial health. Unfortunately, many of the more robust administrative decision support systems are very expensive and require ongoing technology support that many small home care providers cannot afford. In addition, many programs lack the flexibility to incorporate modifications needed for a pediatric or non-Medicare population. It is important, however, that all home care organizations have the information and financial tools necessary to ensure adequate financial planning, correct billing, and timely reimbursement.

An administrative decision support system allows the home care provider to track the expenses and reimbursement related to each patient or procedure.

Enterprise Systems

Enterprise systems are information systems that integrate clinical and administrative data. The nurse enters patient clinical information into a laptop computer in the home, which generates appropriate diagnosis and billing codes in the system. Once the billing information is verified with the physician order, a bill is produced and sent to the payer. Simultaneously, employee time and salary information are captured and made part of the payroll process. This seamless information technology is ideal in the home care setting; however, few home care providers are able to afford or develop such integrated systems.

Patient Monitoring Systems

The use of various patient monitoring systems is increasing in health care. These systems include downloadable patient monitors as mentioned previously, clinical information tracking devices over the Internet, centralized home monitoring stations that allow real-time physiologic monitoring and communication with a nurse, and telemedicine devices with real-time broadband connections to health care professionals.

▶ Downloadable Monitors

The downloadable patient monitors currently available include apnea monitors, cardiac monitors, blood pressure monitors, and peak flow monitors. These monitors record physiologic data and download information over telephone lines or wirelessly to a physician's office or monitoring station. The benefits of such monitoring seem obvious; however, the provider must have a plan for how to deal with this information as it arrives in the office. These information intrusions can be as disruptive as telephone calls or unscheduled visits. Physicians should develop an office plan to deal with the information to ensure a timely response to patients who are in need.

▶ Internet Devices

Similar to the downloadable devices, a new wave of Internet connection devices are available to link patient and provider. These Internet devices can be computers or smart telephones, for example. Once connected to the Internet, a patient is brought to a provider's Web site or menu where clinical information can be input and subsequently evaluated. In addition, patients can order supplies, schedule visits, e-mail questions, or research health-related information. These devices are inexpensive and simple to use and provide an easy solution to monitor a patient's condition. The same concerns about patient confidentiality that are present with clinical information systems apply for Internet devices. Patients should be given access only to secure Web sites that use encryption or other security technology.

▶ Centralized Home Monitors

Centralized home monitoring systems initially were developed for patients at the extremes of life, including neonates being discharged to home after a stay in the neonatal intensive care unit and elderly patients who lacked the mobility or ability to call for help. These monitors, also known as home-assisted nursing care, record physiologic data and transmit them to a central monitoring station where a nurse or other health care professional is available immediately. In addition, there can be two-way voice and video communication so that the nurse can see and talk to the patient or caregiver. Such immediate access may benefit some patients who have a fragile clinical status or who have caretakers who lack the confidence to make good clinical judgments.

▸ Telemedicine

Even while centralized home monitoring systems have not yet had a significant increase in use, a similar type of technology has shown tremendous growth in recent years. Telemedicine is the remote delivery of health care, usually over large distances, through the use of high-resolution monitoring devices over broadband high-speed connections. Telemedicine devices usually incorporate physiologic monitoring equipment, including stethoscopes and cardiac monitors, and two-way audio and video communication. Telemedicine requires the patient and physician to have access to a monitoring device. Through a remote electronic examination, the physician can assess the patient as though they were in the room together, develop a diagnosis, and offer a treatment plan.

Telemedicine programs at larger health care institutions have been growing recently to serve a large population of patients who live a considerable distance from their treating physician. The US military developed a large telemedicine program to give military personnel living abroad access to specialists not available in their area. This same model has been applied in the private sector where pediatric subspecialists are caring for their patients hundreds of miles away with the assistance of telemedicine and the patient's primary care physician. Physicians should research carefully the legal and regulatory implications of this type of telemedicine practice, especially when caring for patients outside of the physician's state or country. As technological advances continue, remote patient monitoring will play a bigger role in the care of patients in the home.

Summary

Facts about home care technology include the following:

- Information and other technologies have been developed to meet the increasing documentation needs of home care and to provide efficiency in caring for patients at home.
- Clinical information systems allow home care providers to capture patient information in the home and transmit the data to the provider's main office. This enables clinical supervising personnel to monitor a provider's care and a patient's outcomes.
- Home care providers using clinical information systems must have policies and procedures in place to protect patient confidentiality when transmitting information.
- Administrative decision support systems allow home care providers to track expenses and reimbursement for each patient and procedure to ensure the financial viability of the organization.
- Enterprise systems integrate clinical and administrative data. These systems are ideal, yet costly for home care providers.
- The use of patient monitoring systems in home care, such as centralized home monitoring, clinical information tracking devices via the Internet, and telemedicine devices, is increasing.

Bibliography

Bujnowska-Fedak MM, Staniszewski A, Steciwko A, Puchala E. System of telemedicine services designed for family doctors' practices. *Telemed J E Health.* 2000;6:449-452

Dahlberg NL, Blazek D, Wikoff B, Tuckwell BL, Koloroutis M. High-tech, high-touch perinatal home care. *Caring.* 1995;14:36-39

Handheld computers are key to improving homecare operations for Colorado provider. *Health Care Cost Reengineering Rep.* 1998;3:5-7

Petit de Mange EA. Pediatric considerations in homecare. *Crit Care Nurs Clin North Am.* 1998;10:339-346

Stanberry B. Legal ethical and risk issues in telemedicine. *Comput Methods Programs Biomed.* 2001;64:225-233

Wagner L. Telemedicine offers promise to long-term care. *Provider.* 2001;27:28-29, 32-33

Chapter 6

Family-Centered Home Health Care

Beverly H. Johnson, Juliette Schlucter

Introduction

The concepts of family-centered home care are based on principles that were first articulated by Shelton, Jeppson, and Johnson in 1987. These concepts served as the foundation for US Surgeon General C. Everett Koop's national agenda for children with special health care needs in the late 1980s. This national effort established family-centered, community-based, and coordinated care as the standard of care for children needing specialized health care.

This chapter describes key principles of the family-centered approach to care and how these principles apply in pediatric home care.

What Is Family-Centered Care?

Family-centered care is a philosophy of medical care that puts the patient and family in the center of medical decision making. It is based on mutually beneficial partnerships between families and health care providers. Family-centered providers recognize the vital role that families play in ensuring the health and well-being of infants, children, and adolescents. They recognize that all families, even those who are struggling with very difficult life circumstances, bring important strengths to health care experiences and to making decisions about the care of their children.

Family-centered providers acknowledge that emotional, social, and developmental support are integral components of health care. A family-centered approach to care builds on individual and family strengths; empowers children and families and fosters their development; supports family caregiving and decision making; respects choices made by families; and involves families in all aspects of the planning, delivery, and evaluation of care. Family-centered systems of heath care link families to community resources and support coordination of care. At the heart of family-centered care are

59

partnerships that allow for formal and informal collaboration and information sharing among families and providers throughout the continuum of care.

Core Concepts of Family-Centered Care

- Respect for each individual and family
- Recognition of strengths in the child and family, even in crises
- Choices for families about approaches to care and support
- Flexibility in policies, procedures, and staff practices, to tailor care to the needs, beliefs, and cultural values of individual families
- Information to help families make choices and assume responsibility for the care of their child
- Provision of formal and informal child and family support
- Collaboration among families and health care personnel in the care of an individual child; in developing and evaluating programs and policies in home care agencies, clinics, and hospitals; and in designing systems of care

---

Family-centered care represents a profound philosophical shift from traditional models of health care — from a deficits-based, problem-oriented model to a strengths-based model of care, from a model in which providers are the only experts to a model that builds on the expertise of families.

Key Principles of Family-Centered Home Care

A family-centered approach to pediatric home care is based on an overall attitude toward care rather than on a specific protocol. Guidelines for practicing family-centered pediatric home care derive from the following key principles.

▶ Conveying Respect for the Child and Family

Changing demographics in American society have transformed the structure and function of families. In respect for the great variation in family structures and methods of functioning, it is essential that home health care providers work within the framework with which each family is comfortable. In family-centered home care, respect is conveyed for each family's values, culture, traditions, and resources, and for how it defines its members.

Having an open, respectful view of the definition of "family" is important during a child's hospital stay. In home care, family may be even more broadly defined, and a variety of individuals may be involved with administering medical regimens and therapies and nurturing the child.

The family may be made up of extended family members, a valued neighbor, other caregivers, or a child's best friend. In family-centered home care, families are viewed as important members of the child's health care team. The roles they choose to assume on the team are respected. It is also acknowledged that these roles may change over time.

▸ Identifying and Building on Family Strengths

With a family-centered approach, providers identify and focus on the child's and family's unique strengths and resources, as well as on the areas in which the family needs the greatest amount of support. Ideally, the identification of strengths and needs begins early in the course of the child's illness and is accomplished as part of a collaborative process with the family. This collaboration should begin before the home care services begin, either prior to discharge from the hospital or before the physician and family discuss and agree to home care. Early and thoughtful collaboration allows for a plan for home care that is respectful of family goals, priorities, and values. Families should participate in discussions concerning discharge and transition planning. A predischarge visit to the child's home and alternative sites of care the family plans to use provides an especially helpful opportunity for health care personnel to get to know the family in the family's own environment. Such visits may include the home of a grandparent or a child care facility where the child will receive care for substantial amounts of time.

▸ Exploring Choices

Realistically, the economics of health care today often dictate the choices and options related to the provision of home care. Insurers' and other third-party payers' constraints may determine when home care begins, as well as how many home visits will be covered, how long they will last, and who will provide them. In the worst-case scenario, families simply are told that "home care is going to happen" and they are not prepared for the consequences. It also is not uncommon that a carefully structured hospital discharge plan goes unused because the home care providers develop plans of their own.

Open dialogue between the family, medical team, and insurers is the best way to minimize the effects of these realities. Strong systems of communication allow the family to share its expectations of home care and to prepare for variables that are beyond its control. The family may need time to explore ways to arrange for care that is not covered through insurance.

To the greatest extent possible, families and providers should explore options and choices concerning the following issues:

- The date when home care will begin
- The roles and responsibilities that parents, siblings, other family members, and nonfamily caregivers will assume
- The days of the week and time of day for home care visits
- The places in the home and community where care will be delivered
- Approaches to care and treatment, including complementary therapies
- Ways to incorporate therapies and other care procedures into family patterns to minimize the disruption of the child's normal activities and family routines
- The involvement of schools, community agencies, and other providers of support services
- Arrangements for respite care
- Benchmarks that will enable family members to feel that their child's health care plan, as well as their caregiving ability, is producing positive results
- Preparation and transition planning prior to the termination of home care

A comprehensive written plan of care should evolve from these discussions. Since many families may not truly understand the issues of care at home until their child is at home, time for follow-up conversations, evaluations, and ongoing planning should be anticipated and planned for.

▶ Coordinating Care

Having a care coordinator who works collaboratively with the family over time is especially important for children with complex health care needs.

The child's primary care physician is often the closest to the home setting and can be a link to community resources; therefore, the primary care physician has an important role to play in coordinating the child's care with the family and the home care agency. Without the support of a primary care physician, the family is often left alone to manage the burden and stress of care coordination. A communication system needs to be established among the primary care physician, subspecialists, home care providers, other community providers, and family.

Involvement of multiple providers is a reality of home care. Efforts must be made to include all individuals and organizations involved in a child's care in the communication network (eg, nurses, therapists, physicians, durable medical equipment suppliers, home care pharmacists, and school or child care personnel).

▶ Service Flexibility

Respecting family privacy is a hallmark of family-centered home care. The comings and goings of home care providers are necessary, but can be potentially disruptive intrusions on the family's normal routines. Families whose children are receiving home care frequently maintain that they feel they are living in a "fishbowl." While they welcome the home care provider's expertise and the opportunity to share caregiving responsibilities, family members may feel uncomfortable if they sense they are being forced to relinquish control in an environment where their wishes should take priority.

For these reasons, it is essential that home care agencies and staff be flexible in the ways they work with families to plan and provide pediatric home care.

▶ Communication, Information Sharing, and Learning

Family-centered providers approach every new child and family with the assumption that the relationship will be a learning experience for everyone involved. The family and child will learn new skills, and home care providers will learn about the family's strengths and needs and how to respond to them. Children and families need information if they are to collaborate confidently in care planning and caregiving. Such information must be shared with families in ways that each family finds most useful and easiest to assimilate. Language may pose a barrier if the provider is not fluent in the language that the family prefers; more subtle difficulties in language (eg, the use of jargon or technical terms) must also be recognized and overcome. Home care providers should make arrangements to have translation services available.

Sharing information "up front" about what families can expect is essential. Home care is still a new concept to most health care consumers. Families have few models or criteria to use to define what constitutes quality home care. What will the home care team do? What will the family be expected to do? Will they be capable of performing a medical procedure? It is very likely that some confusion and miscommunication will occur. Providing clear and specific information about how, who, what, when, and where is critical. Linking families to other families who have experienced similar home care is another important source of information for families.

Documentation procedures and charting forms that are consistent with family-centered principles can capture families' strengths, needs, goals, priorities, and values. Families should have the opportunity to see the agency's home care chart, daily logs, and flow sheets. Written documentation ensures quality; it also fosters communication and collaboration with the family and among all disciplines involved in the child's care. Appropriately designed forms also capture families' questions and observations, which can be of value to the health care team.

Electronic technology has the potential to enhance quality and consistency in pediatric home care and to increase access to information and support for both families and home care providers. In the future, families, primary care physicians, subspecialists, and home care providers should jointly explore creative ways to use information technology (eg, e-mail, electronic charting, telemedicine) to facilitate communication and care coordination.

▶ Ongoing Emotional and Practical Support for Families

Providing medical care in the home for a child with an acute or chronic health condition and working with home care staff are physically and emotionally challenging for many families. Family members may experience an initial flush of success; they are proud to have mastered the skills needed to assume a new role in their child's health care. They rightfully feel that an enormous hurdle has been overcome.

This mood may quickly give way to despair as the family realizes the enormity of its new responsibility. In the hospital, someone else prepared meals, did the dishes, cleaned the room, and did the laundry, in addition to organizing and providing most of the care. In home care, many new medical regimens are added to the family's routine domestic chores and other responsibilities.

Because of the new demands placed upon them and the withdrawal of the support offered by the hospital, families providing home care may need formal and informal support to manage the logistical matters related to running a household and providing the child's care. Communication and coordination with a variety of community agencies, vendors, family members, and friends may be necessary.

Support for the developmental and educational needs of the child is essential. Coordination with child care staff, school nurse, home tutor, athletic coaches, and others is necessary for integrating medical care into the child's daily routines. "Play" is the "work" of children, including those who are seriously or chronically ill. Planning for playmate visits and opportunities for interactions with brothers and sisters is another component of a home care plan.

Planning for playmate visits…is another component of a home care plan.

▶ Family-to-Family Support

The experience of home care can also be emotionally exhausting and very isolating. During hospitalization, social isolation generally is not an issue for families. It is relatively easy to establish informal, supportive relationships with other children and families on the unit, in the playroom, in the family lounge, in the clinic, or in a support group meeting. When caring for a child's special medical needs at home, it can be challenging for families to maintain relationships with friends as well as to meet others in similar circumstances.

To decrease social isolation and enhance support, facilitating opportunities for children and families to connect with others who have had similar experiences is essential. The home care provider can take the initiative by offering the names of other families in similar circumstances who have volunteered to provide parent-to-parent support. Families then can decide whether they wish to avail themselves to this opportunity.

In addition to needing the unique support of a family-to-family network, families receiving home care also have a great need for respite care. Home care staff should help make the family aware of the importance of respite time and the value of respite care for the overall well-being of the family.

Home care staff can support and help facilitate a family seeking respite care services either from a professional agency or from trained friends or relatives.

▸ Support for Home Care Staff

Home care also can be an isolating experience for home care practitioners. They do not have the opportunity for informal daily interactions with colleagues. Colleagues are not immediately available for advice on technical and clinical issues. It also is challenging for home care providers to connect with colleagues for emotional support.

Providing an effective orientation and mentoring program coupled with ongoing staff development sessions and opportunities for reflective practice will help in building the capacity of home care staff. Families who have experienced pediatric home care can help in both planning the educational programming and presenting some of the sessions. Another way to support home care employees is to create time in regularly scheduled staff meetings for candid, supportive discussions about the handling of difficult or challenging situations.

Caring for the caregivers, the front line of a home care agency, is essential to recruiting and maintaining a qualified staff with the skills, attitudes, and energy to practice family-centered care.

Home Care and the Therapeutic Relationship

The nature of the therapeutic relationship in home care is different from that in an office or hospital setting for two primary reasons. First, the caregiving takes place within the privacy of the patient's home. Second, as distinct from the hospital setting, there is neither supervisory support nor professional guidance on site for home care staff as there is in a hospital or clinic.

Lines between health care personnel and family members can get blurred. This can be a source of stress for both the family and home care providers. For this reason, the roles and responsibilities of families and professionals in home care need to be clearly defined. Communication about what constitutes a therapeutic boundary must take place between the provider and the family in a positive and proactive manner.

Family-centered care can provide the framework for families to negotiate and renegotiate roles and responsibilities with home care providers. Family-centered care ensures that providers listen to and respect the family's point of view; as a result, it empowers a family to openly communicate with the health care team. This pattern of communication is the key to creating and maintaining therapeutic relationships in the home, and it naturally provides for periodic evaluation of the care plan.

Summary: Translating the Philosophy Into Systems of Care

To operationalize a family-centered approach in pediatric home care, clinicians, administrators, other staff, and families can begin by asking targeted questions about a home care program's or agency's philosophy and practices. The following questions capture information that indicates, in general terms, whether and how the agency is making a commitment to family-centered practice.

- Does the home care agency's stated philosophy of care reflect the principles of family-centered care?
- Is this philosophy of care communicated clearly throughout the agency, to families, and to others in the community?
- Do families who use pediatric home care services participate as advisors to the agency? Do families participate in the agency's quality improvement initiatives?
- Are the home care agency's policies, programs, and staff practices consistent with the view that families are allies and that they are important to the child's care plan and to his or her health and well-being?
- Does the home care agency have personnel with the appropriate training and experience to meet the technical aspects of pediatric care and provide care in a developmentally supportive, family-centered manner?
- What systems are in place to ensure that families have access, on an ongoing basis, to complete, unbiased, and useful information about their child and the plan of care?
- What systems are in place to ensure that families have access to formal and informal sources of emotional and practical support? Is information about opportunities for peer support shared with families on a regular basis?

- What opportunities are built into the agency's system of care for families to participate in care coordination and the management of transitions? What support is available to families to participate in this planning and decision making?
- How does the child's primary care provider work with the family and the home care agency to coordinate care and facilitate communication about the child and the plan of care? If the primary care provider does not take this role, who will?
- How does the agency's human resources system support the practice of family-centered care? In what ways are families involved in the orientation and education of pediatric home care staff?

Acknowledgment

The authors wish to acknowledge the thoughtful reviews by families and professionals, especially Betsy Anderson, Elizabeth Ahmann, and Connie Lierman; the editorial assistance of Linda Harteker; and the support of the Nathan Cummings Foundation for the development of this chapter and the self-assessment inventory in the Appendix.

Bibliography

Ahmann E. *Home Care for the High-Risk Infant: A Family-Centered Approach.* 2nd ed. Gaithersburg, MD: Aspen Publishers; 1996

Ahmann E. Thinking critically about family-centered home care nursing. *Pediatr Nurs.* 1994; 20:588-590

Ahmann E, Bond NJ. Promoting normal development in school-age children and adolescents who are technology dependent: a family centered model. *Pediatr Nurs.* 1992;18:399-405

Dokken DL, Sydnor-Greenberg N. Helping families mobilize their personal resources. *Pediatr Nurs.* 1998;24:66-69

Hostler SL. Pediatric family-centered rehabilitation. *J Head Trauma Rehabil.* 1999;14:384-393

Institute for Family-Centered Care. Change: it's happening everywhere. *Advances in Family-Centered Care.* 1995;3. Available at: http://www.familycenteredcare.org/adv_issue3.htm. Accessed August 22, 2001

Institute for Family-Centered Care. Family re-union 7 puts family-centered care in the spotlight. *Advances in Family-Centered Care.* 1998;5. Available at: http://www.familycenteredcare.org/adv_issue5.htm. Accessed August 22, 2001

Klug RM. Clarifying roles and expectations in home care. *Pediatr Nurs.* 1993;19:374-376

McKlindon D, Barnsteiner JH. Therapeutic relationships. Evolution of the Children's Hospital of Philadelphia model. *MCN Am J Matern Child Nurs.* 1994;24:237-243

Perrin JM, Shayne MW, Bloom SR. *Home and Community Care for Chronically Ill Children.* New York, NY: Oxford University Press; 1993

Shelton TL, Jeppson ES, Johnson BH. *Family-Centered Care for Children With Special Health Care Needs.* Washington, DC: Association for the Care of Children's Health; 1987

Swanson SC, Naber MM. Neonatal integrated home care: nursing without walls. *Neonatal Netw.* 1997;16:33-38

Thyen U, Kuhlthau K, Perrin JM. Employment, child care, and mental health of mothers caring for children assisted by technology. *Pediatrics.* 1999;103:1235-1242

US Department of Health and Human Services. *Surgeon General's Report — Children with Special Health Care Needs: Campaign '87.* Washington, DC: US Dept of Health and Human Services; 1987

Resource

Moving Toward a Family-Centered Pediatric Home Care: A Self-Assessment In, developed by the Institute for Family-Centered Care, is a comprehensive self-assessment tool that examines whether family-centered principles are applied to policies and practices related to key aspects of home care. This tool is a resource for self-reflection, planning, evaluation, and prioritizing a process for change, and for integrating family-centered concepts within the infrastructure of a home care program or agency.

Chapter 7

Family-Directed Home Health Care

Denise Callarman; Leann Lazzari

Introduction

The current model of home care recognizes the nurse as the key component to care for a child in the home. When nurses are not available to provide care in the home, children who are medically fragile frequently are not offered home care services. As a result, many children are institutionalized and lose the benefits of a loving home environment. Fortunately, family-directed home care is an alternative.

What distinguishes a family-directed model of home care from other models is the recognition of the family as the primary care-giver. To be successful, this model not only requires family-centered care, it demands family-directed care. The professional's role in family-directed care is to pro-vide consultative guidance to ensure that care is delivered appropriately in the home. This best can be achieved when all parties, including physician, family, and support services, agree to work together in partnership.

In this home care model the caregivers (usually parents or guardians) are responsible for coordinating the ongoing needs of the child. The primary caregiver incurs most of the caregiving responsibility. Tasks include, but are not limited to, the following:

- Directing nursing and respiratory care
- Directing physical, speech, and occupational therapy sessions
- Maintaining and modifying the care plan
- Ordering medical supplies
- Keeping adequate inventory
- Attending health care-related appointments
- Participating in rehospitalizations
- Coordinating special educational needs
- Training alternative caregivers
- Coordinating care services
- Maintaining health records and other documentation for health care professionals and payers

Because this model eliminates the nurse as the case manager in the service plan, it is incumbent on the parent to coordinate care with support. Service organizations, churches, schools, emergency care, neighbors, and family become the major support system. To prevent the feeling of isolation after hospital discharge, it is important to include representatives from these community resources during the planning process. The success of this model depends on the motivation and capability of the family to assume its responsibilities. Success results from the family being motivated and committed, adapting well to changing circumstances, and partnering well with other members of the health care team.

How Does a Child Fit Into This Model of Care?

The following are reasons for placing a child in a family-directed home care environment:

- The family cannot find adequate caregiving support in the community because of the medical complexity of the child.
- The child gets reinstitutionalized for nonmedical reasons.
- The professional or nonprofessional primary caregiver becomes seriously ill.
- The physician requests it after assessing the family's willingness and capability.
- To conserve health insurance resources.
- The family wants it.

Because reimbursement for services is becoming more limited and nursing staff is difficult to find, components of this home health care model are more prevalent. If appropriately managed and financially supported, the care model opens an array of services and creative programs for families and physicians. In some cases, this positive alternative may be the only way to ensure families stay together in their homes and community where they belong.

Before agreeing to use this model, families first must be informed of all options, including all models of care and care settings (ie, home, hospital, infusion center, out-of-home child care, etc) to ensure they choose the setting that works best for their particular situation. It is critical that the family-directed model of care not be forced on families because this model requires significant time, energy, motivation, and commitment for success. A sound family-professional-payer partnership is essential for this program to remain safe and cost effective.

A Team Approach

A team approach to management is essential for the success of this model. Parents, medical professionals, community services, and the payer should develop a quality home care plan prior to hospital discharge. The home care plan should acknowledge the additional responsibility the primary caregiver may have to the spouse, siblings, employer, house upkeep, etc. Initially these additional demands may appear unrealistic, but they usually are manageable because of the family's commitment to the child. The plan should include the tasks and responsibilities of the primary caregiver and an explanation of how those tasks will be fulfilled.

Family-directed care should provide for the same ancillary services and ongoing maintenance as nursing-directed home care. The primary caregiver should keep appropriate notes and records for later review. A system to ensure quality care and review should be established by the health care team. Ensuring appropriate medical, spiritual, emotional, educational, and caring support in the home makes for a successful home care program, keeping the child home and the family intact.

▶ The Physician's Role

Without adequate support from resources outside the home, the family or caregiver may experience burnout (causing illness, depression, etc) in a very short time. One of the major responsibilities of a physician in home care is to assess the caregiver's needs and capacities. Physicians should be sensitive to the social dynamics within the home and offer opportunities for conflict resolution, alternative care arrangements, and support. Similarly, primary caregivers should be encouraged to delegate responsibilities so there is time to care for themselves.

Professionals are trained to evaluate the total care needs of a patient when providing medical care, yet they also should evaluate the total home when developing and maintaining an appropriate home care program. The ideal goal of any home care program is to provide a better quality of life for the child and family. For this reason, the child's physician has the responsibility of ensuring that the home care plan is meeting its goal. The family as a whole should be in good physical and psychosocial health to perform the sometimes exhausting task of maintaining a safe home care environment

for a child who is medically fragile. Evaluating the parents, specialists, educators, siblings, visiting nurses (if any), and others within the home care network is appropriate and should be done prior to discharge, 3 months after
discharge, 9 months after the first evaluation, and annually thereafter. This
can be accomplished by a home care physician visit for the purpose of
case management.

▸ Respite Care

If the primary caregiver becomes ill or simply wants to find relief and an
alternative caregiver is not available, a contingency plan must be in place.
The home care plan should have identified options for the child's care
during this period. Alternative care arrangements are imperative to ensure a
better quality of life for the entire family and to ensure this model's success.
Alternative home care plans may include other family members, trained
caregivers, home care nurses, or care outside the home. Consideration of the
following options for caregiver relief allows the program to become more
efficient, cost effective, and, of course, maintain its family-directed focus:

1. **Medical Respite Care** — Respite, meaning "a break from your labors,"
   is an essential part of home health care. It is an alternative of care that
   can offer assistance in the home on an as-needed basis by a trained
   medical professional or outside the home through a community-based
   respite care site. A medical center (ie, hospital) should not be used for
   respite care because families need community support, children become
   exposed to illness, and most children do not like being placed in a hospital. Parents are unlikely to use an institutional model for respite care
   unless it is the only option. Community-based respite care is an ideal
   program for families.

2. **Personal Care Attendants (PCAs)** — These are nonprofessionals
   chosen by predetermined criteria with skills to provide care under the
   supervision of parents and professionals. They are selected and managed
   by the family. A PCA, if properly oriented to a child's care plan and
   trained in home health care, can be a cost-effective, family-centered alternative caregiver for this model of care. A PCA should be employed by
   the family only when the physician and the family agree that the care
   needs of the child do not require a nurse with extensive professional
   training (such as a registered nurse or licensed practical nurse).

3. **Out-of-Home Medical Day Care** — Medical day care is an excellent addition to the care needs of the child. It may be the only way a primary caregiver can work (*see* Chapter 37). Nonmedical inclusive child care also may be an option if supplementary personnel are available to assist the child with special health care needs.

4. **Reinstitutionalization** — In some instances, children have been required to be reinstitutionalized when caregiving options in the community become exhausted. This is certainly the last resort when a family simply cannot continue to safely care for the child at home. Institutional options include
   - Acute hospital
   - Rehabilitation hospital
   - Transitional care settings
   - Long-term care settings (eg, nursing homes)

   This choice is not family centered or cost effective.

Home Care Planning for the Parent

Whether a family chooses to use a family-directed model of home care, health care team members should strive to develop a parent-payer-provider partnership. The goal of such a partnership is to create a coordinated team approach to prevent fragmentation of health care services and to recognize and empower families as integral players within the delivery system.

▸ Create a Parent-Payer-Provider Partnership

In developing the most effective home care delivery model, it is important to create a partnership among all involved parties. The earlier in the process this partnership is formed, the more successful the home care program will be. Ideally, this partnership is formed before a discharge occurs from the hospital. The process should be initiated by a designated staff member of the hospital, usually one of the discharge planners or social workers.

For children who are medically fragile with high-tech needs, an initial meeting should be held to identify the team members, including family members, hospital staff, primary care physician, physician specialists, home nursing, home therapy, durable medical equipment suppliers, payers, school district, and other community resources.

The following are issues that should be discussed among the team:

Organizational

- What are the roles and responsibilities of each team member?
- What is the plan for ongoing communication and decision making?
- What is the best means for exchange of medical information between physicians, families, and nursing agencies?

Medical

- Who is the primary care physician?
- Are any specialists required?
- What services are required for the child?

Social

- What community services are available that could provide some of the required services such as the 0–3 program for children 3 years or younger, Easter Seals, and/or similar programs?
- What support services are available near the family?
- Are there other families in similar situations that the family could meet?

Financial

- What services will be reimbursed by the payer as part of the plan for the child?
- What services may not be reimbursed by payers?
- What is the process for appealing for an exception to the plan coverage to allow for required services?

Educational

- If the child is of school age, what services will the school district provide (eg, physical therapy, occupational therapy, speech therapy, nursing care, classroom aid) and what type of classroom setting is best for the child?
- If the child is younger than school age, what educational services will be offered as part of the child's early developmental program?

▶ Create a Process for Implementing Home Care

The most appropriate method of transition from hospital to home needs to be identified, with consideration given to the child's stability as well as family readiness. The necessary resources must be in place prior to moving a patient back home. The transition process may include a combination of the following:

- Hospital to long-term care facility to home
- Hospital to step-down unit to home
- Hospital to community site to home
- Hospital to home

▶ Create a Home Care Manual

The key to making home care work for families is organization. Every aspect of home care needs to be documented, organized, and communicated to allow for the most optimal outcome. A home care manual should be developed prior to discharge to include the information shown in Table 7-1.

TABLE 7-1. Information to Include in a Home Care Manual

- Directory of all members of the home care team documenting each person's name, particular discipline, address, and phone number
- Diagnosis and reference information about diagnosis
- Specific health care needs and reference information about needs
- Policies and procedures defining the child's specific care and equipment maintenance
- Policies and procedures relating to the family's personal guidelines to be followed within the home
- Section for documenting daily care
- Section for communication
- Time-management section for scheduling daily and weekly care, medications, physician visits, medical procedures, and long-term planning to enable coordination of services when possible
- Use of the Emergency Information Form for Children With Special Needs, developed by the American Academy of Pediatrics (AAP) and the American College of Emergency Physicians (ACEP) (see Appendix)

NOTE: An excellent resource for creating a home care manual is *The Home Care Organizer*, available from State of the Art, Inc (800/790-9267).

▶ Create a Health Care Passport

A health care passport for medical professionals documents the information listed in Table 7-2 and maintains valuable historical health care data. This passport should be kept in the home care manual and be presented when admitted to the hospital because it will educate the staff about the child's history and special health care needs. This passport is convenient for families and, by keeping all important information in one place, results in the relaying of more accurate information when providing the medical history of a child and prevents information that could prove to be important from being left out inadvertently.

TABLE 7-2. Information to Include in a Health Care Passport

- Current picture of child and basic information, including name, date of birth, address, names of parents or guardians with phone numbers, primary care physician's name and phone number, payer information, diagnosis, and health care needs
- Profile summary of child's life, including likes, dislikes, precautions, cognitive ability, means of communication, and other information as appropriate
- Log of all surgical procedures, including date of procedure, name of procedure, reason, outcome, and place procedure was performed
- Log of hospitalizations, including dates, reason, outcome, and name and location of the hospital
- Log of all medications given, including time period, reason, response, and any allergic reactions
- Allergies and other warnings

▶ Monitoring the Home Care Program

A method for monitoring the home care program on an ongoing basis involving all disciplines and members of the team should be created. This monitoring includes the following:

- Monthly status reports distributed by all team members
- Team meetings scheduled at regular intervals
- Teleconferences scheduled at regular intervals

Summary

- The family is recognized as the primary caregiver in family-directed care.
- There are a variety of reasons for placing a child in a family-directed home care environment. It is imperative that families are informed of all options before agreeing to use this model.
- A team approach to management is essential for the success of family-directed care. A parent-payer-provider partnership must be developed and include all involved parties.
- One of the major responsibilities of physicians in home care is to assess the caregiver's needs and capacities. A plan to provide respite care when needed is imperative to ensure a better quality of life for the family and to ensure the model's success.
- A home care manual and home care passport are valuable tools in family-directed home care.

Bibliography

Illinois Department of Public Health. 2 Ill Adm Code 1125 Section 1100.760; Children's Respite Care Center Alternative Health Care Model; November 15, 1996. Available at: http://www.idph.state.il.us/ralesregs/77-1100.htm. Accessed September 25, 2001

Goldberg AI, Alba AA, Oppenheimer EA, Roberts E. Caring for mechanically ventilated patients at home. *Chest*. 1990;98:1543

Goldberg AI, Trubitt MJ. An integrated approach to home health care. *Physician Exec*. 1994;20:45-46

Rehabilitation Institute of Chicago. *What Ever Happened to the Polio Patient?: Proceedings of an International Symposium*. Chicago: Rehabilitation Institute of Chicago; 1982

US Department of Health and Human Services. The Surgeon General Workshop on Self-Help and Public Health. September 20-22, 1987; Los Angeles, CA

PART TWO

Guidelines for Pediatric Home Health Care Programs

Chapter 8

Pediatric Home Nursing and Ancillary Programs

Marion Townsend, RN; Francine Pasek, RN; Catherine Prophet, RN, BSN; Mark McConnell, MD

Introduction

All children who require hospitalization for physiologic monitoring or invasive medical treatments should have the opportunity to have their care initiated or continued in the home environment. In general, children will require ongoing nursing services in the home as long as they have skilled medical needs that cannot be met safely by the family or other health care professional. Additionally, patients at risk for physiologic deterioration should be monitored regularly by trained nursing personnel in the home if frequent physician office visits are not feasible.

Home Nursing Programs

Because nurses are key to a successful home care program, it is important to ensure that the home care nurse is competent to care for children in the home. Pediatric home care nurses should have at least 1 year of acute pediatric or neonatal experience or other comparable pediatric experience. Nurses should possess basic pediatric nursing skills, including independent assessment skills, competency in medication calculation and administration, aseptic technique, and use of specialized home equipment. Nurses should always act under the direction of the attending physician. Nurses should be provided with orientation in agency policies and procedures, specialized home equipment, common home health pediatric nursing procedures, and documentation policy. Pediatric nursing competencies should be evaluated at orientation and annually thereafter and include the following:

- Compliance with standard precautions, and safety and emergency procedures
- Use of documentation on all charting forms in accordance with documentation policy

- Ability to perform an admission according to policy and procedure
- Ability to safely calculate, prepare, and administer intravenous (IV) fluids and other medications
- Ability to care for IV access lines according to written policy and procedure
- Ability to provide nursing care based on disease process, current nursing research, and policy and procedure
- Ability to perform nursing procedures independently or with minimal assistance based on policy and procedure and nursing research
- Ability to safely demonstrate use of specialized equipment necessary for a child's care according to manufacturer's guidelines

Nurses should be supervised by a nursing supervisor who has adequate experience in pediatric home care to serve as a resource to the home care nurse. The nursing supervisor is responsible for ensuring nurse competency on a regular basis. The nursing supervisor also is responsible for overseeing care provided by nursing staff and all disciplines. Visits should be staffed by nurses proficient and competent in providing care that is specific for the patient. For example, a neonatal nurse provides care to premature infants, and an oncology nurse administers chemotherapy.

▶ **Nursing Care Coordination**

A nurse (patient care coordinator or case manager) should be assigned to coordinate the care of the patient. This care management should include the initial assessment, follow-up telephone calls, and coordination of care with other disciplines. The patient care coordinator provides ongoing assessment and reassessment at least every 62 days, according to Centers for Medicare and Medicaid Services (CMS) (formerly Health Care Financing Administration [HCFA]) guidelines, notifies the physician of any changes in patient condition, and coordinates the delivery of skilled care, including patient/family education. Additionally, this nurse should coordinate care with other providers such as durable medical equipment vendors, pharmacies, and other agencies. Indications for home nursing visits and suggested frequency and duration of home nursing care for specific medical problems are listed in Table 8-1.

TABLE 8-1. Indications for Home Nursing Visits

Type of Visit	Frequency	Duration of Care
A. Prematurity	The number of skilled nursing visits will depend on the patient's clinical status, family's ability to provide care, and equipment required. Nursing visits may be needed for patient assessment, weight checks and caregiver instruction on newborn care, feeding technique, and medication administration. Examples would be: preterm newborns with no underlying disease process might require one to two visits, while preterm newborns who are technologically supported with use of apnea/bradycardia monitor, O_2, oximeter, and feeding tubes may require one to six visits. Preterm newborns who are terminal may require weekly or biweekly visits.	Varies according to disease process
B. Phototherapy	Initial visit and daily thereafter for assessment, weight check, and blood draws until bilirubin level is appropriate as determined by physician.	3-5 days
C. Apnea Monitor	Monitor delivered to hospital with instruction by respiratory therapist, initial skilled nursing visit within 72 hours of discharge for assessment, review of equipment instruction, disease process, review cardiopulmonary resuscitation (CPR); additional visits as required (prn).	2 weeks
D. IV Antibiotic Infusion	Initial visit to instruct caregiver on administration, flush, site and line care; second visit to observe competency, two to three additional visits as needed to restart intravenous (IV) catheter, assessment or to provide additional education. Registered nurse (RN) to administer all doses of antibiotics on infants less than 6 months of age.	For duration of therapy
E. TPN/IL Infusion	Initial visit to instruct on set up, organization of supplies, central line care, and flushes. Three to seven additional visits to demonstrate caregiver competency. Additional visits prn for lab draws if indicated.	3-5 days initially and then prn
F. Tracheostomy Care	Caregiver must have already changed tracheostomy prior to discharge from the hospital. Daily visits to instruct on tracheostomy site care, equipment use and care, suctioning, and observe tracheostomy change. Some physicians require children with tracheostomies to have 24-hour nursing care indefinitely because of the small risk of possible obstruction of the tracheostomy tube leading to death.	2 weeks up to indefinitely

TABLE 8-1. Indications for Home Nursing Visits, continued

Type of Visit	Frequency	Duration of Care
G. Shift Care	Provided according to patient/family needs. Can be short- or long-term, 8, 12, or 16 hours/day depending on the needs of the family.	As long as necessary
H. Home Ventilator	Initial hospital evaluation to assess needs, deliver equipment to hospital, then 3-4 days of 24-hour care decreasing daily nursing time to intermittent visits if caregivers are competent and available. Otherwise, continued shift care for 16-24 hours/day – especially while caregivers sleep and/or work.	Per individual patient and family needs
I. Enteral Therapy	One to two visits to instruct on enteral therapy, use of infusion pump (if applicable), safety precautions, skin care, stoma care, preparation of formula, insertion/verification of nasogastric tube (if applicable), replacement of gastrostomy tube (if applicable), and ordering supplies.	2 weeks
J. Asthma	One skilled nursing visit to instruct family on diagnosis, triggers, use of handheld nebulizer, administration of medications, use of peak flow meter, and when to notify physician.	3 days
K. IVIG Infusion	One to three monthly visits to obtain pre- or post-labs as ordered, initiate IV, administer pre-medications, infuse IVIG over recommended time frame (typically 2-4 hours), observe for adverse reaction, and discontinue IV at completion of infusion.	For duration of therapy
L. Subcutaneous Injections (GCSF, Insulin, etc)	One to three skilled nursing visits to instruct parents on proper technique of administration of subcutaneous injection, site rotation, medication rationale, side effects, and adverse reactions. Subsequent visit required to observe parental competency.	1 week

---

Example

Eight-year-old child with IV antibiotics via peripherally inserted central catheter line for 6 weeks. The patient's home care needs include seven RN-level visits for administration of medication, observation of caregiver, education on use of infusion pump, signs and symptoms of site infection, infiltration, medication rationale, side effects, adverse reactions, and flushing of the line. Second visit to observe return demonstration by caregiver. Weekly visits for dressing and cap changes.

▶ Guidelines for Nursing Documentation

Regulatory requirements for home care documentation vary by state, but usually include a consent to treat, patient bill of rights, caregiver responsibilities, emergency plan, advance directives, and home safety evaluation. In addition, initial nursing assessments should include medication profiles, nutritional status, plan of care, and patient/family education plan. Each nursing visit should be documented completely and include a record of interventions and procedures with patient/family response, recommendations for additional skilled services, any communication with physician and office staff, and a report to physician on findings. Ongoing nursing visit notes should include patient reassessment including vital signs and weight, reevaluation of care plan, patient/family education, recommendations for additional skilled services, nursing interventions, and patient response to interventions.

Patient/Family Assessment

An initial assessment should be completed for each patient upon admission to home care service, which includes physical, psychosocial, nutritional, safety assessments, medications, immunizations, and ability and willingness of parents to learn. Based on the initial assessment, a care plan is developed with patient-specific goals. One of the goals of the nurse should be to help the patient and family become independent in the care, although this is not always possible. Further education of the patient or family may be necessary to achieve the goals of the plan of treatment. Reassessment, evaluation, and revision of goals are done at least every 62 days, according to CMS guidelines.

Physician Communication

Because the attending physician is responsible for medical treatment of the patient, the home care nurses should be diligent about communicating any pertinent patient issues with the attending physician. Home care providers should determine ahead of time how a patient's attending physician would like clinical information and questions relayed to him or her. There should be a clear plan on how to contact the physician after hours or in the event of an emergency. Generally, it is the responsibility of the home care nursing staff to develop a plan of care based on the physician's orders and with the physician's input. Once developed, the physician should be diligent about signing the plan of care and returning it to the home care organization within 20 days. Likewise, supplemental orders should be reviewed and signed by the attending physician and returned to the home care provider within 30 days. Repeated failures to obtain timely signatures on orders or plans of care may result in disciplinary actions against the home care provider by government regulators.

Guidelines for Other Home Care Personnel

A licensed vocational nurse (LVN) or licensed practical nurse (LPN) may provide some patient care responsibilities in the home. An LVN/LPN must be a graduate of an accredited school of nursing and should have a minimum of 1 year of prior professional nursing experience preferably in pediatrics. The LVN/LPN should be supervised by a registered nurse, who usually is the nursing supervisor. The LVN/LPN provides services according to agency policies, follows the plan of treatment, evaluates the care plan, participates in patient conferences, completes clinical progress notes, prepares and administers medications, performs venipuncture if certified, and assists patients and families in learning self-care techniques. An LVN/LPN generally is prohibited from admitting a patient on service, developing a care plan, initiating patient family education, and administering intravenous medications.

Home health aids (HHAs) are nursing personnel who assist patients and families with basic care tasks. Home health aids are not regularly used in pediatric home care, but may be used for respite care when custodial care is the only service required. An on-site supervisory visit by a registered nurse must be done every 2 weeks if the patient is receiving other skilled services such as physical therapy. If no other skilled services are being provided, an on-site supervisory visit can be done every 62 days with the home health aid present.

Table 8-2 lists three types of nursing caregivers and care they are trained to provide.

TABLE 8-2. Nursing Care Priveleges by Type of Caregiver

	Level of Caregiver		
Task	Registered Nurse	Licensed Vocational Nurse	Home Health Aide
Ventilator care	When trained	When trained	No
Tracheostomy tube reinsertion	When trained	When trained	No
Central line care	Yes	No	No
IV medication administration	Yes	No	No
Oral/IM/SQ/rectal medication administration	Yes	Yes	No
GT feedings	Yes	Yes	When trained
GT reinsertion	Yes	Yes	No
Initial assessment	Yes	No	No
Initiation of the plan of care	Yes	No	No
Suctioning	Yes	Yes	When trained
Bowel care	Yes	Yes	When trained
Sterile dressing changes	Yes	Yes	No
General wound care	Yes	Yes	When trained
Chart documentation	Yes	Yes	Yes
Physician orders	Yes	Only those which do not apply to IV medications	No
Draw labs	Yes	Only peripheral when trained	No

▶ Physical Therapy

Physical therapists should be graduates of an accredited therapy program licensed by the state. In addition, most therapists complete an internship program and should have at least 1 year of experience working with pediatric patients in an acute care hospital. They should have completed training in basic cardiopulmonary resuscitation. Some therapists may have additional training in specialty areas such as feeding therapy and spinal cord injury. Therapists should receive an orientation on agency policy and procedures, and documentation policy.

Supervision of therapists can be done by a senior physical therapist, but each therapist reports directly to nursing administrative staff. The therapist's supervisor should evaluate competencies at orientation, in the field at the patient's home, and then again on an annual basis.

Therapists are assigned to patients according to their area of expertise. As an example, therapists experienced with patients who have spinal cord injuries would be assigned to patients with spinal cord injuries, and therapists experienced in feeding therapy would be assigned to patients with feeding difficulties. For continuity, it is best to have the same therapist throughout the course of therapy if at all possible. Therapists should make recommendations for frequency and duration of ongoing therapy during the initial evaluation, which is then approved and ordered by the physician.

Home physical therapy is indicated for patients who are homebound due to a considerable and taxing effort to leave the home, for patients who are immunosuppressed, or if therapy would be too exhausting for the patient to perform and complete outside the home. Patients seen most frequently in the home are children with neurodevelopmental delays, prematurity, brachial plexus injuries, or traumatic brain injuries; children who are medically compromised leading to mobility disorders or juvenile rheumatoid arthritis; and children with cardiac problems or feeding issues. Some patients may require therapies that can be delivered either by an occupational therapist or physical therapist. If a patient requires therapy for decreased tone, strengthening, or mobility deficits, either therapist may provide skilled care, rather than having two separate therapists.

Home physical therapy is indicated for patients who are homebound due to a considerable and taxing effort to leave the home, for patients who are immunosuppressed, or if therapy would be too exhausting for the patient to perform and complete outside the home.

If the physical therapist will be the only professional initiating home care, the therapist should collect all necessary clinical and administrative information and document the information similar to the way nursing personnel are required to document. The initial therapy evaluation should include gross motor assessment, developmental assessment, treatment modalities and procedures, short-term and long-term goals, recommendations for frequency and duration of ongoing therapy, and equipment recommendations. The patient should have a reassessment, revision of goals, and medication profile done every 62 days.

Providing the family with a home program is essential to help the family follow through with therapy goals. Evaluation of caregiver participation and revision of the home therapy program are done on an ongoing basis. Therapists should be diligent about documenting their therapy, including treatment modality and patient response to therapy. When goals are met and therapy services are no longer required, the physician is notified and the patient should be discharged from service.

The attending physician is responsible for medical treatment of the patient and development of the plan of treatment in consultation with the therapist and agency staff. The therapist should confer regularly with the physician and report the physical and emotional conditions, response to treatment, and social and/or physical factors in the environment that affect patient care. Therapists should attempt to use community resources whenever possible. Community resources include school districts, state and county services, and outpatient therapy facilities.

▸ Occupational Therapy

Occupational therapists should be graduates of an accredited occupational therapy curriculum, accredited jointly by the Committee on Allied Health Education and Accreditation of the American Medical Association and the American Occupational Therapy Association, or eligible for the National Registration Examination of the American Occupational Therapy Association. Occupational therapists should have completed an internship in pediatric therapy or have experience providing therapy to children. Otherwise, they should have received training, orientation, and a competency evaluation similar to physical therapists.

Supervision of occupational therapy staff can be done by a senior physical therapist, but each therapist reports directly to nursing administrative staff. Competencies are evaluated shortly after orientation, in the field at the patient's home, and then again on an annual basis through their written documentation. Their annual assessments should cover a scope of practice similar to that of the physical therapists.

Occupational therapists are assigned to patients according to their areas of expertise. For the sake of continuity, the patient's best interest is served if the same therapist provides all the therapy whenever possible.

Similar to physical therapists, indications for home therapy are for patients who are homebound secondary to considerable and taxing effort to leave the home, are immunosuppressed, or if therapy would be too exhausting for the patient to perform and complete outside the home. Typical patients requiring occupational therapy include those who have impaired fine motor function or self-care skills; decreased strength, tone, and mobility in upper extremities; and oral motor dysfunction.

Occupational therapists provide the following types of therapies: teaching the activities of daily living program; work simplification and energy conservation; muscle re-education program; perceptual, fine motor/dexterity, and gross motor training; neuro-developmental training; sensory enhancement; arrangement of orthotics/splinting; arrangement of adaptive equipment; teaching caregiver exercises/activities; work capacity evaluation; and feeding therapy.

Recommendations for frequency and duration of ongoing therapy are made during the initial evaluation, then approved and ordered by the patient's attending physician.

In most states, an occupational therapist may not admit a patient to home care or complete an initial screening evaluation. A physical therapist or a registered nurse must initiate admission of a patient to home care. The initial therapy evaluation includes fine motor assessment, developmental assessment, treatment modalities and procedures, short-term and long-term goals, recommendations for frequency and duration of ongoing therapy, and equipment recommendations. Reassessment and revision of goals are completed as often as necessary but not less than every 62 days.

Occupational therapists should provide the family with a home program to help them follow through with therapy goals. Evaluation of caregiver participation and revision of home program should be done on an ongoing basis.

▸ Speech Therapy

Speech therapists should possess a master's degree in speech-language pathology or audiology, and a Certificate of Clinical Competence in Speech from the American Speech and Hearing Association. Speech therapists should have completed an internship or have additional experience in caring for pediatric patients. Otherwise, they should have received training, orientation, and a competency evaluation similar to physical therapists.

The speech therapist is under direct supervision of a senior therapist, but reports directly to the nursing administrative staff. Competencies are evaluated shortly after orientation at the patient's home by a senior therapist, and then on an annual basis through review of the speech therapist's written documentation, recommendations, goals, and outcomes.

Speech therapy in the home is indicated for children who are home-bound and speech or hearing impaired, secondary to congenital disorder, trauma, surgery, brain injury, or medical illness. Children with voice disorders, speech articulation disorders, language disorders, and hearing disorders also benefit from speech therapy. Assessment of patients by a speech therapist should include testing for speech and hearing function, patient compre-hension, physical limitations, and previous level of function. In addition, caregiver's willingness to learn and ability to follow through with home therapy instructions are assessed.

▸ Social Work

A home care medical social worker should possess a master's degree in social work from an approved school, college, or university accredited by the Western Association of Schools and Colleges, the Northwest Association of Secondary and Higher Schools, or a master's degree granted by educa-tional institutions whose programs are approved by the Commission on Accreditation for Marriage and Family Therapy Education, or an essentially equivalent accrediting agency as determined by the board. In addition, social workers should have completed a 2-year internship. Social workers should receive orientation on the home care agency policies and procedures. The medical social worker is supervised by, and reports directly to, the nursing administrative staff.

Each home care organization should have a medical social worker who is available to evaluate a patient and the patient's family. For continuity, the patient and family are best served if the same medical social worker provides each visit if at all possible.

Social services typically are underutilized in pediatric home care. Payers should allow medical social worker intervention as part of a patient's home care benefits. Medical social worker visits are indicated when patients or families have difficult or complicated psychosocial problems. Indications for patient referrals to social services may be an inappropriate or unsafe living situation, an unstable mental condition of patient or caregiver, family conflicts, financial concerns, a need for access to community resources that may not be readily available, an abusive or potentially abusive parent or caregiver, poor compliance with a home care treatment plan, or family grieving issues. Recommendations for frequency and duration of ongoing therapy are made during the initial evaluation, and then approved and ordered by the physician.

A medical social worker's initial patient/family assessment should include demographic data, significant medical history, and a full assessment of family strengths and deficits. Also evaluated are the patient's/caregiver's ability to function physically or mentally, the social situation (including environment, home setting, family dynamics, economic concerns, emotional reaction to illness, treatment regime, and limitations), the social situation's impact on the patient's progress toward treatment goals, the need for community resources, developmental risk factors, safety measures, and vulnerability.

The medical social worker should communicate regularly with the patient's attending physician and report any psychosocial issues affecting patient care. A copy of all documentation and a discharge summary should be sent to the physician.

Summary

- Every child who requires hospitalization for physiologic monitoring or invasive medical treatments should have the option of being cared for at home.
- It is important to ensure that home care nurses possess the skills necessary for caring for children in the home.
- Each home visit should be carefully documented by the nurse and should include a record of procedures, recommendations for additional services, any communication with the physician or staff, and a report to the attending physician.
- A patient/family assessment is imperative before a child is admitted to home care.
- Other certified and/or licensed home care providers include LPNs/LVNs, home health aids, physical therapists, occupational therapists, speech therapists, and medical social workers.

Bibliography

Beacon Health Corporation. *The Conditions of Participation and Interpretive Guidelines.* Mequon, WI: Beacon Health Corporation; 2001

Bello-Jones T. *Vocational Nursing Practice Act.* Sacramento, CA: California Board of Vocational Nursing and Psychiatric Technicians; 1997. Available at: http://www.bvnpt.ca.gov/bnpvn.htm. Accessed September 26, 2001

California Association for Health Services at Home. *Side-by-Side Comparison: Title 22 Regulations — Division 5, Chapter 6 and Medicare Conditions of Participation for Home Health Agencies.* Sacramento, CA: California Association for Health Services at Home; 1998

Terry RA. *Nursing Practice Act With Rules and Regulations.* Sacramento, CA: Board of Registered Nursing; 1994

Chapter 9

Selecting a Home Infusion Company

Robert L. Poole, PharmD; Fred Y. Nishioka, PharmD; John Kerner, Jr, MD

Introduction

Although many home infusion companies provide therapies for pediatric patients, few have the knowledge and expertise to safely and effectively provide the complex therapies required of children with chronic illnesses.

The key elements of a successful pediatric home infusion program include the following: Personnel *specifically trained in pediatrics;* policies and procedures *specific for pediatric patients and their families;* appropriate equipment and supplies *designed to provide therapies safely to a child;* communication systems *to keep physicians, patients, families, and providers informed of all significant clinical issues; and the appropriate use of* alternative infusions sites.

Personnel

A multidisciplinary team of clinicians and administrative support personnel working together to provide family centered care is ideal. While structures may vary, at the core should be a medical director with expertise in pediatric nutrition (enteral and parenteral) and infusion therapy. The medical director must have excellent relationships with referring physicians and be well versed in dealing with insurance issues such as required documentation and statements of medical necessity.

The entire team of clinicians should have significant experience with pediatric home infusion therapies, including recognizing and treating complications resulting from the therapies. Pharmacists must have knowledge of the stability and solubility of solutions with respect to pH and calcium/phosphate solubility, convert physician orders into an accurate compounding formulation, and assess laboratory tests to make appropriate adjustments. Physicians and nurses must be knowledgeable about line access, security of lines, placement of lines, and line infections. Clinical nutritionists work together with physicians and pharmacists to provide adequate nutrition for healing and growth. Personnel records for all clinicians (pharmacists, nurses, and dietitians) should include documentation of competency in caring for the pediatric patient.

Pediatric home infusion pharmacists have inpatient fluid management experience, preferably in the pediatric intensive care unit, the neonatal intensive care unit, and oncology unit. Pharmacists should be knowledgeable about pediatric chronic disease management, including cystic fibrosis, hemophilia, growth hormone deficiency, gastrointestinal disorders (eg, short bowel syndrome, inflammatory bowel diseases, genetic malabsorption syndromes), bone marrow and solid organ transplants, oncologic disorders, infectious diseases, and pain management.

Pediatric home care nurses are responsible for assessing the clinical appropriateness and safety of home care. They also must be experts in vascular access and infusion devices, and in developing pediatric-specific protocols. These nurses will act as the coordinators of family-centered care and be involved with patient, family, and social issues. They will facilitate the transition to family-directed care and self-infusion if required.

▶ Administration

The administrative operations of a home infusion program are critical to its long-term viability. The importance of key reimbursement personnel cannot be overemphasized. From contracting to authorization of services and billing to collections, dedicating the appropriate resources to the financial operation is imperative to ensure that reimbursement will follow the provision of services.

▶ Case Management

Case management plays a major role in the private insurance arena where reimbursement is negotiable. Many private insurance plans pay per diem rates for most therapies. Some plans still reimburse based on fee for service; however, prospective payment or capitation is an important mechanism of payment in the managed care world. It is critical to carve out injectable therapies through managed care contracts and determine who is at risk — the plan, the hospital, or the physician group — during any contractual discussion. The coordination of patient intake by a competent customer service employee facilitates insurance authorization and information gathering with a new patient.

▶ Delivery

The delivery of medications, supplies, and equipment is an important service, especially when dealing with high-cost biotechnology drugs or complex long-term therapies. Home infusion companies should use responsible personnel who are good with children and will instill confidence. Close coordination of scheduled deliveries will greatly help families to live more normal lives. Supply delivery should be coordinated with family schedules and coincide with nursing visits.

Overall, clinical and financial operations should be managed by a director who is well versed in contracting, pharmacy operations, clinical care of patients, and financial and personnel management. Additionally, all home infusion personnel should be familiar with the unique needs of children.

Policies and Procedures

When selecting a provider of home infusion services for pediatric patients, be sure the program has been licensed and accredited. Accrediting agencies, like the Joint Commission on Accreditation of Healthcare Organizations, do a complete review of programs every 3 years and require that providers have quality of care measures in place to review patient outcomes, patient satisfaction, and process improvement.

Home infusion companies caring for children must have pediatric-specific policies and procedures in place. Protocols should address patient/parent teaching, drug administration, vascular access, dressing changes, management of complications, and other pertinent policies. Teaching materials should be available in multiple languages, which can shorten the time for training patients and families to become competent in providing the necessary care.

Care plans should be prepared specifically for each patient and contain the following key elements: problem list, desired therapeutic outcomes/goals, clinical/administrative interventions, disease-specific patient monitoring, and outcomes/resolutions.

An on-call program staffed by pediatric-trained clinicians skilled in telephone assessment must be in place and available 24 hours a day, 7 days a week. On-call personnel should be able to handle any required changes in therapy and triage any reported problems.

Equipment and Supplies

Managing an inventory of high-cost pharmaceuticals to meet the needs of patients and minimize cost to the organization requires special purchasing skills. The use of a group purchasing organization to contract for the procuring of equipment, supplies, and medications for alternate site use can be cost effective if it is a pediatric–product-focused group. Monitoring use patterns will allow "just-in-time" inventory, minimizing inventory-carrying costs.

Over the past decade, a number of high-tech and low-tech devices have been developed to improve the lives of home care patients. Disposable elastomeric infusion devices allow patient mobility while delivering an accurate dose in a specific fluid volume. These low-tech devices do not use electrical or battery power and are easy to operate, with minimal teaching time required. A variety of portable pumps have been designed to fit in backpacks, fanny packs, etc, to allow patient mobility. Low-volume micro-infusion devices are used for continuous subcutaneous infusion of medications (eg, Deferoxamine). Portable enteral feeding pumps are used for continuous nasogastric or naso-jejunal feeds. Multichannel pumps can be used to separate therapies (eg, total parenteral nutrition, fat emulsion, and antibiotics). Many of these pumps can be programmed remotely over the telephone to facilitate changes in therapy. All electronic and programmable pumps and devices must be on a regularly scheduled maintenance program with service checks performed by clinical engineers for safety and accuracy.

Managing an inventory of high-cost pharmaceuticals to meet the needs of patients and minimize cost to the organization requires special purchasing skills.

Regardless of the types of technology used, pediatric home infusion patients require an individualized list of supplies that needs periodic updating and replenishment. A list of commonly used supplies appears in Table 9-1. There also is a current transition toward the use of systems without needles to protect the patient, family, staff, and the environment from exposure to infectious waste. Home infusion companies should provide families with safe containers for disposing of sharps and used tubing along with instructions for disposing of filled containers.

TABLE 9-1. Supply List for a Pediatric Home Total Parenteral Nutrition Patient

Total parenteral nutrition solution

Lipids

Pediatric multivitamin injection

Infusion pumps – two or multichannel

IV pole

Tubing for total parenteral nutrition

Tubing for lipid

Extension sets

Alcohol wipes

Heparin flush syringes

Normal saline flush syringes

Injection connectors without needles

Hypodermic syringes/needles for additives

Site dressing supplies (vary depending on venous access device and protocol)

Dextrose 10% for emergency use

Sharps container

Other supplies as ordered by physician

Communication

Once a patient has been referred for home infusion therapy, it is important to keep the primary physician informed of significant changes in status. A therapeutic plan with desired outcomes (ie, the plan of care) should be developed with significant input from the primary physician. Establishing and developing a positive relationship with the patient and family is critical to caring for a child at home. Teamwork among the home infusion staff is central to a successful program. Home infusion staff often will serve as the communicator between the patient/family and the physician.

Alternative Infusion Sites

Determining the most appropriate site for infusion therapy depends on the family resources, family willingness to participate in care, and nursing assessment of the family's ability to provide home care. Some families do not have sufficient refrigerator space for medication storage, and the purchase of an additional refrigerator is necessary. Other patients may require care outside the home if the family is unable to administer infusion therapy.

In these cases, alternative infusion sites may be appropriate. Alternate infusion sites include infusion centers where patients go to receive hydration therapy, a day-hospital setting where a patient receives chemotherapy and returns home, a Ronald McDonald House or local motel/hotel when transitioning a patient from hospital to home, or an inpatient hospital. Adult patients are able to adapt to most environments, while children may be lost and afraid without their toys, room, pets, and siblings. After all, home is where a child belongs.

Summary

The welfare of the patient remains the physician's concern and responsibility after discharge from the hospital. It is the duty of the physician to initiate home infusion with a home care company that provides safe and adequate care. For these reasons, physicians and discharge planners need to assess home infusion companies. Beyond having adequate mixing, storage, and delivery systems for pediatric home infusion therapies, it is critical that a company have personnel trained and experienced in pediatric needs.

The following are key points to remember:
- Home infusion programs for children should employ pediatric-trained personnel, follow pediatric-focused policies and procedures, and use pediatric-specific equipment and supplies. In addition, the program should have a communication system in place to notify physicians of changes in the patient.
- When families cannot provide a safe environment for home infusion, alternative care sites should be investigated.
- The administrative operations of a home infusion program are critical to its long-term viability. Dedicating appropriate resources to financial operations is particularly important.
- The ideal provider of home infusion services is licensed and accredited.

Bibliography

American Society for Parenteral and Enteral Nutrition. Standards for nutrition support physicians. A.S.P.E.N. board directives. *Nutr Clin Pract.* 1996;11:235-240

Fisher AA, Poole RL, Machie R, et al. Clinical pathway for pediatric parenteral nutrition. *Nutr Clin Pract.* 1997;12:76-80

Mascarenhas MR, Kerner JA Jr, Stallings VA. Parenteral and enteral nutrition. In: Walker WA, Durie PR, Hamilton JR, Walker-Smith JA, Watkins JB, eds. *Pediatric Gastrointestinal Disease.* 3rd ed. Hamilton, Ontario: B.C. Decker; 2000:1705

Misra S, Ament ME, Reyen L. Home parenteral nutrition. In: Baker RD Jr, Baker SS, Davis AM, eds. *Pediatric Parenteral Nutrition.* New York, NY: Chapman & Hall; 1997:354-369

Chapter 10

The Physician's Perspective on Home Infusion Therapy

Marvin E. Ament, MD; Laurie Reyen

Introduction

The use of home infusion therapy in pediatrics has grown remarkably in the past decade. More familiarity with home care therapies, availability of small portable infusion devices, and growth of managed care have increased demand for pediatric home care. The physician must be familiar with the resources needed to make a successful course of home infusion therapy for the patient.

Patient Selection

The optimal candidate for home infusion therapy is the child with a primary disease and/or comorbid condition who has demonstrated therapeutic response to the medication to be used in the home and who is physiologically stable for home care. The therapeutic goals and expected duration of therapy should be established at the outset. Based on the above information, additional criteria for patient selection include the following:

- Caregivers willing and available to provide and participate in care at home
- Adequate resources available to support the proposed care in the home
- Insurance coverage for parenteral medications and solutions, durable medical equipment, home nursing care, and other necessary support services
- Home environment safe and adequate for proposed home therapies
- Vendors available to provide appropriate services and equipment at home
- Child with stable and appropriate vascular access for home infusion therapy

Excellent communication between all members of the medical care team and caregivers, as well as payers and vendors, is essential in selecting and planning for pediatric home infusion therapy.

Contraindications to Home Infusion Therapy

Home infusion therapy is contraindicated if the child's caregivers are unwilling or unable to learn the techniques and procedures to follow when providing home infusion care. This is especially true if the caregiver has a psychological or cognitive impairment that would interfere with safe delivery of infusion therapy. Home therapy also is contraindicated when there is inadequate financial support to reimburse for the costs of necessary care. It also is inappropriate for the child whose home environment or social supports are inadequate to support safe delivery of infusion therapy.

Home Care Company Selection

An ideal home infusion pharmacy is licensed by a state board of pharmacy for mixing parenteral products in an aseptic fashion. This licensure should include documentation of sterile practice in formulating solutions, compounding, labeling, and quality assurance policies and procedures in line with the American Society for Parenteral and Enteral Nutrition (ASPEN) and American Society of Health-System Pharmacists National Advisory Group's guidelines for "Safe Practices for Parenteral Nutrition Formulations." The agency's pharmacists, nurses, and dieticians should have documented competencies in the care of pediatric patients receiving infusion therapy in the home setting and, when available, certification or specialized training. The home infusion pharmacy should be accredited by an appropriate professional organization like the Joint Commission on Accreditation of Healthcare Organizations or ASPEN. In addition, the agency should have financial and billing personnel able to deal with consumer and insurance provider issues in a timely and knowledgeable manner. Prior to the selection of a specific home infusion pharmacy, the agency's ability to provide the needed services to the patient in a prompt and timely manner should be determined.

In communication with members of the referring health care team, the pharmacy should demonstrate prompt response to phone calls by physicians. Communication between pharmacy and physician should happen when the following occur:

- Initiation of service
- Change in prescriptions for parenteral medications and solutions
- Changes in therapy
- Initiation of new therapies
- Service issues

The pharmacy should have the ability to provide parenteral delivery systems appropriate to the patient's age and disease-specific needs, including infusion pumps (pole mount versus portable infusion pumps).

The service capabilities of an ideal home infusion pharmacy should include 24-hour availability of personnel to answer questions about intravenous therapy and infusion systems, and the ability to provide replacement equipment in a timely manner if equipment fails. Nursing personnel should be available directly through the company or through close liaison with certified nursing agencies in the community to provide support and education to patients and families in the administration of home infusion therapies.

The agency should have an established liaison with nursing or phlebotomy services to draw laboratory tests daily, weekly, monthly, or quarterly as necessary for monitoring response to therapy. Online recording of patient's blood chemistries and nutritional parameters on a continuous basis is desirable, along with the availability of personnel with expertise in interpreting lab data and clinical information to alert the physician to potential problems. The agency should be proactive in alerting the physician to problems as they arise. The availability of social service support is helpful to resolve psychosocial issues that may interfere with effective home infusion care.

Responsibilities of the Physician

A successful plan for home infusion therapy must include a designated physician with accountability and responsibility for the home treatment plan and the necessary follow-up care. The physician or physician's designee should be available 24 hours a day and be able to provide timely response to the home care patient and home care pharmacy when changes in the patient's condition or medical emergencies occur.

Responsibilities of the Nurse

The patient's nurse in the inpatient or ambulatory care setting should be
responsible for assessing whether the family and child are ready and appropriate for home care. The nurse provides patient and family education in
preparation for home infusion therapy and serves as a communication link
between the physician, home care provider, and patient's family in the initiation of the home infusion plan of care. The medical social worker may
also play an important role in family assessment and preparation.

Patient and Family Education

Patient and family education for home infusion therapy is key to ensuring
patient family participation and successful outcomes of care. Patient and
family education should include the following information:
- Child's disease state — expected course and rationale for home therapy
- Care procedures and skills
- Safe and effective delivery of medication infusions
- Safe and effective use of medical equipment
- Infection control
- Home safety
- Hazardous waste disposal
- Home monitoring of child's condition, response to therapy
- Emergency care procedures
- Access to follow-up care
- Medical care providers
- Home care pharmacy
- Coping skills

Vascular Access

Vascular access that is stable and appropriate for the specific home infusion
therapy must be established and maintained to achieve successful outcomes.
In determining which venous access device to use, the physician should
consider one that is durable and able to meet the planned home infusion
therapy needs. The device should be as simple and safe as possible and should
be manageable for the parent and child.

There are a variety of vascular access devices available for home infusion therapy. The peripherally inserted central catheter is appropriate for patients with intermediate therapy needs of weeks to months (eg, antibiotic infusions or short-term parenteral nutrition). The child must have adequate peripheral vascular integrity for insertion of the device. The child may experience some limitations in activity and mobility secondary to placement site and the risk of dislodgment.

The tunneled central venous catheter (eg, Hickman or Broviac) is appropriate for patients with long-term, intensive therapy needs from months to years at a time (eg, parenteral nutrition). These devices present fewer limitations in the child's activities and mobility secondary to the stability provided by the cuff in the catheter's subcutaneous tunnel.

The subcutaneous infusion port (eg, Mediport) is appropriate for patients with long-term, intermittent therapy needs, such as patients with cancer, immunodeficiency syndromes, or cystic fibrosis. The port is best used for intermittent access, but can be used for continuous access, as well. When not in use, there is little limitation in activity or mobility because there is no external catheter and no care is required except for a monthly heparin flush. The child may experience discomfort with the skin puncture for port access, although this may be ameliorated by the use of a topical anesthetic. When in use, the child's activity may be limited, as there is a risk of fluid extravasation with port needle dislodgment. All of the devices mentioned are available in single- or double-lumen designs.

Peripheral intravenous catheters rarely are suitable for pediatric home infusion therapy. They are short-term and often highly unstable and pose a higher risk of phlebitis, extravasation, and dislodgment in the home. They may be appropriate in select cases where therapy is planned for an extremely short period of time and there is adequate nursing support available to monitor and maintain peripheral access.

▶ Management of Vascular Access Devices

Vascular access device care should be provided according to standardized policies and procedures. Patient, family, and staff education programs should be designed to reinforce these standards for device care. Ongoing monitoring of device-related outcomes is important in identifying if device care is safe and appropriate. The Centers for Disease Control and Prevention's

"Guideline for Intravascular Device-Related Infections" (*see* Bibliography) is available as a resource for establishing procedures to reduce risk of device-related infections. Device care procedures (catheter dressing change, catheter access, catheter cap change) should be designed to limit risks of device-related infections. Ongoing monitoring and immediate response to signs and symptoms of device-related infections is necessary to prevent undue morbidity or mortality.

The concentrations and volumes of heparin used to maintain vascular access device patency may vary depending on the device, frequency of use, and the size of the child. In the event of catheter occlusion, medical care personnel should be available to provide the appropriate assessment and intervention to restore catheter patency. Equipment and personnel for vascular access device repair should be available as necessary. Parents should be provided with education and anticipatory guidance in device safety and care issues appropriate to their child's developmental level. School personnel should be informed about the child's vascular access device and appropriate emergency care measures.

Summary

The keys to successful home infusion therapy include the following:

- The optimal candidate for home infusion therapy is the child with a primary disease and/or comorbid condition who has been responding to medication and is physiologically stable for home care.
- Home infusion therapy is contraindicated if there is a lack of family support or resources, or if the child's medical condition is such that the burden of infusion therapy outweighs the benefits.
- Successful home infusion therapy must include a designated physician who is accountable and responsible for the treatment plan and follow-up care.
- The patient's nurse provides education in preparation for home infusion therapy and serves as a liaison among the physician, provider, and family.
- Appropriate and stable vascular access must be established and maintained to achieve successful outcomes.

Bibliography

Ament ME. Home total parenteral nutrition. In: Walker WA, Durie P, Hamilton JR, Walker-Smith JA, Watkins J, eds. *Pediatric Gastrointestinal Disease.* Vol 2. Hamilton, Ontario: B.C. Decker; 1991:1676-1688

Colomb V, Fabeiro M, Dabbas M, Goulet O, Merckx J, Ricour C. Central venous catheter-related infections in children on long-term home parenteral nutrition: incidence and risk factors. *Clin Nutr.* 2000;19:355-359

Howard L, Malone M, Murray S, Ellis L. Management of patients on home parenteral and enteral nutrition. In: Shikora S, Blackburn G, eds. *Nutrition Support, Theory and Practice.* New York, NY: Chapman & Hall; 1997:563-587

Misra S, Ament ME, Reyen L. Home parenteral nutrition. In: Baker R, Baker S, Davis A, eds. *Pediatric Parenteral Nutrition.* New York, NY: Chapman & Hall; 1997:354-369

Public Health Service, US Department of Health and Human Services, Centers for Disease Control and Prevention. Guideline for prevention of intramuscular device-related infections. Available at: http://www.cdc.gov/ncidod/hip/IV/IV.htm. Accessed August 14, 2001

Puntis JW. Nutritional support at home and in the community. *Arch Dis Child.* 2001;84:295-298

Vargas JH, Ament ME, Berquist WE. Long-term home parenteral nutrition in pediatrics: ten years of experience in 102 patients. *J Pediatr Gastroenterol Nutr.* 1987;6:24-32

Chapter 11

Home Parenteral and Enteral Nutrition

Donald E. George, MD

Introduction

As a general rule it is important to use the gut for feeding whenever possible. However, when a child is unable to meet metabolic demands orally or via enteral feedings, parenteral nutrition via central venous catheter (CVC) is required. Parenteral nutrition has the greatest risk of morbidity and mortality of all nutritional support modalities because of the increased risk of liver dysfunction and risk of infection from chronic indwelling venous access devices.

Parenteral Nutrition

Whenever possible, children who require parenteral nutrition also should receive enteral feeding even in low, seemingly insignificant volumes to help promote gut adaptation and immune function and minimize bacterial translocation in the gut. Infants and toddlers receiving parenteral nutrition also should receive speech therapy and small-volume oral feedings of differing tastes and textures to promote normal oral motor development and prevent food refusal. Pediatric nutritional and fluid requirements are based on body weight and underlying disease process. Parenteral nutrition should not be used for rehydration.

▶ Discharge Requirements

Well before discharge, a home assessment should be completed to ensure necessary criteria for the discharge have been met. Caregivers need to room-in and demonstrate competency in skilled care prior to discharge. Equipment and supplies should be delivered to the home prior to discharge. At a minimum, a skilled pediatric nurse should visit the home at initiation and termination of the infusion for the first 24 hours. Timing for discontinuation of nursing home visits is determined by caregiver competency. If caregivers are not fully comfortable providing care, additional nursing visits may be necessary.

▶ Home Environment

A home assessment should be done prior to discharging a child who requires parenteral nutrition. Electricity, running water, refrigeration, and access to a telephone are necessary to safely provide parenteral nutrition at home.

▶ Caretakers

Two adult caretakers should be identified prior to the child's discharge from the hospital. These caretakers should be trained in the following areas: care of the vascular access device, pump operation, storage and hanging of parenteral nutrition and lipids, adding medications to the parenteral nutrition bag, signs and symptoms of sepsis, signs and symptoms of metabolic disturbances associated with parenteral nutrition and lipid administration, recognition/prevention of mechanical complications associated with CVCs, and recognition and appropriate response to potentially life-threatening complications of parenteral nutrition and CVCs. Two trained adult caretakers are preferable so that someone is always available to intervene if problems occur and one caretaker is not available.

▶ Home Care Company Requirements

To provide parenteral nutrition successfully to a child at home, it is important for the family to have a single pharmacy and supplies contact person. The home care company should employ a nursing staff with experience in nutritional support and the care of central venous access devices. The pharmacy providing the parenteral nutrition should be accredited and employ a pharmacist who has experience mixing parenteral nutrition for children. The home care company should provide 24-hour on-call clinical staff. The family should have a single contact person for pharmacy, nursing, and supplies. The home care provider should develop emergency preparedness plans with the family.

▶ Medical Equipment

Appropriate durable medical equipment (DME) is important for the safe delivery of parenteral nutrition in the home setting. The infusion pump must be programmable, have the ability to ramp infusions, have a lockout on the face of the pump, and have a low occlusion pressure (less than 10 psi). It is important for the home care company to provide pharmaceuticals, equipment replacements, or supplies within a time frame that does not jeopardize the care, health, or welfare of the child. This may mean that the family is provided with a backup pump and an extra bag of dextrose-containing solution. In addition, the home care company needs to provide for biohazardous waste disposal.

▶ Patient Requirements

The child should demonstrate appropriate growth and biochemical stability on the total parenteral nutrition (TPN) admixture. The rate of infusion with an appropriate period of time off TPN infusion each day should be fixed 48 hours prior to discharge. The window, or time off TPN, should be sufficient to allow the family to accomplish tasks of daily living. It is imperative that the child has intact, patent central venous access in place prior to discharge.

▶ Parenteral Nutrition Admixture

Solutions should include pediatric vitamins and pediatric trace elements. The TPN solutions may be mixed as a three-in-one admixture or as a two-in-one admixture with lipid infusion, depending on need. Trophamine should be used as the amino acid component in infant TPN formulas.

▶ Monitoring Children on Parenteral Nutrition

At a minimum, a fingerstick blood glucose should be obtained with hookup and disconnect for the first 24 hours at home and then as needed. A complete blood count with differential, electrolyte panel, magnesium, carbon dioxide, and liver enzymes are obtained weekly for the first 2 weeks at home, then biweekly for a month, and then monthly. Routine labs usually are drawn by the home care nurse and ideally are coordinated with the routine cap change on the venous access device. Labs also will be drawn when there is a change in admixture or with signs/symptoms suggestive of metabolic disturbance or infection. Additional labs that may be necessary include zinc, copper, magnesium, manganese, iron studies, and vitamin levels.

The febrile child with a central venous access device must receive immediate evaluation in an attempt to identify the potential infection. If no source of infection is identified, the child is assumed to have central catheter associated sepsis and should be evaluated for hospital admission.

A physical examination in the physician's office is completed biweekly for the first month and monthly or as needed thereafter if questions about metabolic or septic complications arise. A complete history and physical examination including height, weight, weight-to-length ratio, and skinfold thickness measurements should be completed with each visit. Adequacy of nutritional intervention is determined based on the child's response to treatment. With growth, specifics of nutritional therapy need to be calculated, including free water in mL/kg, nonprotein kcal/kg, grams of protein/kg, and nonprotein calorie-to-nitrogen ratio. Adjustments to rate and admixture are made when clinical picture, physical exam, or laboratory data indicate a need for a change in therapy.

▸ Administration of Parenteral Nutrition

Parenteral nutrition must be administered by infusion pump through a central venous access catheter. Non-implantable single lumen venous access devices are the best choice for infants and young children receiving parenteral nutrition at home. Implantable venous access devices, such as MediPort, require frequent subcutaneous access for daily administration of TPN and may be less desirable. Effective topical anesthetic does not negate the need to restrain a young child during access of the implantable device. In adolescents, an implantable venous access device may be more cosmetically acceptable.

Children on home parenteral nutrition should be given a period of time off each day from TPN infusion to allow the family to accomplish necessary tasks of daily living and to allow the child a maximum amount of time to achieve developmental milestones (fine and gross motor skills, explore the environment, attend school or social functions, etc). The infusion rate should be ramped up and down to prevent iatrogenic episodes of hyperglycemia and hypoglycemia.

The parenteral admixture should not be infused cold. This is particularly important in infants and small children where it may cause life-threatening bradycardia or hypothermia. An aseptic technique should be used whenever the CVC or infusion system is accessed. Tubing should include appropriately sized in-line filters when administering parenteral nutrition or lipids. The tubing should be changed with each cycle of parenteral nutrition. All tubing connections must Leur-lock to maintain line integrity. Concomitant medication administration with parenteral nutrition may result in precipitation and line occlusion. Unless compatibility is well documented, parenteral nutrition should not be administered simultaneously with other medications.

▶ Care of the Non-implantable Central Venous Access Catheter

All infusions through a venous access device need to be regulated by an infusion pump. Aseptic technique needs to be strictly observed whenever the catheter is accessed. Care should be organized in such a manner as to limit the number of times the line is accessed. The fewer times the line is opened the fewer the associated complications. Recessed valves should be changed with each access of the line. Non-recessed valves should be changed every 7 days. If the venous access device is used to withdraw blood, the recessed valve and cap or the non-recessed valve should be changed. If lipids are infused, the recessed valve is changed every 24 hours. If parenteral nutrition is cycled, the recessed valve should be changed each time it is hung. Acetone-free alcohol is used on the line to preserve long-term integrity of the catheter. Transparent dressings should be changed once a week or immediately if the dressing becomes wet, soiled, or loose. Non-transparent dressings should be changed three times a week. Two-percent chlorhexidine is used to clean the exit site during a dressing change.

It is important to secure the catheter and dress the child in clothes that prevent grabbing hold of the catheter and pulling it out. It is helpful in infants who have developed a grasp to have the non-implantable catheter tunneled over the shoulder to exit on the back. This simplifies catheter care for the parent and reduces the incidence of catheter dislodgment. If the catheter exits on the chest wall, coiling the catheter and taping it securely is helpful. Dressing infants in one-piece outfits also is helpful in preventing the grabbing and dislodging of the catheter. It is important to keep the catheter taped securely so the injection cap is not in the diaper area or used for teething.

Catheters should be flushed with normal saline before and after each infusion and medication administration. The volume of the flush should be approximately a minimum of five times the catheter volume. Between infusions, the catheter should be locked off with heparin flush of 10 units/mL at a volume slightly in excess of the catheter volume. Assiduous flushing with saline is vital to prevent fibrin sheath formation with subsequent clot development and line occlusion. Use of 5-mL or greater volume syringes for flushing is recommended. Never force anything through the catheter. A smooth edge clamp should be easily accessible in case of catheter leakage or break. Catheter occlusions should be assessed and treated in a clinical setting.

Enteral Feedings

When a child is malnourished because of inadequate oral intake to meet metabolic demands and the child does not have intestinal malabsorption, persistent vomiting, or inability to protect the airway, enteral feedings via nasogastric or gastric tube is the nutritional modality of choice. If the child is unable to protect the airway or has a significant degree of gastroesophageal reflux, enteral feedings via jejunal tube or gastric feedings after completion of Nissen fundoplication are the nutritional modalities of choice.

Children's nutrient requirements vary based on age. Any underlying disease process also must be given consideration in determining appropriate intake. As a general rule, adult enteral formulas should not be used in children younger than 10 years. Fluid and nutrient requirements are calculated based on body weight and underlying disease process. The effectiveness of enteral therapy should be evaluated with frequent weight checks and appropriate blood work. In children who receive all feedings enterally, it is critical to calculate not only caloric and nutrient requirements, but also ensure they are receiving adequate fluids. The adequacy of the prescribed feeding regimen needs to be assessed frequently and changed based on growth and/or biochemical indices.

The effectiveness of enteral therapy should be evaluated with frequent weight checks and appropriate blood work.

Enteral feedings disrupt the development of hunger-satiety sequence and oral motor development; therefore, these children are at high risk for developing food refusal. Infants and toddlers with normal oral motor coordination who are receiving nutrition via enteral access should receive speech therapy and receive small-volume oral feedings of differing tastes and textures to promote normal oral motor development and prevent food refusal. In addition, infants who are enterally fed should be given the opportunity for nonnutritive sucking (ie, pacifier) during the enteral feeding. Nonnutritive sucking promotes increased weight gain and quickens the transition to oral feedings in infants who are receiving nutrition via enteral access.

Jejunal feeds often are appropriate for children who have significant gastroesophageal reflux or difficulty protecting the airway. All jejunal feedings must be regulated by a pump. Bolus feeds into the jejunum will cause dumping syndrome. Naso-jejunal and gastro-jejunal tubes are difficult to maintain and are not the best choice for home care.

▶ Home Environment

A home assessment should be done prior to discharging a child who requires enteral feedings. Electricity, running water, refrigeration, and access to a telephone all are necessary to provide enteral feedings safely at home.

▶ Caretaker Requirements

Two adult caretakers should be identified prior to the child's discharge from the hospital. These caregivers should be trained in the following areas: the preparation and storage of formula, pump operation (when appropriate), specific feeding regimen, care and maintenance of the enteral access feeding device, care and cleaning of the enteral feeding supplies, recognition of signs and symptoms of mechanical, infectious, and metabolic complications associated with the enteral access device or feeding regimen, and prevention of mechanical complications associated with enteral feeding devices. When enteral feedings are administered via nasogastric tube, caregivers should be proficient in placing the tube and checking placement after insertion. When enteral feedings are administered via gastrostomy tube/low-profile device, caregivers should be proficient in intubating the gastrostomy stoma with a foley catheter to maintain its patency pending tube replacement and recognize the signs and symptoms of tube dislodgment or migration of the tube into the surgical tract. When enteral feedings are administered via jejunal tube, the caregivers should be competent in checking tube distal tip placement, recognizing signs and symptoms of tube dislodgment, and understanding the necessity of never bolus feeding into the small bowel. It is important to stress that two individuals be trained in the care of the child to allow for respite for the primary caregiver.

▶ Home Care Company Requirements

To successfully provide enteral feeding to a child at home, it is important
that the family have a single contact person for DME and supplies. The
family should have 24-hour access to on-call clinical staff with expertise in
pediatric nutritional support. The home care company must provide appropriate DME. For example, an enteral pump used to feed a child should be
programmable to allow incremental increases in volume of 1 mL/hour. A
lockout on the face of the pump is mandatory. If the infant is being fed for
more than 12 of 24 hours, a portable pump is necessary to allow the family
to accomplish essential tasks of day-to-day living and to allow some degree
of physical mobility for the child, thus promoting motor development. The
home care company must provide equipment replacement or supplies
within a time frame that does not jeopardize the care or health of the child.

▶ Patient Requirements

The child must be stable, hydrated, and gaining weight on enteral feedings
prior to discharge from the hospital. In addition, duration of enteral feedings
should be limited as much as possible to allow the family to accomplish
tasks of daily living. Infants younger than 1 year and children who are
neurologically impaired and receiving feedings via a nasogastric tube should
be placed on an apnea or cardiorespiratory monitor when they are not
directly observed by a caregiver to monitor for tube dislodgment and
prevent aspiration.

▶ Nasogastric Tubes

For long-term nasogastric tube feedings, a polyurethane radiopaque tube
is recommended. Many of these tubes come with a stylet. Because of the
risk of perforation, caregivers are instructed to remove the stylet prior to
placing a tube at home. The tube can remain in place for 4 to 6 weeks.
Infants and children have fragile skin and securing the tube with zinc oxide-
impregnated tape, then using colloidal skin barriers such as DuoDerm and
transparent adhesive dressings, often are helpful. Proprietary velcro securing
devices can be used to stabilize the tube. It is important to determine the
appropriate length of tube to be inserted for proper placement. Proper
placement should be determined radiographically. Once the proper insertion
length has been determined, the tube is marked with indelible ink where it

exits the nares. The caregiver is instructed to insert the tube to the mark when reinsertion is necessary. If the nasogastric tube is dislodged, it can be cleaned thoroughly with soap and water, rinsed well, and reinserted. It is important to evaluate tube insertion length in the growing child.

Tube placement should be checked before each feeding and before giving medications. Litmus paper (pH range 1 to 12 with color chart) can be used to help determine distal tip tube placement. Tube aspirate with a pH of less than 4 is indicative of gastric placement. If the tube aspirate pH is greater than 5, the tube may be in the small bowel. This technique must be modified if the child is on a hydrogen receptor antagonist or a proton pump inhibitor because both may cause an elevated pH reading. Auscultation alone may be unreliable in a small child or infant.

▶ Gastrostomy Tubes

Low-profile gastrostomy devices (eg, gastrostomy button) often are cosmetically and functionally superior to a gastrostomy tube. It is important that caregivers are educated to recognize signs of balloon breakage or migration into the tract. The button should freely rotate. If a child is placed on antibiotics, concomitant treatment with nystatin suspension is helpful to prevent candidal growth around the button device. When administering bolus feedings to an infant, it is important to burp the infant or, for infants with a Nissen fundoplication, to vent the gastrostomy for 30 minutes after each feed. This allows the infant to dispel gas and reduce discomfort from gastric distention. Leakage of formula or drainage from around the tube, erythematous changes in the skin around the tube, or the development of granulation tissue around the stoma requires evaluation. A replacement tube should be readily available should the gastrostomy tube come out. The gastrostomy tube can be replaced at home after the tract is mature (8 to 12 weeks); prior to this time, there is a risk of placing the tube into subcutaneous tissues.

Routine stoma care includes the use of equal parts of hydrogen peroxide and water applied and rinsed twice a day. Should the skin around the stoma become irritated from leakage of formula or stomach contents, barrier ointments or powders to protect the skin often are effective. Leakage from around the gastrostomy indicates a mechanical problem with the gastrostomy tube, such as a ruptured balloon or a change in the size of the stoma that

necessitates a change in the diameter or stem length of the device. Leakage
from the low-profile device itself indicates a malfunction of the one-way
valve, necessitating replacement. Bleeding from the gastrostomy tube may
be secondary to mechanical trauma to the stoma or the stomach lining,
migration of the balloon or retention device into the tract, or a gastrointestinal bleed. Bleeding from the gastrostomy tube requires evaluation by a
physician to rule out a clinically significant gastrointestinal hemorrhage.

▸ Jejunal Tubes

Jejunal feedings can be administered through a naso-jejunal tube, gastro-
jejunal tube, or surgical jejunostomy. In all instances the feedings must be
administered by pump at a rate that is well tolerated by the child. Bolus
feedings or feedings at an excessive rate may result in dumping syndrome.

   Naso-jejunal and gastro-jejunal tubes are difficult to maintain. If a
transpyloric tube is used, it is important to check distal tip placement prior
to feeding through the tube. Tube aspirate checked with litmus paper
(pH range 1 to 12 with color chart) should have a pH greater than 5.

▸ Maintaining the Patency of Enteral Tubes

Any form of enteral feeding tube must be flushed prior to and after each
feeding and medication administration to prevent obstruction. There are
certain medications that are incompatible with formulas and can occlude
the feeding tube when administered concomitantly. Because it is difficult
to know if a particular medicine is compatible with formula, it is safe to
assume that it is not compatible and that mixing with the formula in the
feeding tube can contribute to blockage. The tube should be flushed with
15 to 30 mL of water before and after the medication is given, which will
prevent formula in the tube from mixing with the medicine and hopefully
prevent tube occlusion. Clearing an occluded tube may be attempted with
cola, pancrelipase mixed with bicarbonate of soda, or special mechanical
devices developed specifically for clearing occluded enteral tubes. The wire
stylet used for placing gastrostomy tubes should not be reinserted into the
tube in an attempt to clear a blockage because doing so may cause a perforation of the esophagus or stomach.

▶ Cleaning Enteral Feeding Equipment

All feeding bags and connecting tubing should be cleaned thoroughly with soap and hot water immediately after a feeding is completed. Once the bag has been rinsed, it is left hanging with the clamp open until dry and then stored in the refrigerator until the next use. If formula residue remains, it can be removed by filling the bag with a solution of equal parts of vinegar and water, leaving the solution in the bag for at least 5 minutes, and rinsing twice with water. If properly cared for, feeding bags and tubing can be reused as long as they remain clean and are working well.

Summary

Important facts about parenteral and enteral nutrition include the following:
- When a child is unable to meet metabolic demands orally or via enteral feedings, parenteral nutrition via CVC is required.
- If possible, a child receiving parenteral nutrition also should receive low volumes of enteral feedings to promote gut adaptation and immune function and to minimize bacterial translocation in the gut.
- For both parenteral and enteral feeding, a home assessment should be conducted prior to discharge to ensure the patient's home has electricity, running water, refrigeration, and a telephone.
- Parenteral and enteral feeding require two trained caregivers so that someone is always available.
- Pharmacies supplying enteral and parenteral nutrition should be accredited and employ a pharmacist experienced in preparing nutrition for children.

Bibliography

American Society for Parenteral and Enteral Nutrition. Standards for nutrition support physicians. A.S.P.E.N. board directives. *Nutr Clin Pract.* 1996;11:235-240

Collins E, Lawson L, Lau MT, et al. Care of central venous catheters for total parenteral nutrition. *Nutr Clin Pract.* 1996;11

Frankel EH, Enow NB, Jackson KC, Kloiber LL. Methods of restoring patency to occluded feeding tubes. *Nutr Clin Pract.* 1998;13

Orr M. Vascular access device selection for parenteral nutrition. *Nutr Clin Pract.* 1999;14

Chapter 12

Pediatric Chemotherapy Guidelines

Edward Korycka, RN, CRNI, OCN

Introduction

The following guidelines were developed to assist the clinician in meeting the needs of the pediatric patient receiving chemotherapy in the home. This chapter will discuss setting the stage for chemotherapy at home, review chemotherapy agents used at home, and discuss preventing or treating the often-debilitating side effects. In addition, the nutritional needs of the pediatric patient on chemotherapy and emergency scenarios that may occur in the home are discussed.

Setting the Stage

For a trusting relationship to be built, children need honesty, and clinicians delivering chemotherapy need to be attentive to the clinical and personal needs of the patient. A child receiving chemotherapy will realize quickly that the truth has not been explained when "unexpected" side effects from the therapy are experienced. Clinicians and caregivers must answer patient questions and offer explanations about side effects in an age-appropriate manner. Whenever possible, written explanations of the protocol should be provided to parents because it is difficult to remember details during a crisis-laden time period. Home care providers also should provide patient teaching materials on vascular access devices, chemotherapy agents, and nutrition to families prior to hospital discharge so that they know what to expect. Table 12-1 shows a sample teaching sheet.

Chemotherapy in the Home Environment

Planning prior to hospital discharge should include identification of the chemotherapeutic protocol and the type of vascular access device to be used in the home. An initial home care

TABLE 12-1. Example of a Basic Teaching Sheet*

Practical Guide for Eating

- **Give food a chance.** Remember that what sounds unappealing today may sound good tomorrow.
- **Take advantage of the up times.** When you feel well, take advantage of it by eating well. It is important to eat foods with good nutritional value; many nutrients can be stored in your body for later use.
- **Discuss your eating problems with your doctor and your health team.** Before you try home remedies, be sure your problems are not symptoms of needing medical attention. Do not hesitate to ask questions and to tell the doctor what seems to be bothering you even if you think it is unimportant.
- **Avoid foods that do not interest you.**
- **Atmosphere does make a difference.** Eating with friends, having music at dinnertime, or varying the place in the house where you eat can be helpful in providing a pleasant atmosphere.
- **Stay away from raw eggs and raw meats** if your treatment or condition makes you susceptible to infection.
- **Make use of time savers.** Take advantage of foods that are easy to prepare, that heat easily in a microwave, or that are prepared easily in other appliances.

*Source: *Eating Hints for Cancer Patients: Before, During & After Treatment*. National Institutes of Health, National Cancer Institute; 1997. NIH publication 98-2079

assessment done prior to discharge should focus on the appropriateness of the vascular access device and the family's ability to participate in the patient's care.

▶ The Initial Home Care Assessment

Before the first home treatment, the home care nurse and pharmacist gather relevant clinical information that will facilitate the evaluation of the patient's overall clinical status and meet the goals of therapy. An accurate baseline assessment will assist in evaluating the patient's ability to tolerate the current therapy and the implementation of needed interventions. The following points should be addressed in the initial home care assessment:

- Record the patient's health history that is especially relevant to the planned chemotherapeutic protocol (eg, a history of cardiac or pulmonary disease, allergic reactions, previous radiation treatments).
- Review immediate and delayed side effects of planned chemotherapy.
- Evaluate the patient's past history with chemotherapy administration.

- Teach the patient/caregiver about the administration procedure and side effects for the planned chemotherapy.
- Give the patient/caregiver written information about the planned therapy, side effects, and good nutrition.

▶ Role of the Primary Family Caregiver

The home care company provides nurses to administer the actual chemotherapeutic agent but the family is taught to provide some basic care needs (eg, flushing the vascular access device, changing catheter dressings, and even giving subcutaneous injections). A primary family caregiver should be identified so that the home care nurses can give consistent instructions to that person and measure that person's ability to provide the therapy independently. The primary caregiver also communicates the patient's supply and equipment needs to the home care nurse. Other family members may want to be involved in the care of the child, but one person must take the primary caregiver role. Outcomes in pediatric home chemotherapy improve if the caregivers are educated about the therapy and its side effects.

▶ Role of the Home Care Provider

Chemotherapy in any environment should be administered only by clinicians trained to do so. Ensuring nursing competency will improve patient outcomes. Allowing personnel who do not have training or competency to administer chemotherapeutic medications is unsafe for the provider and patient. Basic guidelines should be considered before a home care provider assumes the responsibility of administering home chemotherapy.

- Intravenous chemotherapeutic agents are administered only by trained registered nurses.
- Registered nurses certified for chemotherapy administration also are trained in intravenous therapy.
- The nurse is observed by a trained chemotherapy practitioner before being allowed to administer chemotherapy independently.

A properly trained nurse is a helpful extension to the physician treating a pediatric home care patient who requires chemotherapy.

▶ Coordinating Protocol Therapies

Before administering the first treatment, the nurse and pharmacist review the physician's order and a copy of the specific protocol, if applicable. If the patient is on a protocol, it is critical to maintain the correct timing of each dose and laboratory draw. Where and when the laboratory specimens are obtained should be discussed with the patient's caregivers. To coordinate specific protocol therapies, the home care agency will need the following information:

- Patient's name
- Patient's height and weight
- Drug name(s)
- Dosage/m^2, total dose, and cumulative dose of each drug
- Rate of administration
- Route of administration
- Allergies
- Antiemetics, with dose, route, and frequency (as needed)
- Vascular access device (with specific flush orders)
- Hydration orders (as needed)
- Pretreatment or rescue (eg, granulocyte-colony stimulating factor) regimens (as needed)

Posttreatment assessment begins right after the drug is administered and continues until the patient's white blood cell count reaches nadir and recovers. The nurse and caregiver should be well informed about the expected side effects of the drug and any anticipated treatments. A complete systems assessment should be performed at each home care visit and any unusual or anticipated reactions should be reported to the physician.

▶ Policies and Procedures

Home care companies that administer chemotherapy agents should have the following policies and procedures in place:

- Chemotherapy administration
- Management of extravasation of chemotherapy agents
- Hazardous waste disposal of chemotherapeutic agents
- Management of cytotoxic spills
- Accessing central access venous devices

The following sample policy may be used as a template for developing a more specific policy for the administration of home chemotherapy.

Chemotherapy Administration

Policy: It is the policy of _____(this nursing agency)_____ to accept and provide service to medically stable clients requiring chemotherapy under the direction of the prescribing physician with a written prescription for the chemotherapeutic agent.

Performed by a registered nurse who demonstrates competency in intravenous (IV) therapy and who has been oriented to _____(this nursing agency's)_____ policies and procedures on chemotherapy administration, extravasation, and cytotoxic spill.

1. Criteria for patient selection.

   A. Patients selected for home chemotherapy will meet specific selection criteria in addition to the standard admission policies of _____(this nursing agency)_____ .

   B. Patients needing continuous infusions of vesicants (tissue-irritating chemotherapy agents) require a central venous access device for administration.

   C. If the patient's venous access is questionable, the chemotherapy is not to be administered.

   D. The patient must meet the following criteria:
   - The patient must be medically stable and meet physiologic criteria specified in each drug policy.
   - Baseline laboratory tests will be obtained prior to therapy and periodically throughout the course of therapy as ordered by the physician. Laboratory results must be documented on the patient's chart.
   - Any patient not meeting these criteria will not be accepted for service without concurrence of the director of operations or designee, the nursing manager, the pharmacy manager, and medical director.

2. A first cycle of chemotherapy will be given in a medically supervised setting, not in the home, whenever possible.

3. A signed physician order is required and a copy must be in the home at the time of administration. The order will include, but is not limited to, the following: the specific drug to be infused including absolute dosage (mg/kg or mg/m^2), dilution, route of administration, frequency, explicit number of doses, and length of infusion.

Chemotherapy Administration, continued

   A. A separate order must be obtained for each course
      of treatment.

   B. The physician may order the specific lumen/port of
      an access device that is to be used for chemotherapy
      administration.

   C. The nurse will note that the patient's body weight and
      body surface area are documented on the prescription
      correctly.

4. Only drugs included in _____(this nursing agency's)_____
   Policy and Procedure Manual may be administered.

5. Procedure.

   A. Any chemotherapeutic agent, vesicant or non-vesicant,
      to be administered by IV push will be administered via a
      free-flowing IV.

   B. During administration of chemotherapy, the peripheral site
      is to be exposed for easy assessment.

   C. If vesicant chemotherapeutic agents infiltrate,
      _____(this nursing agency's)_____ policy
      for management of extravasation is to be followed.

   D. Vesicant continuous infusions require a central venous
      access device for administration on a pump. A pump
      will NOT be used to administer chemotherapy via
      peripheral access.

   E. The use of body protection techniques, including gloves
      and a chemotherapy gown, are to be employed during
      the administration of chemotherapy unless medication is
      delivered via cassette. Only gloves are required when
      handling cassette medication.

   F. Each patient will be issued a kit for hazardous waste
      disposal. All drug waste will be collected and returned to
      _____(this nursing agency)_____ for proper
      disposal. Under no circumstances should these hazardous
      substances be disposed of by pouring or flushing them down
      a drain. In the case of a cytotoxic drug spill, this nursing
      agency's procedure for cytotoxic spills is to be implemented.

Chemotherapy Administration, continued

G. Equipment.
  • Gloves and gown (if indicated)
  • Plastic-backed pad
  • Sterile gauze pads
  • Alcohol pads
  • Chemotherapy needles/waste container
  • Chemotherapy spill kit
  • Intravenous tubing, pump, ancillary supplies as needed
  • Heparinized and normal saline flushes as ordered
    by doctor
  • Equipment needed to access central venous device or initiate peripheral access per _____(this nursing agency's)_____ policy

H. Administration steps.
  • Determine appropriate area to perform procedure.
  • Explain procedure to patient/caregiver and review physician orders.
  • Wash hands.
  • Don gloves and gown (if indicated).
  • Gather and assemble all supplies. Place all syringes, bags, and cassettes on plastic-backed pad. A plastic-backed pad also should be kept under the device while administering IV bolus chemotherapy.
  • Prime all IV tubing. Tubing being primed with cytotoxic drugs should be primed into a gauze pad that has been placed inside of a plastic bag. The bag then is disposed of in the chemotherapy waste container.
  • Access central venous device or initiate peripheral IV as per _____(this nursing agency's)_____ policies.
  • If chemotherapy is to be administered via bolus, initiate primary infusion as ordered by doctor; cleanse access port of IV tubing with alcohol pad and allow alcohol to dry; while IV solution is infusing, administer ordered premedications and chemotherapy at ordered infusion rates via access port; and after chemotherapy administration, discontinue primary infusion and flush access device per _____(this nursing agency's)_____ policy. Remove peripheral IV per _____(this nursing agency's)_____ policy.

Chemotherapy Administration, continued

- If chemotherapy is to be administered via continuous infusion, review infusion pump settings; administer premedications as ordered by doctor if indicated; initiate continuous infusion via pump with central venous access; and when discontinuing continuous infusions, flush central venous access device as ordered by doctor and de-access device per _____ (this nursing agency's) _____ policy.

- Place all contaminated syringes, tubing, bags, bottles, and cassettes into chemotherapy needles/waste container to be discarded by _____ (this nursing agency's) _____ personnel. All other used supplies may be discarded in a plastic bag.

- Remove apron (if indicated) and gloves; if contamination is suspected, place in chemotherapy needles/waste container.

I. Documentation should include, but not be limited to, site of IV insertion (if peripheral); type, size, and gauge of access device; presence or absence of blood return; therapy administered including dose, route, and rate of infusion; patient's response to procedure and therapy; patient education, including possible side effects and adverse reactions; nursing interventions; and physician contacts.

Side Effects of Chemotherapy

Chemotherapy can cause serious problems throughout the body. The more evident side effects occur in the rapidly dividing cells of the skin, gastrointestinal, and hematopoietic systems. Table 12-2 lists common side effects associated with chemotherapy and suggestions for counteracting those effects.

▸ Treating Nausea and Vomiting

Nausea and vomiting are frequently associated with the administration of chemotherapeutic agents. It is important to address the emetic potential of these side effects before they cause nausea and vomiting so that the patient does not form an association with the emetic effects and the drug. Once this distress begins, the patient may be less inclined to complete therapy. In addition, the actual physiologic effects of anorexia, dehydration, aspiration pneumonia, and weight loss may halt the progress of the therapy. Table 12-3 is a quick reference to help determine the emetic potential of a drug so that the clinician may decide on the appropriate antiemetic.

▶ General Guidelines for Antiemetic Therapy

When administering antiemetic therapy, be sure to abide by the following guidelines:

- Rule out other causes of nausea and vomiting before prescribing an antiemetic. Antiemetics may impede diagnosis of other, more serious conditions.
- Consult manufacturer's product information before use, especially in children.
- Use of antiemetics in children is not recommended for uncomplicated vomiting.
- Antiemetics should be used in conjunction with appropriate fluid and electrolyte therapy.

Maintaining Nutrition During Chemotherapy

The profound negative effects chemotherapy has on the gastrointestinal system, such as anorexia, diarrhea, and nausea (Table 12-2), ultimately affect the patient's nutrition. Table 12-4 lists suggestions for alleviating gastrointestinal symptoms and improving a patient's nutrition.

Chemotherapy and Home Safety

The home care provider is responsible for determining hazardous materials policies for the protection of clinicians and patients from exposure to chemotherapeutic agents. The patient not only runs the risk of being exposed to these agents topically, but also through extravasation. Consider the following in any home administration of chemotherapeutic agents:

- Is there informed consent to administer hazardous drugs/chemicals or vesicants in the home?
- Are there orders from the physician about what to do in case of extravasation?

TABLE 12-2. Chemotherapeutic Side Effects and Suggested Actions

System	Side Effects	Suggested Actions
Hematological	Myelosuppression	Monitor patient's blood counts.
	Neutropenia	Administer granulocyte-colony stimulating factor.
	Nadir	During nadir, screen visitors to avoid contact with people who have colds or other infections.
	Thrombocytopenia	Watch for signs of bleeding.
	Anemia	Patient may need platelets or packed red blood cells.
Gastrointestinal	Anorexia	Encourage high-calorie, protein-rich foods.
	Stomatitis	Frequent small meals may be tolerated better than three large meals.
		Avoid spicy or acidic foods and liquids while mouth is sore. Maintain good oral hygiene.
	Nausea/vomiting	Avoid fluids with meals; have fluid between meals.
	Diarrhea	Use antidiarrheal as necessary, avoid foods that irritate the gastrointestinal tract. Increase fluid and potassium intake.
	Constipation	Use natural laxatives (ie, prune juice) for constipation, increase fluids and exercise (as tolerated).
Hair and skin reactions	Alopecia	Consider buying a wig, scarf, or hat prior to hair loss.
	Photosensitivity	Other reactions cannot be prevented but early recognition and treatment may help decrease discomfort. The patient/caregiver may call 800/395-LOOK to contact the American Cancer Society and the National Cosmetology Association.
	Transient erythema	
	Urticaria	
	Hyperpigmentation	
	Telangiectasis	
	Ulceration	
	Radiation recall	
Cardiac	Cardiac arrhythmia	Instruct the patient/caregiver about symptoms such as dyspnea, ankle edema, cough, rales, cyanosis, or change in mental status. These should be reported to the nurse or physician immediately.
	Congestive heart failure	
Genitourinary	Impaired renal function	Patients should receive hydration orally or intravenously before and after administration of agents that can cause renal and bladder problems.
	Hemorrhagic cystitis	
	Sterility	
Pulmonary	Dry hacking cough, pain on inspiration	Consider pulmonary function tests. Teach the patient about long-term effects and recognizing appropriate symptoms. Some cytotoxic changes may not be apparent for months or years.
	Pulmonary infection	

TABLE 12-3. Relative Emetic Potential of Antineoplastic Drugs

Emetic Potential	Antineoplastic Agent	Emetic Potential	Antineoplastic Agent
High	Azacitidine	Low	Androgens
	Carboplatin		Asparaginase
	Carmustine		Bleomycin Sulfate
	Cisplatin		Busulfan
	Cyclophosphamide		Chlorambucil
	Cytarabine		Cladribine
	Dacarbazine		Corticosteroids
	Dactinomycin		Cyclophosphamide
	Doxorubicin		Docetaxol
	Irinotecan		Estrogens
	Mechlorethamine Hydrochloride		Etoposide
	Melphalan		Floxuridine
	Streptozocin		Fludarabine Phosphate
	Thiotepa		Fluorouracil
Moderately High	Altretamine		Gemcitabine
	Carboplatin		Hydroxyurea
	Cisplatin		Leucovorin Calcium & 5-FU
	Cyclophosphamide		Levamisole Hydrochloride & 5-FU
	Cytarabine		Melphalan
	Dacarbazine		Mercaptopurine
	Daunorubicin Hydrochloride		Methotrexate
	Doxorubicin		Paclitaxel
	Estramustine		Pentostatin
	Idarubicin Hydrochloride		Progestins
	Ifosfamide		Teniposide
	Mitomycin C		Thioguanine
	Mitoxantrone Hydrochloride		Topotecan Hydrochloride
	Plicamycin		Vinblastine Sulfate
	Procarbazine Hydrochloride		Vincristine Sulfate
	Thiotepa		Vinorelbine

Adapted with permission from the Pharmacy and Therapeutics Committee, Fox Chase Cancer Center, Philadelphia, PA.

TABLE 12-4. Symptom-Specific Guidelines for Nutrition

Anorexia	Offer small, frequent, high caloric-density feedings. Adjust meal size to appetite.
	Enhance or minimize food odors.
	Create a relaxed, pleasant eating atmosphere.
Alterations in taste/smell	Avoid offensive foods.
	Experiment with seasonings and food combinations.
	Enhance or minimize food odors.
	Serve foods at room temperature.
Nausea/vomiting	Eat dry, bland foods (eg, crackers, toast) before meals.
	Minimize food odors.
	Shorten food preparation time.
	Consume larger portions when nausea subsides.
	Eat bland, easy-to-digest meals several hours before treatment.
	Eat and drink slowly.
	Identify highly tolerated foods; avoid poorly tolerated foods such as fatty, spicy, overly sweet, or strongly flavored foods.
Stomatitis/mucositis	Avoid acidic, salty, or spicy foods.
Diarrhea	Use low-residue diet during acute phase.
	Increase fluid consumption.
	Increase potassium intake.
	Avoid gas-producing foods and beverages.
	Adjust lactose intake to level of tolerance.
Constipation	Increase residue as tolerated.
	Increase fluid consumption.
Dysphagia/odynophagia (painful swallowing)	Modify foods to a soft consistency.
	Avoid highly seasoned, spiced, or acidic foods.
	Adjust food temperature to tolerance.
Mouth dryness	Modify foods to a more liquid or pureed consistency.
	Use artificial saliva.
	Add sauces, gravies, and juices.
	Serve liquids with meals.
	Experiment with food temperature.

- Is there a chemotherapy spill kit in the home?
- Is there an anaphylaxis kit in the home in case of reaction?

Other points to consider include the following:

- Nurses administering chemotherapy should be skilled at the procedure.
- Technical expertise at initiating the venous access site is mandatory to preserve access and avoid complications.
- Do not administer vesicants over a bony prominence (ie, wrist) in the antecubital fossa, over tendons, or near neurovascular bundles.
- Hazardous chemicals or vesicants should be administered only via central line or through a newly started IV site via a running IV.
- The IV site must be assessed frequently while the hazardous chemical is infused.
- Because of the possibility of aerosolization, chemotherapeutic agents should be mixed in a clean area under a hood.
- The fluid volume in children must be monitored carefully because less fluid is administered than in an adult.

The Cytotoxic Spill Procedure template on the following page may be used to develop procedures for cytotoxic spills.

Summary

Chemotherapy in the home is a very involved process. The following must provide a foundation for its use:

- The home care provider or clinician referring a patient to home care is responsible for developing a comprehensive plan that starts with setting the stage for therapy and making sure that the patient and caregiver understand the therapy and possible side effects.
- Administration should be done by experienced and qualified clinicians.
- After administration of these agents, the clinician must ensure that the patient is observed adequately for side effects and toxicities.
- Goals of the plan should be evaluated for the success of the therapy and the quality of life that has been achieved.

These steps provide the basis for safe and effective administration and monitoring of chemotherapy agents in the home.

Cytotoxic Spill Procedure

Policy: It is the policy of _____(this nursing agency)_____
to provide a standard procedure for the safe, accurate, and competent removal of cytotoxic drug spill.

Performed by a registered nurse employed by ___(this nursing agency)___
who have been oriented to the cytotoxic spill procedure.

Equipment

(1) Chemotherapy drug spill kit, containing
    (2) Pair gloves
    (1) Pair safety goggles
    (1) Respiratory mask
    (4) Spill mats (plastic-backed absorbent pads)
    (1) Chemotherapy caution label
    (2) Red waste container bags
    (1) Semipermeable chemotherapy safety gown
    (1) Pair shoe coverings

Procedure

1. Limit access to area until spill has been eliminated.
2. Open the spill kit or the equipment gathered.
3. Don gown, double gloves, shoe coverings, and goggles.
4. Limit the spread of spilled fluid by placing absorbent pads over the spill after allowing aerosols to settle.
5. Remove glass particles using spill kit box as scoop. Empty glass into cardboard or plastic waste container.
6. Remove saturated absorbent pads and place in red bag labeled "Biohazard/Infectious Waste."
7. Clean contaminated area with detergent (non-germicidal) and rinse with equal amount of clean water.
8. Fully dry area with absorbent towel.
9. Place contaminated equipment into bag provided in kit. Remove outer pair of gloves and dispose with contaminated waste.
10. Place bag with contaminated equipment into second bag, along with gloves, goggles, mask, and shoe coverings.
11. Close bags and apply chemotherapy caution label.
12. Wash hands.
13. Call agency for immediate pickup of contaminated materials. DO NOT DISCARD IN HOUSEHOLD TRASH.

Bibliography

Borison HL, McCarthy LE. Neuropharmacology of chemotherapy-induce emesis. *Drugs.* 1983;25(suppl):8-17

Murphy GP, Lawrence W Jr, Lenhard RE Jr, and the American Cancer Society. *Textbook of Clinical Oncology.* 2nd ed. Atlanta, GA: The American Cancer Society; 1995

Terry J, Baranowski L, Lonsway RA, Hedrick C, eds. *Intravenous Therapy: Clinical Principles and Practice.* Philadelphia, PA: W.B. Saunders Co; 1995

Tortorice PV, O'Connell MB. Management of chemotherapy-induced nausea and vomiting. *Pharmacotherapy.* 1990;10:129-145

Wong DL. *Whaley & Wong's Essentials of Pediatric Nursing.* 5th ed. St Louis, MO: Mosby; 1997

Wujcik D. Chemotherapy administration. *Cancer Nurs.* 1987;10:53-64

Chapter 13

Home Intravenous Immunoglobulin Therapy for Children Infected With Human Immunodeficiency Virus

Stephen Arpadi, MD

Introduction

Intravenous immunoglobulin (IVIG) has been used extensively for treatment of children with primary and acquired immunodeficiencies. It was one of the earliest therapies provided to children infected with human immunodeficiency virus (HIV). Soon after the first case reports of acquired immunodeficiency syndrome (AIDS) in children, successful clinical experiences with IVIG were reported. The efficacy of IVIG for decreasing recurrent bacterial infections has been demonstrated in a multicenter randomized placebo-controlled trial. It also has proven beneficial and important in some children for treatment of primary idiopathic thrombocytopenic purpura (ITP), and for pediatric HIV infection.

In properly selected patients, IVIG can be given in the home safely and effectively, usually at a significant cost reduction compared with a hospital-based infusion center.

Clinical trials performed prior to the development of currently available, highly active antiretroviral therapies demonstrated that monthly IVIG infusions reduced episodes of serious bacterial infections. The effect was not apparent in children with CD4 counts less than 200/dL and there was no effect on mortality. Intravenous immunoglobulin also appears to decrease episodes of febrile illnesses in general as well as illnesses due to some viral pathogens.

Idiopathic thrombocytopenic purpura, which occurs with increased frequency in children infected with HIV, also may be treated with IVIG. Patients infected with HIV experience an increase in platelet count within 2 to 5 days of receiving a course of IVIG.

Indications for Initiation of Intravenous Immunoglobulin Therapy

Conditions indicating the need for IVIG therapy include the following:
- Children with HIV with recurrent (serious) bacterial infections
- Children with HIV with hypogammaglobulinemia
- Children with primary ITP
- Children with HIV with chronic ITP
- Children with primary hypogammaglobulinemia

Dosage and Administration

For children with HIV with prior documented recurrent bacterial infection, IVIG therapy may be indicated. The recommended dosage is 400 mg/kg of body weight administered at intervals of 4 weeks. Shorter intervals may be required for children who experience "breakthrough" infections.

For treatment of acute ITP, IVIG is administered at doses of 1 to 2 g/kg of body weight for 2 to 5 days. In the majority of patients with HIV, the effect of therapy is transient and repeat infusions within 3 to 4 weeks are required. Dosing of 400 to 1,000 mg/kg of body weight at intervals of 2 to 4 weeks has been used for maintenance infusions for patients with chronic ITP.

Intravenous immunoglobulin should be administered in a separate line by itself, without mixing with other intravenous solutions or medications. Initial doses should be provided under conditions that allow for monitoring and management of adverse experiences. Initial IVIG infusions should be given in a hospital or clinic with access to emergency equipment. Subsequent doses can be given at home. The initial infusion rate should be 0.01 to 0.02 mL/kg body weight per minute for 30 minutes; if well tolerated, the infusion rate may be gradually increased to a maximum of 0.08 mL/kg per minute. Once tolerance has been established, additional infusions may be started at the maximum rate. Some patients benefit from pretreatment with diphenhydramine and acetaminophen. Medications and equipment should be available in the home to treat adverse allergic reactions, including normal saline bolus, diphenhydramine, and epinephrine.

Home Administration

Most often, IVIG has been administered in clinics and hospital-based infusion centers, but it can be safely administered at home. As with other intravenous therapies, the initial dose should be administered in a more controlled environment. If that dose is well tolerated, home administration can be undertaken. A nurse present in the home during the infusion monitors for adverse reactions such as allergies or hypertension. Epinephrine, diphenhydramine, and IV fluids should be available if needed. Universal pretreatment with diphenhydramine or acetaminophen is reserved for individuals who have previously experienced adverse reactions.

Monitoring and Managing Adverse Reactions

In general, IVIG is well tolerated by children. Potential reactions include anxiety, flushing, wheezing, abdominal cramps, myalgia, arthralgia, and dizziness. Many of these adverse reactions are related to the rate of infusion and resolve with a reduction in this rate. Rashes have been reported rarely, as has anaphylaxis. Renal adverse reactions, including renal failure, also have been reported in association with IVIG. Physicians contemplating IVIG for children with conditions that appear to increase the risk of renal adverse reactions, including preexisting renal insufficiency, diabetes mellitus, hypovolemia, sepsis, and coadministered nephrotoxic drugs, are advised to administer IVIG at the lowest practical rate. Special precautions are required if IVIG is to be administered to individuals with prior history of allergic reaction to intramuscularly administered immunoglobulin.

Formulations and Preparations

Several preparations of IVIG are available for intravenous administration. Because of limitations in supplies of some IVIG preparations, the choice of products often is dictated by availability. Some products (Polygam and Panglobulin) are prepared from concentrate or reconstitution of lyophilized powder that may provide benefit over premixed mixtures (Gamimune N 5%, Gamimune N 10%, Sandoglobulin 10%, Venoglobulin-I 5% and 10%) in children who cannot tolerate large-volume infusions.

Summary

Additional aspects of IVIG therapy include the following:

- Although IVIG administration at home is most common in the HIV population, it can be offered to children with other disease entities.
- The principles outlined for initiation of IVIG at home for patients with HIV also apply to any other disease state that requires repeated administration of IVIG (eg, hypogammaglobulinemia).
- Using the home environment for these lengthy treatments can benefit the child and family by avoiding the disruption of school and work that a clinic-based infusion program entails.

Sample Policy

Administration of IV Immune Globulin

Purpose:

To administer Immune Globulin at home to prevent or modify acute bacterial or viral infections in patients with iatrogenically induced or a disease-associated immunity.

Responsible Party:

Registered nurse who has demonstrated competency in performing this procedure.

General Information:

- There is a worldwide shortage of IVIG. There are eight different preparations of IVIG in the United States. All eight are approved for use in primary immunodeficiencies, five are for idiopathic thrombocytopenia, and one is for chronic lymphocytic leukemia.

- IVIG is a human serum product. Parent/caregiver must be informed of the risks.

- Adjuvant Medications:
    - ~ Drugs must be kept at the bedside at all times in case the child has an adverse reaction.
        - ‹ 0.01 mg/kg (0.1cc/kg) Epinephrine 1:10,000 IV and/or Benadryl 1 mg/kg IV.

Administration of IV Immune Globulin, continued

‹ Tigan suppository (<14 kg, 100 mg, 14-45 kg, 100-200 mg) in the case of nausea/vomiting.

‹ Additional IV fluid (normal saline) should be available during the infusion to be utilized to clear IV line of IVIG in case of a reaction.

‹ If ordered, premedicate thirty minutes before dose with the following medications:

‹ Tylenol 10-20 mg/kg/dose (maximum of 650 mg) PO or PR.

‹ Benadryl 0.5-1 mg/kg/dose (maximum of 50 mg) PO, IV, IM

~ Adverse Reaction:

‹ **If patient experiences the following decrease IVIG administration rate by ½ and notify the physician:** headache, fever, chills, nausea, vomiting, joint/muscle/ back pain, chest tightness, palpitations, dizziness, sweating, itching rash, flushing or irritation at the needle site.

‹ **If patient experiences the following stop the IVIG infusion, maintain patency with D5W or Normal Saline and notify the physician or active EMS:** Drop of B/P equal to or over 20% of baseline, shortness of breath, dyspnea, wheezing, sneezing, hives.

Equipment:

- Antibacterial soap
- Disinfectant spray
- Protective barrier
- Premedications if ordered (see above)
- 500 cc bag of Normal Saline or D5W
- Topical anesthetic cream if indicated for peripheral IV start, or Implanted VAD access
- IV start kit or Huber needle and supplies for implanted VAD access
- Retractable needle removal device for Huber needle if applicable
- IVIG premixed or with needle transfer set if applicable
- Adjuvant medications in case of adverse reaction (see above)
- Normal saline multidose vial if applicable
- Heparin (100 units/cc) multidose vial if applicable

Administration of IV Immune Globulin, continued

- Normal saline syringes, or prefilled syringes with needleless access adapters
- Heparin syringe or prefilled syringe with needleless access adapter
- Gloves
- Electronic blood pressure machine
- Infusion pump and tubing
- Alcohol pads
- Cotton ball or gauze pad
- Plastic adhesive bandage
- Sharps disposal container
- Laboratory supplies for blood draw if indicated

Procedure:

1. If a peripheral IV or implanted VAD access is required, apply topical anesthetic cream at least 1 hour before procedure. Parent/caregiver may be instructed to perform this task before the nurse's arrival.
2. Identify patient and inform patient (at age-appropriate level) and parent/caregiver rationale for procedure. Inform parent/caregiver of side effects and adverse reactions.
3. Clean work area with a detergent-disinfectant.
4. Place protective barrier over clean surface.
5. Wash hands with antibacterial soap.
6. Gather equipment, medication and place on protective barrier.
7. Give premedications as ordered.
8. Check dosage and medications with physician orders.
9. Calculate drug dosage. Double-check calculation to reduce risk of error.
10. Inspect bottle visually for discoloration or particulate matter. If noted, do not use and inform pharmacist.
11. Establish IV or insert Huber needle per procedure if applicable.

Administration of IV Immune Globulin, continued

12. Spike bag of IVIG with spike end of infusion set.

13. Prime tubing.

14. Flush IV line with normal saline to check patency.

15. Attach tubing pump. Program pump as ordered.

16. Take a set of vital signs prior to starting IVIG (Temperature, Pulse, Respiration, and Blood Pressure).

17. Flush IV line for patency.

18. Connect IVIG tubing to patient.

19. Start pump.

20. Increase rate as ordered.

21. Monitor vital signs as ordered during the infusion and at completion. Assess for adverse reactions, see above.

22. Draw labs per procedure before, and/or after infusion if ordered.

23. When IVIG is completed, flush line with normal saline and heparin if applicable.

24. Withdraw needle while applying slight pressure with gauze or cotton ball over the insertion site. If using needle with safety device, activate needle protection assembly. If removing Huber needle, use retractable needle removal device.

25. Secure and cover needle at insertion site.

26. Discard needle, and supplies into sharps disposal container. Make sure that bag and tubing are completely empty and discard in wastebasket.

27. Document procedure, vital signs, patient current weight, Implanted VAD insertion or IV insertion including size, site, number of attempts, medications administered including dosage, route, length of infusion, patient tolerance of infusion, flushes, any adverse reactions or side effects, parent/caregiver education and response to all teaching provided on clinical nursing note.

Used with permission from Building Block Pediatric Home Health Services, Inc; 2001

Bibliography

Bussel JB, Haimi JS. Isolated thrombocytopenia in patients infected with HIV: treatment with intravenous gammaglobulin. *Am J Hematol.* 1988;28:79-84

Calvelli TA, Rubenstein A. Intravenous gamma-globulin in infant acquired immunodeficiency syndrome. *Pediatr Infect Dis.* 1986;5(suppl 3):S207-S210

Ellaurie M, Burns ER, Bernstein LJ, Shah K, Rubinstein A. Thrombocytopenia and human immunodeficiency virus in children. *Pediatrics.* 1988;82:905-908

Mofenson LM, Moye J Jr, Bethel J, Hirschhorn R, Jordan C, Nugent R, and the National Institute of Child Health and Human Development Intravenous Immunoglobulin Clinical Trial Study Group. Prophylactic intravenous immunoglobulin in HIV-infected children with CD4+ counts of 0.20×10⁹/L or more. Effect on viral, opportunistic, and bacterial infections. *JAMA.* 1992;268:483-488

National Institute of Child Health and Human Development Intravenous Immunoglobulin Study Group. Intravenous immunoglobulin for the prevention of bacterial infections in children with symptomatic human immunodeficiency virus infection. *N Engl J Med.* 1991;325:73-80

Wood CC, McNamara JG, Schwartz DF, Merrill WW, Shapiro ED. Prevention of pneumococcal bacteremia in a child with acquired immunodeficiency syndrome-related complex. *Pediatr Infect Dis J.* 1987;6:564-566

Chapter 14

Home Antibiotic Therapy

Lourdes R. Laraya-Cuasay, MD

Introduction

Home intravenous (IV) therapy for children generally has been accepted as safe, effective, and more cost-effective than similar therapy in the hospital. Having access to home IV therapy can improve the quality of life of patients, lower school absenteeism, and prevent loss of wages. The use of home IV therapy has increased because of the availability of antibiotics requiring once- or twice-daily administration; improved vascular access and infusion devices; increased acceptance of home IV therapy by patients, parents, caregivers, and health personnel; and availability of structured services for home care. Infusion of antimicrobials in the home can be safe and effective if done appropriately. It has become a generally accepted medical practice that can reduce treatment costs, improve patient satisfaction, and reduce the psychologic effects of prolonged hospitalization for ill children.

Preparation for Home Intravenous Therapy

The safe and effective administration and delivery of antibiotics, antifungals, and antivirals (anti-infective agents) in the home require a coordinated team approach with many disciplines. Close cooperation among nurses, pharmacists, physicians, social workers, discharge planners, parents, and patients is necessary to achieve a good outcome. A successful transition to home infusion requires an individualized plan based on the developmental level of the child. The proper infusion pump must deliver the particular anti-infective through the prescribed route using the best intravascular access for the individual patient. A home infusion pharmacist must review the drugs for stability at the concentrations and for the length of time required for home therapy. A reliable on-call service for all disciplines is necessary.

Patient Selection

Not every hospitalized patient with an infection is a candidate for home IV therapy. The pediatrician, with advice from the nursing team and social worker, must assess if home IV therapy is beneficial for the individual patient and family. An infectious diseases specialist may be consulted. The pediatrician with experience in home IV therapy can be very helpful in the evaluation. The physician responsible for monitoring the patient while at home must be identified early. Pre-discharge planning allows the family and home care providers to prepare for home care and provide appropriate education. The pediatrician should consider the following guidelines when selecting patients for home IV therapy:

▶ **Guidelines to Patient Selection**

1. The disease requires treatment beyond the anticipated period of hospitalization. No alternate routes of drug delivery are feasible and there is reasonable expectation of control of infection.
2. The patient is physiologically stable and does not require ongoing hospitalization for other reasons.
3. The patient must have adequate IV access.
4. Initial response to therapy is deemed satisfactory.
5. No acute allergic reactions to drugs have occurred or, if the patient was on a desensitization regimen, all reactions are under control. The first dose of an anti-infective agent has been given in the hospital or other controlled clinical setting.
6. An accredited acceptable home care/nursing company is on call for problems or emergencies.
7. The home setting is safe and has electricity, running water, a working phone, and an area for proper storage of medications, such as a refrigerator.
8. A health care facility for therapy-related emergencies is available.
9. The parent or caregiver is capable of safe and effective delivery of parenteral anti-infectives, compliant with the recommended treatment as demonstrated by previous behavior, and able to participate in the proposed therapy. The ability of the caregivers to understand and perform the required treatments must be considered.
10. Reimbursement issues have been addressed and found satisfactory or acceptable to all parties concerned.
11. The physician responsible for the care of the patient in the home has been identified.

A variety of infections have been successfully treated in the home care setting. Clinicians select patients based on their assessment of clinical stability and their comfort level with the available provider. The patient should be afebrile with stable vital signs. The infection should be reasonably stable and nonprogressive. Any concomitant condition, such as pulmonary, cardiac, or renal disease, also should be stable. The prognosis of the condition should be predictable and the diagnosis firmly established. There is published experience of home IV therapy for abscess, cellulitis, cytomegalovirus retinitis and other human immunodeficiency virus (HIV)-related infections, endocarditis, Lyme disease, meningitis, osteomyelitis, pelvic inflammatory disease, pneumonia with or without empyema, infectious exacerbation in cystic fibrosis, postoperative wound infections, pyelonephritis, septic arthritis, and skin and soft tissue infections, but critical evaluation of the outcomes of such therapy is not yet available. Home IV antibiotic therapy in the treatment of pulmonary exacerbations in cystic fibrosis and in febrile neutropenic patients have published guidelines.

▶ Contraindications to Home Intravenous Therapy

Patients not considered candidates for home IV anti-infective therapy are those with severe infections, poor compliance, lack of IV access, and a poor social situation. Patients who are likely to abuse an IV system are not desirable candidates, although computerized IV pump technologies reduce the likelihood of tampering. The presence of a drug- or alcohol-abusing family member in the home may dictate continuation of therapy in a hospital or subacute facility.

Drug Selection and Dosing

The severity of infection and patient factors determine whether outpatient parenteral anti-infective therapy will be required. Anti-infective selection depends on the clinical presentation, likely organisms, pharmacodynamics, pharmacokinetics, and drug stability. It is a complex decision involving factors that relate to the patient, disease, pathogen, anti-infective agent chosen, and facilities available in the home.

Drug selection should be based on antimicrobial susceptibility testing, when available. Ability to self-administer is another determinant of the choice of drug. The choice of anti-infective agent should be individualized based on the disease, the patient's clinical and social situation, caregivers ability to provide care, drug stability, and home care services available.

Some flexibility in the dosing schedule may be allowed by the physician to reduce family and work conflicts and to ensure adequate patient and parent rest. In addition, the expertise of the physician and the pharmacist must be combined to ensure a safe and therapeutically effective program. Drug dosages may need to be modified for renal or hepatic impairment, poor nutritional status, or when other drugs are being used that may have interactions. Table 14-1 lists anti-infective agents commonly used in home care.

TABLE 14-1. Anti-infective Drugs Used in Pediatric Home Intravenous Therapy

Generic Names

Acyclovir	Fluconazole
Amikacin Sulfate*	Foscarnet Sodium
Amphotericin B	Ganciclovir
Amphotericin B Liposomal	Gentamicin Sulfate*
Ampicillin Sodium*	Imipenem-Cilastatin Sodium*
Ampicillin/Sulbactam	Meropenem
Aztreonam*	Metronidazole Hydrochloride
Cefamandole*	Mezlocillin Sodium
Cefazolin Sodium*	Minocycline Hydrochloride
Cefepime Hydrochloride*	Nafcillin Sodium*
Cefonicid Sodium*	Netilmicin Sulfate*
Cefoperazone Sodium*	Oxacillin Sodium*
Cefotaxime Sodium*	Penicillin G Potassium
Cefotetan Disodium*	Penicillin G Procaine*
Cefoxitin Sodium*	Pentamidine Isethionate
Ceftazidime*	Piperacillin Sodium
Ceftizoxime Sodium*	Piperacillin/Tazobactam
Ceftriaxone Sodium*	Polymyxin B Sulfate*
Cefuroxime Sodium	Rifampin
Cephalothin Sodium*	Ticarcillin Disodium
Cephradine*	Ticarcillin/Clavulanate Potassium
Chloramphenicol Sodium Succinate	Tobramycin Sulfate*
Ciprofloxacin	Trimethoprim/Sulfamethoxazole
Clindamycin Phosphate*	Trimetrexate Glucuronate
Colistimethate Sodium*	Vancomycin Hydrochloride
Doxycycline Hyclate	Vidarabine
Erythromycin Gluceptate	Zidovudine (AZT)
Erythromycin Lactobionate	

*Has intramuscular preparation also.

Drug stability is an important factor to consider when choosing an anti-infective agent for home IV therapy. A stable drug is defined as one that, when in solution, retains 90% or more of its original concentration for a minimum of 24 hours at room temperature (25°C) and for 4 to 7 days under refrigeration at 3°C to 5°C. Temperature, pH, and final concentration affect drug stability. When a patient carries the drug reservoir very close to the body, the drug solution may reach temperatures near 37°C. Body heat, blankets, and thick clothing may increase environmental temperature close to the solution. This can be corrected by having an insulated pouch, with two frozen gel packs, hold the infusion pump and drug reservoir. Drugs that are stable for less than 24 hours are not ideal choices for home IV use (eg, ampicillin, imipenem-cilastatin, doxycycline, and trimethoprim-sulfamethoxazole). Unstable drugs are best given intermittently.

Drug Delivery

Several drug delivery systems are available for pediatric use. These include elastomeric devices, which restrict flow rate by using tubing with a calibrated diameter; gravity drip systems; portable pumps; electronic syringe pumps; and electronic stationary pumps. An elastomeric infusor device is a popular choice for ambulatory patients, especially children who want to continue school attendance, because they are small and lightweight and often can be carried in a pocket.

The following are factors to consider in the selection of the delivery method:

1. Pharmaceutical factors — drug or therapy type, dosage and dosage interval, labor or compounding time, age and weight of child
2. Financial reimbursement — number of drugs, duration of therapy and type of IV line, distance from provider
3. Nursing considerations — availability of home care, home environment, competence of parents or caregivers, caregiver preference, activity level of child
4. Psychosocial factors — family/patient ability to comply to schedule of therapy prescribed, ability to learn techniques of IV administration, clinical diagnosis

Syringe pumps range in capacity from 5 to 60 mL, and drugs administered in this manner are highly concentrated. Rate-restricted systems have varying reservoir sizes from 50 to 500 mL. Gravity bags can be of any size. Compact portable infusion pumps have reservoir cassettes of 50, 150, or 250 mL. External reservoirs of any size can be accommodated.

Manufacturer's recommendations for dilution of antibiotics for IV use sometimes are not appropriate for pediatric patients because of the unsuitably large volume of fluid for the desired infusion time. Pharmacists and home infusion nurses should calculate the volume of fluid required to dilute any anti-infective agent carefully to ensure that the patient will not develop fluid overload. The volume of diluent is critical in neonatal patients receiving home IV therapy. Awareness of fluid volume issues in home IV therapy highlight the importance of having pediatric-trained pharmacists and nurses available to provide home IV therapy to pediatric patients.

▸ Intravenous Access Methods

The choice of IV access method is determined by age, experience of the patient and caregivers, expected length of therapy, and anticipated frequency of future IV therapy. Patients of all ages have had successful home IV therapy.

Intravenous access for home IV therapy can be done using a variety of catheter types. Semipermanent devices are available for home IV access use. The peripheral IV catheter is noninvasive, has a low infection rate and low cost, and is easy to remove, but is used only for short duration therapy because IV restart sites may become limited. The streamlined catheter is soft and can last longer than standard peripheral catheters in some patients. The peripherally inserted central catheter (PICC) and midline catheters are longer peripheral catheters with increased longevity potential that can last for repeated courses of therapy. They are more costly and have the potential for infection. Sometimes they may not last longer than standard peripheral catheters.

Surgically implanted catheters have an extremely long life in some cases and can be used for total parenteral nutrition. Infection, thrombus formation, pulmonary embolism, pneumohydrothorax, or pneumohemothorax can occur. These catheters can be placed subcutaneously like the MediPort, or tunnel and exit from the skin at a distal site such as the Hickman or Broviac catheters. Each catheter has its advantages and disadvantages.

▶ Drug Monitoring

Monitoring of therapeutic drug levels on home IV therapy patients should be done as in the hospital. Periodic audiologic testing should be done for repeated users of aminoglycoside, such as patients with cystic fibrosis. Liver function should be monitored for drugs reported to have hepatotoxicity. Periodic urinalyses and blood urea nitrogen and creatinine determinations may be necessary to monitor nephrotoxicity. Serum creatinine levels should be checked twice weekly for patients receiving aminoglycosides or vancomycin hydrochloride. Weekly complete blood count is recommended for those on beta-lactamase and vancomycin hydrochloride.

▶ Follow-up

Physicians should monitor patients on a weekly or biweekly basis to assess clinical response and observe any related adverse events, such as IV line problems, rash, diarrhea, hematologic reactions, or adverse drug reactions. More frequent visits are required for patients at high risk.

Documentation

At the onset of home IV therapy, the pediatrician should give a written prescription for each chosen drug containing the route of administration and the duration of therapy to the home care pharmacist. The home nurses should complete a home assessment and initial patient assessment. A medication log or register should be developed and a copy should be left with the family. The nurses should provide education for the family and ensure competency with the prescribed treatments.

Potential significant adverse drug reactions (ADRs) should be discussed with the family and the home care nurse. Should any ADR occur, the physician must be notified and the home care nurse should perform a physical assessment. Depending on the severity of the ADR, a physician visit or rehospitalization may be required. The home care record should properly document the occurrence of the ADR, the onset and end of therapy, dosage prescribed, the catheter type used, method used for flushing catheters, any line changes, and comments at nursing visits. The report is sent to the prescribing physician at the end of the therapy.

Patient/Parent Education

Education on home care must start in the hospital. Protocols for care should be shared with the patient and caregivers. The caregivers should be given ample time to learn techniques involved in home IV therapy prior to discharge. Education on identification of ADR and signs and symptoms that require reporting to the nurse is a must. Access to a subcutaneous epinephrine dispenser, such as an EpiPen, should be available for patients who have previously demonstrated allergic reactions.

Complications

Home IV therapy presents the potential for complications. Reported line infections from central catheter and PICC lines are numerous. Rehospitalization may be required for those with severe complications. Intravenous access problems include trauma, kinking, catheter leaks, thrombosis, site infection, or bacteremia. Some complications may require catheter removal or rehospitalization.

Other potential problems with home IV therapy include patient or parent noncompliance, interrupted therapy, drug delivery delays, equipment malfunction, and natural disasters. The many disciplines involved in home care must have written shared protocols and an emergency preparedness plan to address complications when they occur.

Summary

Ways to create successful home antibiotic therapy include the following:
- Through a good working relationship among multiple disciplines, anti-infective therapy in the home can lead to a successful outcome.
- Physician direction and participation, after appropriate patient selection, will help ensure success.
- Cost savings of home infusion therapy can be significant. Maintaining the safety of therapies delivered in the home is a continuing responsibility for all.
- Quality improvement practices contribute to better home care and quality of life for the children being served.

Bibliography

Anastasi JM. Innovations in care: neonatal home antibiotic infusion therapy. *Neonatal Netw.* 1998;17:33-38

Andes D, Craig WA. Pharmacokinetics and pharmacodynamics of outpatient intravenous antimicrobial therapy. *Infect Dis Clin North Am.* 1998;12:849-860

Cystic Fibrosis Foundation. *Clinical Practice Guidelines for Cystic Fibrosis.* Bethesda, MD: Cystic Fibrosis Foundation; 1997

Dahlgren AF. Adverse drug reactions in home care patients receiving nafcillin or oxacillin. *Am J Health Syst Pharm.* 1997;54:1176-1179

de Groot R, Smith AL. Antibiotic pharmacokinetics in cystic fibrosis. Differences and clinical significance. *Clin Pharmacokinet.* 1987;13:228-253

Draft guideline for prevention of intravascular device-related infections, 60 *Federal Register* 49977 (1995)

Gilbert DN, Dworkin RJ, Raber SR, Leggett JE. Outpatient parenteral antimicrobial-drug therapy. *N Engl J Med.* 1997;337:829-838

Gilbert DN, Moellering RC, Sande MA. *The Sanford Guide to Antimicrobial Therapy.* 29th ed. Dallas, TX: Antimicrobial Therapy Inc; 1999

Hoffmann-Terry ML, Fraimow HS, Fox TR, Swift BG, Wolf JE. Adverse effects of outpatient parenteral antibiotic therapy. *Am J Med.* 1999;106:44-49

Hughes WT, Armstrong D, Bodey GP, et al. 1997 guidelines for the use of antimicrobial agents in neutropenic patients with unexplained fever. *Clin Infect Dis.* 1997;25:551-573

Johnson KA, Hagen JC, Bender TW. Multidisciplinary approach to improving pediatric home infusion. *Am J Health Syst Pharm.* 1999;56:473-474

Joint Commission on Accreditation of Healthcare Organizations. *1997-1998 Comprehensive Manual for Home Care.* Oakbrook Terrace, IL: Joint Commission on Accreditation of Healthcare Organizations; 1997

Leaver J, Radivan F, Patel L, David TJ. Home intravenous antibiotic therapy: practical aspects in children. *J R Soc Med.* 1997;90(suppl31):26-33

Nelson JD. *1998-1999 Pocket Book of Pediatric Antimicrobial Therapy.* 13th ed. Baltimore, MD: Williams & Wilkins; 1998

1999 Drug Topics Red Book. Montvale, NJ: Medical Economics Co; 1999

Nolet BR. Patient selection in outpatient parenteral antimicrobial therapy. *Infect Dis Clin North Am.* 1998;12:835-847

Williams DN, Rehm SJ, Tice AD, Bradley JS, Kind AC, Craig WA. Practice guidelines for community-based parenteral anti-infective therapy. *Clin Infect Dis.* 1997;25:787-801

Chapter 15

Pain Management at Home

Bruce P. Himelstein, MD; Jean B. Belasco, MD

Goals of Pain Management

Many pediatric conditions are associated with acute or chronic pain. Pain is defined as an unpleasant sensory and emotional experience associated with actual or potential tissue damage, or described in terms of such damage. The goal of therapy in the home is to achieve pain control safely and effectively, addressing the physical and emotional components of pain. Although there is some debate about indications for home infusion pain control management, palliation for terminal disease is the one clear indication for home infusion management of pain. Severe pain in terminal disease should be treated emergently.

Indications for home infusion of strong opioids include the ineffectiveness of weaker opioids to control pain, the inability of a patient to tolerate strong opioids by mouth or sublingually, or a need to titrate opioids rapidly. Home infusion of a strong opioid does not obviate the need to continue to use adjuvant pharmacological, physical, and emotional pain management tools.

The pediatrician, in collaboration with the patient and family, must carefully weigh the potential risk of sedation, respiratory depression, and addiction versus the anticipated benefit of comfort in terminal disease. This risk/benefit assessment must be made in the context of the primary goal of home infusion therapy, which is optimization of patient comfort.

Managing pain by infusion at home requires special skills and extraordinary teamwork. Generalists and subspecialists are strongly advised to consult with pain specialists, palliative medicine specialists, or a multidisciplinary home care team with expertise in home infusion for pain to develop a comprehensive care plan.

Objectives

The following are objectives of home pain management:

▶ Demonstrate Pain Relief Verbally or Nonverbally

Regardless of how carefully plans are made for home pain management, they are only as good as the ability to continually assess and reassess whether they are working. Effective pain relief must be shown and documented. Lack of good pain relief should be discussed immediately with the primary physician so that the care plan can be revised.

▶ Standardize Pain Assessment

Good pain management demands consistent and accurate assessment. The earlier in the course of management a child and family are exposed to assessment tools, the smoother pain management will proceed. Ideally, parents and children can be instructed in the use of assessment tools so that reliable reports can be assessed in person or by phone. Self-reporting is the best measure of pain, when possible.

▶ Maintain Age-Appropriate Level of Consciousness

Sedation is a common side effect seen with initiation of opioid therapy. Many patients will experience a decrease in sedation over the first days of treatment. However, as doses are increased as a result of increasing pain or tolerance, or as potentially sedating adjunct medications such as phenothiazines, antihistamines, or benzodiazepines are added, sedation may occur again. Although families may be comfortable with sedation depending on the state of disease, treatment should strive to maximize level of consciousness at most times.

▶ Maintain Age-Appropriate Respiratory Function

Respiratory suppression is a common side effect with opioid therapy. Tolerance to this side effect usually develops, but management plans must be in place should it develop at home. This usually means administration of supplemental oxygen or reversal of narcosis if indicated.

▶ Minimize Side Effects

In addition to sedation and respiratory suppression, opioids are associated with many potential side effects that require aggressive therapy. Many of these effects are preventable and/or easily treatable if anticipated in advance, and are particularly critical in the home setting. Tolerance to many of the effects develops. Side effects respond to dose reduction but, depending on pain relief, this may not be possible. The addition of adjuncts may permit some dose reduction. Specific side-effect management is discussed later in this chapter.

▶ Maximize Participation in Activities of Daily Living

Participation in care is critical to the success of pain management. These activities should be encouraged, and staff should promote patient and family participation as much as possible.

▶ Demonstrate Understanding of Pain Therapy

Patients and families need to understand what the plan of care involves and why each intervention is being carried out. Further, many families require education about the concepts of tolerance and addiction.

▶ Maintain Medication Supply

Maintenance of medication supply reflects the overall philosophy of pro-active planning for adequate home management. Sufficient medication must be on hand in the home to keep a continuous supply, particularly for children on constant infusions. This may require storing extra medication cartridges/bags in the house in case the pump malfunctions, or having an alternative means of administration, such as a subcutaneous needle, on hand. Also, medications for the treatment of side effects should be in the home, such as antihistamines, nalbuphine hydrochloride, and laxatives.

Equipment Required

- Pain assessment tools
  - ~ For verbal children 7 years of age and older who are able to cognitively understand numbers and rank, a simple visual analog scale or anchored verbal 0-10 scale can be used, assuming that other factors have not altered the developmental ability of an older child to use such a tool. Appropriate anchors might include 0 being no pain and 10 being the worst pain you could imagine.
  - ~ For verbal children aged 3 to 7 years, several scales have been validated including the Wong-Baker faces scale, the poker chip tool, the Oucher scale, or the Eland color scale.
  - ~ For children under age 3 or older children who are nonverbal or cognitively impaired, there are several behavioral scales, including the Children's Hospital of Eastern Ontario Pain Scale or the Gauvain-Piquard scales.
- Infusion equipment
  - ~ Portable for mobile patients
  - ~ Easy to operate for staff and family
  - ~ Cannot be reset accidentally
- Documentation
  - ~ Should include all assessments and interventions

Procedures

▶ Intake

The primary physician, home care coordinator, pharmacist in consultation with pain specialists, specialist in palliative medicine, or a multidisciplinary home care team with expertise in home infusion for pain assess the current pain status, including detailed medical, psychosocial, and medication history. Determination of appropriateness for home management must include assessment of the family and child's ability to perform self-care.

▶ Pain Assessment

A comprehensive pain assessment in pediatrics is dependent on the age and developmental capacity of the child. Pain assessment scales only assess pain intensity. A comprehensive evaluation should include, but is not limited to, the following:

- Quality of pain
- Location of pain
- Severity of pain
- Duration of pain
- Past experience with pain
- Context of pain (distractions, environmental factors)
- Meaning of pain
- Provocative and palliative factors
- Coping skills
- Reaction of family and friends
- Potential for secondary gain
- Culture and ethnicity
- Patient personality
- Affective state

▶ Plan of Care

A comprehensive plan of care should be developed that incorporates the following:

- Intake assessment
- Medication profile
- Hospital discharge instructions, if applicable
- Presence or absence of intravenous (IV) access
- Pain assessment
- Physician orders
- Input from other home care team members such as the pharmacist or nursing staff
- Side-effect prevention and management plan
- Patient/family preference
- Cognitive-behavioral intervention plan
- Physical and rehabilitative intervention plan where appropriate
- Emergency plans, including contacts for family

▶ Pain Management

Analgesic Interventions

Analgesic interventions include any physically or emotionally based therapy with pain relief as its primary intention. These guidelines do not mandate their use but list the interventions as potential components to overall plans of care for home management of pain. These include, but are not limited to, the following:

- Analgesic medications
- Behavioral interventions (hypnosis, relaxation, biofeedback, desensitization, psychotherapy, distraction, play therapy, comfort measures)
- Anesthetic agents (local, regional, general)
- Neurosurgical techniques
- Neurologic techniques (transcutaneous electrical nerve stimulation, acupuncture)
- Rehabilitative interventions (physical and occupational therapy, orthopedic intervention, exercise)
- Cognitive intervention (education, demystification, symptom diary)
- Supportive (financial, social, spiritual)

Comfort measures should be included universally in pain management plans, even for patients on high-dose opioid infusions. These relatively simple, but often neglected, measures are effective adjuncts to overall pain management. Such measures include, but are not limited to, the following:

- Reposition or use age-appropriate positioning devices such as bumpers or supports.
- Apply warm blankets.
- Apply warm or cool compresses.
- Massage.
- Reduce environmental stimulation.
- Familiarize surroundings.
- Encourage family presence and interaction.
- Encourage/teach age-appropriate comfort techniques — for infants, pacifier, rocking, swaddling, music; for older children, television, music, books, movies, video games, relaxation, imagery techniques.

Analgesic Medications

Pain management should follow World Health Organization (WHO) guidelines. The following are general principles:

- The administration of a medication should be appropriate to pain nature and severity.
- Medications should be administered regularly to maintain constant plasma levels.
- The oral route is preferred.
- Doses of strong opioids must be titrated to clinical effect.
- Anticipate and manage side effects.
- Strive for sleep at night.
- Reassess frequently.
- Discuss the regimen with the patient and family.

Analgesic medications fall into several classes, including

- Non-opioid peripheral acting agents (acetaminophen, nonsteroidal anti-inflammatories)
- Mild opioids (codeine, tramadol hydrochloride)
- Strong opioids (morphine, hydromorphone, fentanyl citrate, methadone hydrochloride)
- Adjuvants

Indications for home infusion of strong opioids include the ineffectiveness of weaker opioids to control pain, the inability to tolerate strong opioids by mouth or sublingually, or a need to titrate opioids rapidly. For ease of use as well as decreased demand on parents to administer bolus medication, continuous infusion or patient-controlled analgesia (PCA) is recommended. Morphine is recommended as a first-line agent, while hydromorphone is second. Fentanyl citrate typically is reserved for patients who have intolerable side effects from morphine or hydromorphone, and may be appropriate for patients previously stabilized on a regimen including transdermal fentanyl citrate. There is no current indication for the use of parenteral meperidine hydrochloride.

Suggested starting doses must be based on a conversion from previous oral opioid therapy and should be developed in collaboration with a pain specialist, palliative medicine specialist, or a multidisciplinary home care team with expertise in home infusion for pain management.

Although the IV route is preferred, morphine, hydromorphone, and fentanyl citrate all can be given by the subcutaneous route for which special catheters are available. Stock concentrations of opioids may be higher for administration by this route to reduce infused volume.

For patients not previously exposed to narcotics, suggested starting PCA settings are listed in Table 15-1.

TABLE 15-1. Starting Patient-Controlled Analgesia Settings

Parameter	Morphine	Hydromorphone	Fentanyl Citrate
Basal infusion	0.01-0.02 mg/kg/h	0.001-0.002 mg/kg/h	1 µg/kg/h
Bolus dose	0.02 mg/kg	0.002-0.004 mg/kg	1-2 µg/kg
Lockout time	8-10 min	8-10 min	8-10 min

Additional medications that should be provided in the home for patients receiving opioid infusions are listed in Table 15-2.

TABLE 15-2. Medications for Patients Receiving Home Opioid Infusions

Medication	Dose	Interval	Maximum	Indication
Diphenhydramine	0.5-1.0 mg/kg IV	Every 6 hours	50 mg	Itching
Nalbuphine hydrochloride	0.025-0.05 mg/kg IV	Every 6 hours	2.5 mg	Itching Urinary retention
Naloxone hydrochloride*	0.1 mg/kg in 25-50 mL saline SLOW IV	Every 2 to 3 min	2 mg	Severe Respiration Suppression

*Given the risk of acute withdrawal and/or pulmonary edema, use of naloxone hydrochloride in the home should be reserved only for severe respiratory suppression clearly due to opioid overdose unresponsive to other measures. Use of naloxone hydrochloride rarely is warranted in the terminal care setting as it may also precipitate a severe pain crisis.

Many adjunct pain medications, including anticonvulsants, steroids, nonsteroidal drugs such as ketorolac tromethamine, anxiolytics, sedatives/ hypnotics including general anesthetics, and clonidine hydrochloride, are available for parenteral use. Indications, dosing, and schedule should be discussed with pain specialists.

▶ Side-effect Management

• Sedation
  ~ Reduce the narcotic dose, if possible.
  ~ Use stimulants (eg, methylphenidate hydrochloride, dextroampheta-
    mine, amphetamine combination preparations) if opioid doses cannot
    be reduced.
• Respiratory suppression
  ~ Reduce the narcotic dose, if possible.
  ~ Stimulate the patient.
  ~ Use naloxone hydrochloride only if absolutely necessary; rapid
    administration may precipitate life-threatening withdrawal and
    pulmonary edema. Dilute the dose in 25 to 50 mL of saline and
    administer slowly, titrating to effect.
• Tolerance
  ~ Increase narcotic dose.
  ~ Add adjuvant treatment.
  ~ Consider switching opioids (opioid rotation).
• Pruritus
  ~ Antihistamine (diphenhydramine, hydroxyzine, cetirizine).
  ~ Low-dose nalbuphine hydrochloride.
  ~ Alternative analgesic (fentanyl citrate may be associated with less
    histamine release than morphine or hydromorphone, particularly
    at lower doses).
  ~ Preliminary studies suggest that there may be a role for serotonin
    antagonists such as ondansetron hydrochloride for pruritus associated
    with systemically administered opioids; given relative cost and the
    lack of evidence of significant improvement over other agents,
    however, its use cannot be recommended uniformly.
• Nausea/vomiting
  ~ Low-dose phenothiazines (chlorpromazine, prochlorperazine, pro-
    methazine hydrochloride).
  ~ Droperidol.
  ~ Metoclopramide hydrochloride.
  ~ Scopolamine (IV or transdermal).

~ Preliminary studies suggest that there may be a role for serotonin antagonists such as ondansetron hydrochloride for nausea and vomiting associated with systemically administered opioids; given relative cost and the lack of evidence of significant improvement over the antiemetics, however, its use cannot be recommended uniformly.

- Urinary retention
  ~ Physical measures such as warmth and ambulation.
  ~ Low-dose nalbuphine hydrochloride.
  ~ Intermittent catheterization.
- Constipation
  ~ Therapy should start concurrently with initiation of opioid.
  ~ Bulk agents alone usually are insufficient.
  ~ Stimulants/cathartics such as senna, lactulose, bisacodyl, or magnesium hydroxide may be appropriate.
- Dysphoria
  ~ May respond to addition of benzodiazepines or phenothiazines.
- Myoclonus
  ~ May respond to benzodiazepines or anticonvulsants (eg, valproic acid, which may be a helpful adjunct for neuropathic pain).

▶ Continuous Reassessment

Response to therapy and side effects should be assessed with each home visit or by telephone follow-up on a regular basis. Assessment includes the following:

- Vital signs
- Pain behavior
- Pain scale score with trend over time
- Pain score before and after any intervention, including analgesic medication
- Satisfaction of child/family with pain relief
- Current medications, route, frequency of administration, and use since last assessment
- Level of sedation
- Other side effects
- Current activities of daily living child is able to perform
- Nonmedication therapy in use for pain

The home care clinician should discuss findings with the patient's primary physician and change the care plan accordingly. All results of pain assessment and intervention should be documented in a home care visit, and a review of the plan of care with patient and family should be included.

▶ Function and Activity

- Encourage appropriate levels of activity and function.
- Give positive reinforcement to patient and caregiver for attempts at normal activity.
- Promote child and family participation and independence in all aspects of pain management.

▶ Patient/Family Education

Items to be covered educationally include, but are not limited to, the following:
- Analgesic interventions, including comfort measures
- Pain medications, including name, dose, route, and schedule
- Pump operation, if applicable
- Administration of rescue medication
- Pain assessment tools
- Meaning of, and distinction between, addiction (habitual physiologic and psychologic dependence) and tolerance (decreased responsiveness over a period of continued exposure)
- Plan for safe medication storage
- What to do in an emergency

Summary

When considering home infusion pain management, the following are important points to keep in mind:
- The goal of pain management in the home is to achieve pain control safely and effectively through the use of medication and other intervention techniques.
- The objectives of home pain management are to standardize pain assessment, to maintain an appropriate level of consciousness and respiratory function, to minimize side effects, and to document verbal or nonverbal indications of a patient's pain.

- Equipment required for home pain management includes assessment tools, infusion equipment, and a documentation system.
- Providing home pain management begins with an intake and pain assessment, which is then used to develop a care plan.
- Patient and family education are integral.

Bibliography

Barrier G, Attia J, Mayer MN, Amiel-Tison C, Shnider SM. Measurement of post-operative pain and narcotic administration in infants using a new clinical scoring system. *Intensive Care Med.* 1989;15(suppl1):S37-S39

Beyer JE, Aradine CR. Content validity of an instrument to measure young children's perceptions of the intensity of their pain. *J Pediatr Nurs.* 1986;1:386-395

Borgeat A, Stirnemann HR. Ondansetron is effective to treat spinal or epidural morphine-induced pruritus. *Anesthesiology.* 1999;90:432-436

Davies PR, Warwick P, O'Connor M. Antiemetic efficacy of ondansetron with patient-controlled analgesia. *Anaesthesia.* 1996;51:880-882

Dresner M, Dean S, Lumb A, Bellamy M. High-dose ondansetron regimen vs droperidol for morphine patient-controlled analgesia. *Br J Anaesth.* 1998;81:384-386

Eland JM. The child who is hurting. *Semin Oncol Nurs.* 1985;1:116-122

Gauvain-Piquard A, Rodary C, Rezvani A, Lemerle J. Pain in children aged 2–6 years: a new observational rating scale elaborated in a pediatric oncology unit—preliminary report. *Pain.* 1987;31:177-188

Hester NK. The preoperational child's reaction to immunization. *Nurs Res.* 1979;28:250-255

International Association for the Study of Pain, Subcommittee on Taxonomy. Pain terms: a list with definitions and notes on usage. *Pain.* 1979;6:249

Kyriakides K, Hussain SK, Hobbs GJ. Management of opioid-induced pruritus: a role for 5-HT3 antagonists? *Br J Anaesth.* 1999;82:439-441

McGrath PJ, Johnson G, Goodman JT, Schillinger J. The development and validation of a behavioral pain scale for children: the Children's Hospital of Eastern Ontario Pain Scale. *Pain.* 1984;(suppl2):S24

Miller MG, McCarthy N, O'Boyle CA, Kearney M. Continuous subcutaneous infusion of morphine vs hydromorphone: a controlled trial. *J Pain Symptom Manage.* 1999;18:9-16

Tramer MR, Walder B. Efficacy and adverse effects of prophylactic antiemetics during patient-controlled analgesia therapy: a quantitative systematic review. *Anesth Analg.* 1999;88:1354-1361

Watanabe S, Pereira J, Hanson J, Bruera E. Fentanyl by continuous subcutaneous infusion for the management of cancer pain: a retrospective study. *J Pain Symptom Manage.* 1998;16:323-326

Wong DL, Baker CM. Pain in children: comparison of assessment scales. *Pediatr Nurs.* 1988;14:9-17

Yee JD, Berde CB. Dextroamphetamine or methylphenidate as adjuvants to opioid analgesia for adolescents with cancer. *J Pain Symptom Manage.* 1994;9:122-125

Chapter 16

The Baclofen Pump

Edward Korycka, RN, CRNI, OCN

Introduction

One of the most widely used drugs for the treatment of spasticity is baclofen (Lioresal). When administered orally, baclofen does not cross the blood-brain barrier, easily; it requires adjustment in dosing to achieve an optimal decrease in spasticity. Once the drug crosses the blood-brain barrier, it is distributed equally between the brain and spine. The spasticity is then relieved via the spinal cord. The distribution to the brain causes the side effects of drowsiness, dizziness, confusion, and possibly respiratory depression. An ideal way to overcome these side effects is with the use of an implanted intrathecal pump.

The following are advantages of this type of delivery:

- Baclofen is delivered directly to the site of action for effective reduction of spasticity.
- Drowsiness, the most commonly reported side effect of antispasmodics, becomes less frequent.
- All vital links for motor control are preserved because ablative procedures and chemical neurolysis are unnecessary.
- Flexibility is maintained to take advantage of future treatment options because the therapy, treatment, and administration system are not permanent.
- Dosage can be adjusted precisely to individual needs.
- A consistent cerebrospinal fluid drug level is maintained.

Baclofen Delivery System

The pump is implanted subcutaneously. A catheter is tunneled from the pump to the first lumbar interspace in the lumbar subarachnoid space. The pump is accessed through the skin into a port on top of the medication reservoir. The pump contains a 0.22 μm filter to prevent contaminants from reaching the subarachnoid space.

Patient Management

Patient management when placing the pump includes the following:
1. Patient selection
2. Screening
3. Surgical phase
4. Postoperative care
5. Long-term care

The long-term care of the implanted pump is usually shared by the physician's office and a home care agency. The amount of care depends on the level of monitoring required and the mobility of the patient. The goal of this phase is to maintain safe and effective therapy. The clinician should understand that the following interventions will take place:
1. The pump will be refilled every 4 to 12 weeks (the larger the dose, the sooner the refill).
2. Dose adjustments will be made based on spasticity assessment and functional capacity.
3. Experienced clinicians should handle the refill process to avoid programming and overdose errors.
4. Assess the delivery system using an external programmer to measure accuracy and remaining reservoir output at scheduled intervals.
5. Identify new factors that may interfere with baclofen efficacy.
6. Assess for concomitant drug interactions.
7. Evaluate and help the patient adjust goals.
8. Assess for tolerance as indicated by a return in spasticity. Consider a baclofen holiday and use instead intrathecal morphine sulfate.
9. Provide written and verbal education to the patient and family.

Complications

Signs of overdose include depressed respiration, somnolence, and coma. Overdoses should be treated with physostigmine (1 to 2 mg intravenously over 5 to 10 minutes). Ventilatory support may need to be provided for serious overdoses.

Summary

The use of baclofen for the treatment of spasticity is supported by the following facts:

- Intrathecal baclofen is a successful alternative to oral medications and neural ablative surgical procedures.
- Clinicians have a vital role throughout all phases of this treatment.
- Understanding the basic operation of the pump, the intrathecal actions of baclofen, and the continued parameters for monitoring will ensure a safe course of therapy for the patient.

Bibliography

Albright AL. Intrathecal baclofen in cerebral palsy movement disorders. *J Child Neurol.* 1996; 11(suppl1):S29-S35

Albright AL, Barron WB, Fasick MP, Polinko P, Janosky J. Continuous intrathecal baclofen infusion for spasticity of cerebral origin. *JAMA.* 1993;270:2475-2477

Albright AL, Cervi A, Singletary J. Intrathecal baclofen for spasticity in cerebral palsy. *JAMA.* 1991;265:1418-1422

Coffe Y Jr, Cahill D, Steers W, et al. Intrathecal baclofen for intractable spasticity of spinal origin: results of a long-term multicenter study. *J Neurosurg.* 1993;78:226-232

Gianino JM, York MM, Paice JA. *Intrathecal Drug Therapy for Spasticity and Pain: Practical Patient Management.* New York, NY: Springer; 1996

Gianino JM, York MM, Paice JA, Shott S. Quality of life: effect of reduced spasticity from intrathecal baclofen. *J Neurosci Nurs.* 1998;30:47-54

Lazorthes Y, Sallerin-Caute B, Verdie JC, Bastide R, Carillo JP. Chronic intrathecal baclofen administration for control of severe spasticity. *J Neurosurg.* 1990;72:393-402

Middel B, Kuipers-Upmeijer H, Bouma J, et al. Effect of intrathecal baclofen delivered by an implanted programmable pump on health related quality of life in patients with severe spasticity. *J Neurol Neurosurg Psychiatry.* 1997;63:204-209

Ochs G, Struppler A, Meyerson BA, et al. Intrathecal baclofen for long-term treatment of spasticity: a multi-centre study. *J Neurol Neurosurg Psychiatry.* 1989;52:933-939

Penn Rd, Savoy SM, Corcos D, et al. Intrathecal baclofen for severe spinal spasticity. *N Engl J Med.* 1989;320:1517-1521

Chapter 17

Home Mechanical Ventilators and Equipment

Sally L. Davidson Ward, MD; Thomas Keens, MD

Introduction

Infants and children may require chronic ventilatory support because of the failure of neurologic ventilation control, ventilatory muscle weakness or fatigue, or increased respiratory loads. Once the decision has been made to institute long-term mechanical ventilation in an infant or child with a stable or progressive disorder of the respiratory system, the caretakers should consider the impact of a prolonged hospitalization or institutionalization on the life of the child and family. Chronic ventilatory support in the home is a safe and relatively inexpensive alternative for many patients that optimizes overall health, rehabilitative potential, psychosocial development, and family well-being. Successful home mechanical ventilation requires the selection of appropriate home care equipment.

Modalities of Providing Chronic Ventilatory Support in the Home

Because the goals of ventilator therapy for children with chronic respiratory failure in the home are different than for children with acute respiratory failure in hospitals, the ideal ventilators for home use are also different. Infants and children can be ventilated at home using one of the following five basic types of assisted ventilation: portable positive-pressure ventilation via tracheostomy, noninvasive positive-pressure ventilation, negative-pressure chest shell (cuirass) ventilation, other negative-pressure ventilation (tank, Port-a-Lung, and Pulmo-Wrap), and diaphragm pacing.

▶ Portable Positive-Pressure Ventilation via Tracheostomy

A portable positive-pressure ventilator is the most common method of providing assisted ventilation for infants and children in the home (Table 17-1). Commercially available home electronic positive-pressure ventilators are relatively portable, thus maximizing mobility. Positive-pressure ventilators powered by compressed air are considerably less portable, and not desirable for home use.

177

TABLE 17-1. Home Respiratory Equipment for the Child Assisted by a Ventilator

---

- Electronic portable positive-pressure ventilator with
  - ~ Two cascades and bracket for cascades
  - ~ One cover and jar assembly
  - ~ Two circuits (intermittent mandatory ventilation and oxygen)
  - ~ Flex tubing
  - ~ Infant or pediatric exhalation manifold
  - ~ Automobile battery adaptor for car use
- Backup ventilator
  - ~ Essential for patients living long distances from medical and technical support
- Car battery (80 A) with case and cables for operation of the ventilator and battery charger
- E-cylinder of oxygen with stand and regulator for emergency use
  - ~ Supplemental oxygen system, if necessary
- Aerosol delivery system with
  - ~ Aerosol set-ups
  - ~ Draeger bags
  - ~ Two tracheostomy adapters
  - ~ Two 22/15 cm connector/adapters
- Portable suction machine with battery pack, connecting tubing, appropriate-sized tracheal suction catheters, and tonsil fine-tip catheters
- Child-size resuscitation bag with appropriate-size mask and tracheostomy adaptor
- Infant apnea/bradycardia monitor with portable battery pack, belt, and electrodes

---

Portable positive-pressure ventilators are not as powerful, technologically sophisticated, or versatile as larger hospital ventilators. Most commercially available home positive-pressure ventilators are volume-preset ventilators without the capability of providing continuous flow of inspired gas. Thus, positive end-expiratory pressure (PEEP) and pressure-support ventilation cannot be achieved. In traditional hospital practice, a set delivered tidal volume of 8 to 10 mL/kg is used for mechanical-assisted ventilation in infants, children, and adults. However, because children assisted by a ventilator generally have uncuffed tracheostomies, a portion of the ventilator-delivered breath escapes in the leak around the tracheostomy. In some older children and adolescents, this leak is relatively constant and a higher tidal volume setting can be used to compensate for the leak and achieve adequate ventilation at home. This tidal volume setting must be derived empirically because there is no way to predict the portion of a ventilator-delivered breath that escapes through the leak. In infants and smaller children, the tracheostomy leak is relatively large and variable, and it rarely can be compensated for by a single tidal volume setting. In this situation, using the ventilator in a pressure-plateau mode can compensate for the tracheostomy leak.

Some commercially available portable positive-pressure ventilators have a high-pressure limit adjustment that is separate from the high-pressure alarm. The pressure limit is adjusted down to the desired peak inspiratory pressure (PIP). A large tidal volume setting then is set. The ventilator will function similar to a time-cycle, pressure-limited ventilator. When the pressure limit is reached, the remainder of the ventilator tidal volume will be delivered to the room, rather than to the patient. If there is a large tracheostomy leak one moment, a large portion of the tidal volume will be delivered through the ventilator, but the lungs will be inflated to the desired PIP. If there is a small tracheostomy leak the next moment, a lesser portion of the tidal volume will be delivered through the ventilator, but the lungs will still be inflated to the desired PIP, and the pressure pop-off valve maintains the pressure at this level until the end of the breath (pressure plateau). In pressure-limited ventilation, the breath is terminated once the pressure limit is achieved. The pressure plateau technique is very successful in home ventilation of infants and small children. It also is useful in older children or adolescents who have large or variable tracheostomy leaks.

Home positive-pressure ventilators have the advantage of being relatively portable...

Some home ventilators are capable of providing continuous flow of inspired gas, which permits the delivery of PEEP and pressure-support ventilation. These ventilators are especially useful in infants and children who cannot be weaned from PEEP, and who have such high resting respiratory rates that they exceed the capabilities of volume-preset ventilators without continuous flow. Because uncuffed tracheostomies with relatively large leaks are used, a modified pressure-plateau mode of ventilation may need to be used despite the availability of continuous flow.

Home positive-pressure ventilators have the advantage of being relatively portable, having the capability for battery operation, being easy to use, and not hindering access to the patient. Positive-pressure ventilation is the method of choice for providing chronic ventilatory support for most children.

▶ Noninvasive Positive-Pressure Ventilation

Positive-pressure ventilation via nasal mask can be used in some infants and children who require nocturnal ventilatory support only. It is inappropriate for children requiring full-time ventilation because it interferes with a normal lifestyle in active, awake patients. The most common technique for noninvasive ventilation is bi-level positive airway pressure (BIPAP). The BIPAP device delivers a continuous flow of gas. Inspiratory and expiratory positive airway pressures can be selected to provide adequate minute ventilation and overcome upper airway obstruction. Patients with adequate spontaneous respiratory rates may be ventilated in the spontaneous mode (assists spontaneous breaths only) or in the spontaneous/timed mode (assists spontaneous breaths with a backup rate). Patients with inadequate ventilatory effort can be ventilated in the timed mode (control mode; set rate and inspiratory duration).

The patient interface can be a nasal mask, nasal pillows, or a full-face mask. The choice of interface depends on patient preference and anatomy. The device is not battery operated.

▶ Negative-Pressure Chest Shell (Cuirass) Ventilation

The chest shell ventilator uses a dome-shaped shell that is fitted over the anterior chest and upper abdomen. A negative pressure is generated inside the chest shell, which expands the chest. The ventilator rate and the negative pressure can be selected. In a properly fitted chest shell, the higher the negative pressure, the higher the tidal volume. This technique can provide effective ventilation in some older children and adolescents without a tracheostomy. However, because the upper airway anatomy of the infant and young child is different from that of the adult or older child, airway occlusion can occur when breaths are generated by a negative-pressure ventilator during sleep. Sometimes, upper airway obstruction can be improved using lower negative-inspiratory pressures and/or longer inspiratory times. Similarly, increasing upper airway caliber by adenotonsillectomy may decrease upper airway obstruction and facilitate negative-pressure ventilation. Chest wall deformities, such as severe scoliosis, restrict chest wall movement and render negative-pressure ventilation ineffective.

Negative-pressure chest shell ventilators are less powerful and less versatile than portable positive-pressure ventilators. Thus, they are not useful in children who require higher ventilator rates, tidal volumes, or distending pressures, as is the case with many cardiorespiratory disorders. For negative-pressure chest shell ventilators to provide adequate ventilation, the chest shell must be fitted closely to the chest to avoid large leaks that dissipate the negative pressure and cause little chest expansion to occur. Currently, the smallest commercially available chest shell fits children of approximately 4 years of age. The chest shell needs to be changed and refitted as the child grows. This technique is useful only for children whose need for ventilatory support is limited to when they are asleep.

Negative-pressure chest shell ventilators are not as portable as electronic positive-pressure ventilators and they are not battery operated. Some patients have difficulty sleeping in a chest shell. Irritation can occur when the chest shell rubs on the skin. However, this usually can be avoided by having the child sleep with a T-shirt under the chest shell and by using cornstarch on the skin. Although not useful for infants or most small children, this technique may be ideal for some older children with neuromuscular disorders and less rigorous ventilator requirements in whom a tracheostomy may be avoided.

▶ Other Negative-Pressure Ventilators (Tank, Port-a-Lung, and Pulmo-Wrap)

The negative-pressure (tank) ventilator, also known as an iron lung, places the child in a metal cylinder, or tank, below the neck. A more portable tank ventilator is made of fiberglass (Port-a-Lung). A negative-pressure wrap (Pulmo-Wrap) ventilator uses a jumpsuit worn by the patient with a metal cage supporting the suit away from the patient. These devices generate a negative pressure around the chest and abdomen that expands the lungs. Ventilator rate and negative pressure can be controlled. Tidal volume is proportional to the negative pressure generated. This technique can provide effective ventilation in some older children or adolescents without a tracheostomy. Infants and young children may develop airway occlusion during sleep and may not be candidates for this technique.

▶ Diaphragm Pacing

Diaphragm pacing generates breathing using the child's own diaphragm as the respiratory pump. The technique involves surgical implantation of electrodes around the phrenic nerves; the electrodes are connected to receivers implanted subcutaneously. The phrenic nerves are electrically stimulated transcutaneously from an external power source (power is transmitted in a manner similar to radio transmission). Pacer rate and electrical current can be controlled, which determine the respiratory frequency and size of each breath. Tidal volume is proportional to the electrical current used in each breath. Effective ventilation can be generated using simultaneous bilateral diaphragm pacing in infants, children, and adults if the phrenic nerves and diaphragms are functional. Because phrenic nerve stimulation causes diaphragmatic contraction, diaphragm pacing is contraindicated in patients with primary phrenic nerve damage or primary diaphragm myopathy. This technique has been successful in patients with central hypoventilation syndromes and with high spinal cord injury. It is particularly useful in providing ventilatory support to ambulatory children during wakefulness.

Some children do not require a tracheostomy with diaphragm pacing. Other patients require a tracheostomy to prevent upper airway occlusion during sleep. Diaphragm pacing has the advantage of being small, light, and easily portable, since it is battery operated. It may be beneficial to select groups of children with central hypoventilation syndromes or high cervical spinal cord injury.

Modes of Ventilation

Positive-pressure ventilators have a variety of modes that can be used to provide assisted ventilation. Different types of patients benefit from different modes. Intermittent mandatory ventilation (IMV), synchronized IMV (SIMV), and PEEP are popular techniques for hospital ventilators used in the management of acute respiratory failure. Older home ventilators did not deliver these modes of ventilation because a continuous flow of gas was not available. Newer portable home ventilators are capable of generating a continuous gas flow using blowers. Children requiring chronic assisted ventilation, who are unable to be weaned from PEEP or unable to be switched from IMV/SIMV to a control or assist mode prior to discharge home, can benefit from home ventilators capable of delivering continuous gas flow.

Most infants and young children can be ventilated in a control ventilator mode. When continuous-flow ventilators are not used, the ventilator circuit should be designed so that the child can take spontaneous breaths through as little dead space as possible. This allows the child to take extra breaths when desired and provides an ability for spontaneous breathing in the event of ventilator malfunction.

Ventilator Circuits

A circuit is required to deliver air from a positive-pressure ventilator to the patient. Gas from the ventilator passes through a heated humidification system. Ventilator gas should be humidified for infants and children at least part of the time. Humidification is impractical when children travel outside the home, but can be used more easily during sleep at night. For most infants and young children, humidification during sleep is desirable. The desired temperature range is 26°C to 28°C (80°F to 85°F). Condenser humidifiers are not as effective as heated humidifiers, but can be used for travel or for short periods of time. An in-line thermometer is placed in the circuit to monitor humidifier temperature. For ventilators without continuous flow, dead space tubing should be minimized because excessive dead space raises PCO_2. Inspired gas may also be warmed and humidified for noninvasive positive-pressure ventilation.

Two circuits generally are provided for home care and are changed three times per week. The circuits (tubing, valve, and cascade) should be cleaned with mild soap and water when not in use, then rinsed in a disinfectant (such as 10% alkyl dimethylbenzol ammonium chloride) and dried.

Power Sources for Ventilators

Portable positive-pressure ventilators used in the home are electrically powered. These ventilators should have an internal battery capable of operating for at least 1 hour. External batteries should be provided for emergency use, portability, or for times when electrical power is not immediately available. Ideally, a fully charged deep-cycle external battery could power the ventilator for 6 to 8 hours. While traveling, an adapter for an automobile battery is also important.

Noninvasive positive-pressure ventilators and negative-pressure ventilators have no internal battery and cannot run on direct current from an external battery. Because of this, their use in patients who are completely dependent on a ventilator can be argued against, especially if electrical power service is interrupted frequently. Diaphragm pacers are powered by batteries only.

Monitoring Systems

All positive-pressure ventilators should have a low-pressure, or disconnect, alarm that sounds in the event that a minimally acceptable pressure level is not being achieved. Most portable positive-pressure ventilators also have alarms for high pressure, incorrect timing, and power failure. Patients who are completely apneic without ventilator support may also benefit from having a chest wall impedance apnea and bradycardia monitor. Tracheostomy tubes less than 6 mm internal diameter may have sufficient resistance to airflow so that a low-pressure alarm will not sound in the event of accidental decannulation. Thus, infants and small children with these tracheostomies should also use transthoracic impedance apnea monitors.

Home Respiratory Equipment Vendor

All mechanical equipment is subject to breakage and malfunction. Unfortunately, ventilators are no exception to this rule. When home respiratory equipment vendors make frequent home visits to perform preventive maintenance and check on ventilator function, emergency calls due to ventilator malfunction are reduced. It is recommended that home respiratory equipment vendors make home visits monthly. On each visit, positive-pressure ventilators should have filters checked. Tidal volume, rate, oxygen concentration, pressures, and alarms should be calibrated and their function checked. Overall function of the ventilator also should be assessed.

Oxygen Delivery

Supplemental oxygen can be introduced to the intake port of positive-pressure ventilators. For patients requiring continuous supplemental oxygen, a liquid oxygen system with a portable unit enhances mobility. Whether they require supplemental oxygen chronically, all children dependent on a ventilator should be provided with an E-cylinder of oxygen with regulator and stand, and a reinflatable bag and mask in the event of emergencies.

Summary

The following are important points to remember when considering home mechanical ventilation equipment:

- Chronic ventilatory support in the home is a safe alternative to hospital care that provides many benefits to patients and families.
- There are five basic types of assisted ventilation — portable positive-pressure ventilation via tracheostomy, noninvasive positive-pressure ventilation, negative-pressure chest shell (cuirass) ventilation, other negative-pressure ventilation (tank, Port-a-Lung, and Pulmo-Wrap), and diaphragm pacing.
- A ventilator circuit consisting of tubing, a valve, and a cascade is required to deliver air from a positive-pressure ventilator to the patient. Two circuits usually are provided for home care and are changed three times per week.
- Portable positive-pressure ventilators are electrically powered. Batteries also can be used in an emergency or for portability.
- Noninvasive positive-pressure ventilators and negative-pressure ventilators are electrically powered. They do not have internal batteries and cannot run on external batteries. This precludes their use for patients who are completely dependent on a ventilator.
- Diaphragm pacers operate on batteries only.
- All positive-pressure ventilators should have a low-pressure or disconnect alarm.
- Equipment vendors should make frequent home visits to provide routine maintenance of ventilator equipment.
- All children dependent on a ventilator should be provided with an extra supply of oxygen.

Bibliography

Gilgoff IS, Peng RC, Keens TG. Hypoventilation and apnea in children during mechanically assisted ventilation. *Chest.* 1992;101:1500-1506

Hartmann H, Samuels MP, Noyes JP, Southall DP. Negative extrathoracic pressure ventilation in infants and young children with central hypoventilation syndrome. *Pediatr Pulmonol.* 1997;23: 155-157

Hillberg RE, Johnson DC. Noninvasive ventilation. *N Engl J Med.* 1997;337:1746-1752

Make BJ, Hill NS, Goldberg AI, et al. Mechanical ventilation beyond the intensive care unit. Report of a consensus conference of the American College of Chest Physicians. *Chest.* 1998;113(5suppl):289S-344S

Splaingard ML, Frates RC Jr, Jefferson LS, Rosen CL, Harrison GM. Home negative pressure ventilation: report of 20 years of experience in patients with neuromuscular disease. *Arch Phys Med Rehabil.* 1985;66:239-242

Weese-Mayer DE, Hunt CE, Brouillette RT, Silvestri JM. Diaphragm pacing in infants and children. *J Pediatr.* 1992;120:1-8

Chapter 18

Home Oxygen Equipment and Aerosol Therapy

Mark O'Gwynn, RRT, MPH

Introduction

Current advances in the technology available to home care providers have allowed for the safe and effective discharge of many pediatric patients. In the past, extensive hospital stays, coupled with high-technology support, was necessary for children to fully recover. Managed care can be partially credited with the emphasis on the economy associated with caring for patients at home. The National Association for Home Care cites impressive comparative figures between long-term institutional care and home care. The average monthly cost for an infant dependent on oxygen in the hospital averages $12,090, compared to $5,250 for services provided in the home.

Oxygen therapy is one of the most often-used services in home care for the pediatric patient. Some of the more common diagnoses that require home oxygen services are bronchopulmonary dysplasia, cystic fibrosis, asthma, bronchiectasis, and various spinal cord injuries. As with most home therapy, benefits include quality of life issues centering around the holistic care of the patient. With respect to pediatrics, additional benefits include faster weight gain and improvement in cognitive function and feeding patterns. It also has been proposed that home therapy (in particular, oxygen) may result in improved schoolwork and attendance in patients with cystic fibrosis.

Goals of Oxygen Therapy

While the frequency and duration of therapy varies with pathology, the common goal of home oxygen services is to relieve hypoxemia. Indications for therapy, as established by the American Academy of Pediatrics, for infants more than 28 days old are documented hypoxemia with $PaO_2 \leq 55$ torr or oxygen saturations less than or equal to 88% on room air. In addition, the patient should be medically stable, feeding appropriately, and growing well.

Once the decision has been made to discharge the patient home with
oxygen, several key factors should be considered. Because oxygen is considered a medication, an objective assessment of the patient's pulmonary status
should be completed to determine the correct liter flow. Oxygen saturation
should be monitored while the infant is clothed appropriate to the home
environment. Also, a compatible delivery device to that which is used in the
hospital should be used. For most infants, a liter flow of 0.25 to 0.50 L per
minute (LPM) usually is adequate to provide desirable saturation values.
However, oxygen therapy should be titrated using pulse oximetry to achieve
the optimum benefit. Some infants may require oxygen therapy while sleeping or eating, so frequency and duration of oxygen therapy also should be
prescribed consistent with the need for therapy.

Oxygen conservation devices, which stop the flow of oxygen during
exhalation, can extend the duration of oxygen delivery from small tanks of
compressed or liquid oxygen. Some of these devices also contain an apnea
alarm, designed to sound if the device does not sense an inspiratory effort
after a predetermined interval. Such an alarm can be useful to detect inadvertent displacement of a nasal cannula or other delivery device, but experience with such devices in pediatric patients is extremely limited.

Delivery Devices

Oxygen delivery devices are divided into two categories: high-flow devices
and low-flow devices. High-flow devices deliver oxygen flow rates that are
high enough to meet the patient's entire inspiratory demands. Examples of
high-flow devices are incubators and oxygen hoods. These devices are used
primarily in the institutional setting during the acute treatment phase. The
flow and pressure demands of this classification of equipment make them
difficult to replicate in the home setting.

Oxyhoods or oxygen tents rarely are used in the home setting. They
limit mobility and visibility of the patient, and carbon dioxide retention can
occur if flow rates through them are inadequate. An inverted bed tent has
been said to avoid these complications, but like the hood or tent, it can be
used only when the child is in bed. Children with tracheostomies receive
supplemental oxygen by tracheostomy collar or T-piece. Transtracheal oxygen
can be administered by a special "micro-tracheostomy" (a 9F catheter), placed

percutaneously into the trachea in older children with bronchopulmonary dysplasia who do not require an artificial airway. This method of oxygen administration is associated with fewer inadvertent displacements of the oxygen source and a lower required oxygen flow rate compared with nasal cannula administration. Thus, transtracheal oxygen therapy is considered an oxygen conservation device because it can substantially increase the duration of gas delivery by portable oxygen sources and, therefore, the time a patient can be away from the home source of oxygen. The catheter requires frequent changing and intermittent cleaning, but it can be reused for up to several months. This interface should be reserved for use in children who require 24 hours per day of supplemental oxygen and who have caregivers motivated to learn the technique.

Low-flow devices are the choice for oxygen delivery in home care. They supply flow rates that are lower than the patient's inspiratory demands. Examples include nasal cannulas, partial, and non–re-breather masks. The most common low-flow device in pediatric home care is the nasal cannula (Figure 18-1). The cannula is constructed from two fused pieces of flexible tubing that taper into nasal prongs that deliver flow into the nares. It is held in place by wrapping a portion of tubing around and behind the patient's ear. Special cannulas are available for all ages of pediatric and neonatal patients. The nasal cannula can be secured to the face using tape or transparent occlusive dressings.

FIGURE 18-1. Infant and Pediatric Nasal Cannula

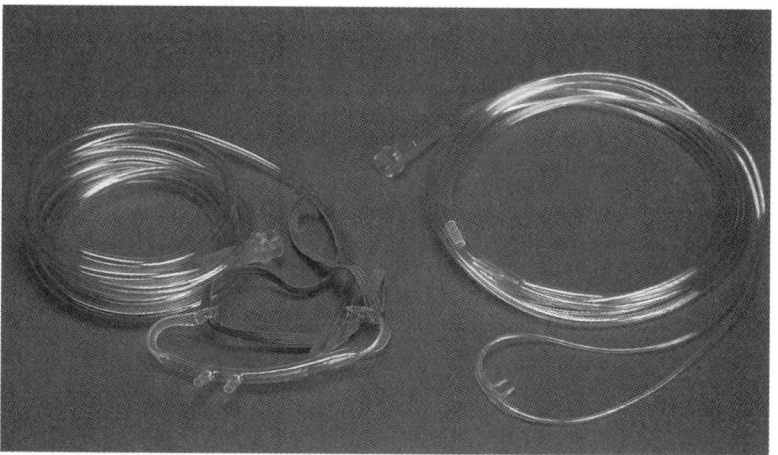

The original patient interface through which oxygen was administered to infants with bronchopulmonary dysplasia at home was a feeding tube placed in the nasopharynx. This method of oxygen administration minimizes inadvertent displacement of the catheter, but it is associated with several complications, including nasopharyngeal irritation, sinusitis, and blockage of the tube by nasal secretions. The nasal cannula is the most common type of patient interface for delivery of supplemental oxygen. It allows for continuous oxygen delivery without sacrificing patient mobility, and oxygen can be administered during feedings. The cannula can be displaced easily, however, and it is also associated with nasal irritation and epistaxis. Nasal congestion or obstruction can hamper oxygen delivery, and infants who experienced negative facial stimulation in the newborn nursery may not tolerate wearing the cannula. Inadvertent displacement of the cannula can be reduced by taping it to the cheeks or to Duoderm or Tegaderm patches affixed to the cheeks. Nasal cannulas used continuously should be changed weekly.

Oxygen Systems

There are three classifications of oxygen systems that are used for home care: oxygen concentrators, compressed gas systems, and liquid oxygen systems. Each offers distinct advantages based on individual need and environment. Factors such as cost, efficiency, portability, and ease of operation should be considered when choosing a system. In infants, make certain that the system of choice will make it easy for the patient to be nurtured and does not inhibit bonding. A reputable medical equipment provider should be consulted to determine which systems are available and assist in determining patient need.

▶ Oxygen Concentrator

The oxygen concentrator is an electrically powered, compact unit that extracts inert gases from room air and concentrates the oxygen until therapeutic ranges (usually 85% to 90%) are attained. It is about the size of a small end table and weighs from 30 to 50 pounds. Concentrators are best suited to liter flows that are less than 6 LPM. The concentration of oxygen starts to decline when higher liter flows are used. The distinct advantage of this system is that it produces its own oxygen and therefore does not require routine refills. This unit is efficient and requires minimal maintenance.

There are several disadvantages of concentrators related to the pediatric population that warrant discussion. Oxygen concentrators are not very portable and restrict the movement of the infant and family. Because the unit is electrically powered, an increase in the family utility use will be noted. Oxygen delivery is dependent on an electric power supply; therefore, the concentrator will not work if the house loses electric power. Patients should always have access to a compressed oxygen source in case of an emergency.

▶ Compressed Oxygen

Compressed medical gases are also employed to provide oxygen in the home. These are the familiar green cylinders that often are used in the hospital setting. Compressed gas cylinders are an excellent backup source to an electrically powered system or where minimal oxygen use is prescribed. There is virtually no chance of product loss as long as the cylinder remains intact. However, this system is cumbersome and offers little opportunity for the patient and family to venture outside the home.

Oxygen stored in tanks of compressed gas can be used for patients who require continuous supplemental oxygen therapy, and they are ideal for infants and children who require only intermittent therapy. They can be sealed so that oxygen can be stored for extended periods without leaking or evaporating. Tanks come in a variety of sizes to facilitate mobility. Tanks of compressed oxygen require the use of a pediatric flowmeter so that liter flow can be adjusted in small increments. Table 18-1 calculates the amount of oxygen remaining in oxygen cylinders based on the liter flow and tank pressure.

▶ Liquid Oxygen

Liquid oxygen is currently the most popular oxygen delivery system for the pediatric population. This system includes a stationary, or base, unit and a small portable unit that can be worn around the shoulder. The design of this unit is based on the thermos. The internal tank, which holds the liquid oxygen, is separated by insulation that prohibits the liquid product from warming (which activates the liquid-to-gas conversion process). A system of coils and one-way valves allows the liquid oxygen to progress through the unit and warm, thus creating oxygen in gas form. The flow is controlled by

TABLE 18-1. Cylinder Size, Liter Flow, and Time

H-TANK CHART
CALCULATED ON CONTINUOUS USAGE

LITER FLOW	200	400	600	800	1000	1200	1400	1600	1800	2000	2200
						PSI					
1	10 HRS 24 MIN	20 HRS 54 MIN	1 DAY 7 HRS 12 MIN	1 DAY 16 HRS 48 MIN	2 DAYS 2 HRS 26 MIN	2 DAYS 8 HRS	3 DAYS 1 HR 12 MIN	3 DAYS 11 HRS 30 MIN	3 DAYS 21 HRS	4 DAYS 7 HRS	4 DAYS 16 HRS
2	5 HRS 12 MIN	10 HRS 24 MIN	15 HRS 52 MIN	20 HRS 54 MIN	1 DAY 2 HRS	1 DAY 7 HRS	1 DAY 12 HRS	1 DAY 16 HRS 48 MIN	1 DAY 21 HRS	2 DAYS 3 HRS	2 DAYS 7 HRS
3	3 HRS 24 MIN	6 HRS 54 MIN	10 HRS 24 MIN	13 HRS 54 MIN	17 HRS 24 MIN	20 HRS 54 MIN	1 DAY 9 HRS 36 MIN	1 DAY 3 HRS	1 DAY 7 HRS	1 DAY 9 HRS	1 DAY 12 HRS
4	2 HRS 36 MIN	5 HRS 12 MIN	7 HRS 48 MIN	10 HRS 24 MIN	13 HRS	15 HRS 16 MIN	18 HRS 18 MIN	20 HRS 54 MIN	23 HRS 30 MIN	1 DAY 2 HRS	1 DAY 4 HRS
5	2 HRS	4 HRS 6 MIN	6 HRS 12 MIN	8 HRS 18 MIN	10 HRS 24 MIN	12 HRS 30 MIN	14 HRS 36 MIN	16 HRS 42 MIN	18 HRS 48 MIN	20 HRS 54 MIN	23 HRS
6	1 HR 42 MIN	3 HRS 24 MIN	5 HRS 12 MIN	6 HRS 54 MIN	8 HRS 42 MIN	10 HRS 24 MIN	12 HRS 12 MIN	13 HRS 54 MIN	15 HRS 42 MIN	17 HRS 24 MIN	19 HRS
7	1 HR 24 MIN	2 HRS 54 MIN	4 HRS 24 MIN	5 HRS 54 MIN	7 HRS 24 MIN	8 HRS 54 MIN	10 HRS 24 MIN	11 HRS 54 MIN	13 HRS 24 MIN	14 HRS 54 MIN	16 HRS 24 MIN
8	1 HR 18 MIN	2 HRS 36 MIN	3 HRS 54 MIN	5 HRS 12 MIN	6 HRS 30 MIN	7 HRS 48 MIN	9 HRS 6 MIN	10 HRS 24 MIN	11 HRS 42 MIN	13 HRS	14 HRS 24 MIN

TABLE 18-1. Cylinder Size, Liter Flow, and Time, continued

E-TANK CHART
CALCULATED ON CONTINUOUS USAGE

LITER FLOW	PSI 200	400	600	800	1000	1200	1400	1600	1800	2000	2200
1	54 MIN	1 HR 48 MIN	2 HRS 48 MIN	3 HRS 42 MIN	4 HRS 36 MIN	5 HRS 36 MIN	6 HRS 30 MIN	7 HRS 24 MIN	8 HRS 24 MIN	9 HRS 18 MIN	10 HRS 12 MIN
2	24 MIN	54 MIN	1 HR 24 MIN	1 HRS 48 MIN	2 HRS 18 MIN	2 HRS 48 MIN	3 HRS 12 MIN	3 HRS 42 MIN	4 HRS 12 MIN	4 HRS 36 MIN	5 HRS 6 MIN
3	18 MIN	36 MIN	54 MIN	1 HR 12 MIN	1 HR 30 MIN	1 HR 48 MIN	2 HRS 6 MIN	2 HRS 24 MIN	2 HRS 48 MIN	3 HRS 6 MIN	3 HRS 24 MIN
4	12 MIN	24 MIN	42 MIN	54 MIN	1 HR 6 MIN	1 HR 24 MIN	1 HR 36 MIN	1 HR 48 MIN	2 HRS 36 MIN	2 HRS 18 MIN	2 HRS 30 MIN
5	10 MIN	21 MIN	30 MIN	42 MIN	54 MIN	1 HR 6 MIN	1 HR 18 MIN	1 HR 24 MIN	1 HR 36 MIN	1 HR 48 MIN	2 HRS
6	9 MIN	18 MIN	27 MIN	36 MIN	45 MIN	54 MIN	1 HR	1 HR 12 MIN	1 HR 24 MIN	1 HR 30 MIN	1 HR 42 MIN
7	7 MIN	15 MIN	21 MIN	30 MIN	42 MIN	48 MIN	54 MIN	1 HR	1 HR 12 MIN	1 HR 18 MIN	1 HR 24 MIN
8	6 MIN	13 MIN	3 HRS 54 MIN	27 MIN	36 MIN	42 MIN	48 MIN	54 MIN	1 HR	1 HR 6 MIN	1 HR 12 MIN

a network of reducing valves and restrictors. Most brands of liquid oxygen systems have the capability to use regulators that will provide the low flow necessary for pediatric therapy.

This design allows the portable unit to be filled from the base system. When full, the portable unit weighs less than 10 pounds and is transported easily. When filled to capacity, the portable unit will last approximately 6 hours depending on the prescribed flow rate. The stationary unit can last from 5 to 7 days and must be refilled on a regular basis.

This system requires that the family be motivated and responsible during the course of therapy. While not difficult, using this type of unit does require a minimum level of dexterity on the part of the caregiver. Care should be given to fill the portable only when needed because there is a certain level of evaporation that occurs routinely. The family must commit to being accessible to the medical equipment provider for scheduled service and fills.

Liquid oxygen systems are not appropriate for the patient who requires supplemental oxygen only intermittently, as the liquid oxygen will evaporate from the base refrigeration unit and cannot be stored for prolonged periods. The flowmeter, which is an integral component of the portable unit, represents another limitation of the liquid oxygen system because it is not calibrated for flows below 0.25 LPM.

Complications

Certain complications are inherent with the provision of oxygen therapy. These are best discussed in an exhaustive review of pediatric and neonatal care. However, in the home setting, most complications are minor and can be reduced or eliminated with proper family education and support. These are primarily related to safety, environmental, and psychosocial issues. Routine medical supervision throughout the course of therapy should be encouraged with the caregiver or support network.

Aerosol Therapy

The pediatric patient at home can be treated with a number of different aerosol generators. The type of equipment used is based on the goals of therapy and special needs of the patient. The primary diagnoses associated with aerosol therapy are asthma, cystic fibrosis, and chronic lung disease.

▶ Compressor Nebulizers

Compressor nebulizers are small, portable flow generators used to deliver aerosolized medications to the airway. These units come in a variety of brands and styles. The concept of operation uses Bernoulli's principle to create the aerosol. The prescribed medication is placed in a chamber and a regulated flow of air or oxygen is introduced to the mixture. This flow breaks the medication particles into a size that can be inhaled by the patient.

Several manufacturers offer systems with external battery capability, custom colors, and video instruction tapes. The type of unit prescribed to the patient should be based on individual need, special circumstances, and reimbursement.

▶ Large-Volume Compressors

Children with tracheostomies have special needs with respect to home medical equipment. Because an artificial airway is present, a device that generates a high volume of aerosol is needed to humidify the airway and aid in the clearance of secretions. This is accomplished through the use of a unit that combines a large-volume nebulizer and a high-output compressor. If needed, oxygen may be added via the outlet port of the nebulizer. This system will provide flows of up to 50 psi with variable adjustment.

Suction Equipment

Suction equipment must be provided to the pediatric patient who is unable to clear secretions via the normal cough response. The need to suction is due to the presence of an artificial airway or a condition that has damaged or destroyed the normal cough reflex. Home suction equipment is manufactured to be portable and simple to use. Most units have primary and secondary systems for power. It is recommended that two machines be placed in the home of each pediatric patient in the event that one fails. At least one of these units should have the capacity to operate from an external battery source. This alternate power source should ensure that adequate pressure and time requirements are present in the event of an emergency.

The physician, on a regular basis, should assess the continued need for home medical equipment. This can be accomplished by regular office visits or in conjunction with the local home care provider. At a minimum, routine saturation checks and equipment maintenance should be completed. A multidisciplinary and cooperative approach to the care of the infant at home will ensure that all goals are met.

Summary

There are various important aspects of home oxygen therapy, including the following:

- Oxygen therapy is one of the most used services for pediatric patients at home. Common conditions treated include bronchopulmonary dysplasia, cystic fibrosis, and asthma.
- Oxygen is considered a medication, so assessment of the patient's pulmonary status should be completed to determine the correct liter flow.
- Oxygen is delivered by high-flow devices, such as incubators and oxygen hoods, or low-flow devices, such as nasal cannulas and masks.
- Three types of home oxygen delivery systems are oxygen concentrators, compressed gas systems, and liquid oxygen systems. The system used depends on the individual needs and environment of the patient.
- The complications of oxygen therapy are primarily related to safety, environment, and psychosocial issues and are usually minor.

Bibliography

Burstein L. Home care. In: Bernhardt S, Cazervinske J, eds. *Perinatal and Pediatric Respiratory Care.* Philadelphia, PA: W. B. Saunders; 1995:1-37

Cairo JM, Pilbeam SP. *Mosby's Respiratory Care Equipment.* 6th ed. St Louis, MO: Mosby; 1999

Turner J, McDonald G, Larter N. *Handbook of Adult and Pediatric Respiratory Home Care.* St Louis, MO: Mosby-Year Book; 1994

Chapter 19

Diagnostic Testing in the Home: pH Probes, Sleep Studies

Mark O'Gwynn, RRT, MPH

Introduction

Accurate in-home diagnostic testing is necessary to keep pace with the early discharge of the infant who is dependent on technology. The most common diagnostic procedures used in home care are apnea/ bradycardia monitoring, ambulatory esophageal pH testing, and multichannel sleep testing.

Each of these evaluations shares the common goal of recognizing disordered breathing. The presence of life-threatening events such as sudden infant death syndrome (SIDS) underscores the need for accurate diagnostic and preventive procedures. Sudden infant death syndrome still remains the leading cause of death in infants between 1 week and 1 year of age. It is only through the early recognition of key risk factors and appropriate clinical intervention that the incidence of SIDS can be decreased.

Apnea/Bradycardia Monitoring

The past decade has seen a virtual explosion in the development of highly sensitive technology to aid in the detection of pediatric apnea. All apnea/bradycardia monitoring devices share the common goal of alerting the caregiver when the infant's respiratory efforts fall below a prescribed standard.

Clinical indications for home apnea monitoring include an event that results in prolonged apnea of 20 seconds or greater, family history of SIDS, or a pathology related to immaturity (such as apnea of prematurity or bronchopulmonary dysplasia) that may cause apnea. The typical period of therapy ranges from 3 to 10 months, at which time the monitor can be discontinued safely.

Apnea devices measure heart rate and respiratory effort by using a technology known as impedance pneumography. Small electrodes are placed on the infant's thorax and held in place with a belt. These electrodes measure differences in the chest rise and interpret these movements as respiration. When normal chest excursion fails to occur, as would be the case

197

during a central apneic event, the device is alerted and an alarm sounds. It should be stressed that this technology simply acts to indicate the occurrence of an event. Parents of high-risk infants who require this type of monitoring should be properly trained in appropriate emergency medical procedures (eg, cardiopulmonary resuscitation, stimulation, etc) prior to discharge from the hospital. All infants should be sent home with memory monitors to facilitate early withdrawal of monitoring.

Microchip technology has allowed many new devices to actually record events during the course of monitoring. A report can be generated or downloaded and evaluated on a regular basis. This allows the prescribing physician to track compliance and number of events, and in many cases, to review the actual waveforms associated with each event. This can be particularly valuable when attempting to evaluate the length of monitoring.

Apnea monitors are poor diagnostic testing devices. Documentation of apnea, or differentiating between different types of apnea, should be done using polysomnography. A more detailed discussion of managing infants with apnea at home appears in Chapter 31.

Ambulatory Esophageal pH Testing

Another common cause of disorganized breathing is gastroesophageal reflux. It is characterized by a variety of symptoms, ranging from wheezing to apnea.

Definitive diagnosis of gastroesophageal reflux can be confirmed by conducting an ambulatory pH study. This involves guiding a small pH-sensitive probe through the nares to rest just above the lower esophageal sphincter to test for pH levels in the esophagus. Placement of the tip of the probe is critical and should be confirmed by radiography. The probe should be taped adequately to prevent dislodging of the catheter. A grounding wire should then be attached to the abdomen. Ambulatory pH studies can be conducted safely in the home.

Careful and thorough instruction should be provided by the home care provider to the caregiver. A complete diary should be kept for the duration of the study, noting infant position, feeding times, type of formula/juice, and any documented events such as regurgitation or apnea. Breast milk or formula can buffer the esophageal pH leading to some inaccuracies in interpretation of the test. The best choice for feeding during the study period is apple juice or another clear liquid. For optimal results, the study should be conducted over a 24-hour period.

According to Johnson and Demeester (*see* Bibliography), evaluation of the tracing and corresponding diagnostic information should provide the reflux index, number of episodes with pH less than 4.0, number of reflux episodes greater than 5 minutes with pH less than 4.0, and the duration of the longest episode with pH less than 4.0. There is considerable debate in the literature regarding definitive interpretation of the data.

Multichannel Sleep Testing

Often, ambulatory pH testing is performed in conjunction with a multichannel sleep study, or polysomnography, which will confirm associated apnea. There are a variety of manufacturers who supply multichannel sleep testing equipment. The goal of this diagnostic procedure is to provide the clinician with as much information as possible about the child's cardio-respiratory status. Each channel typically represents a different physiologic function including electrocardiogram, electroencephalogram, oral and nasal air flow, body position, and oxygen saturation. These physiologic parameters provide comparative information when attempting to rule out various forms of apnea or differentiating sleep apnea from obstructive apnea.

Multichannel systems allow the clinician to view, in real time, many different events that contribute to the overall pathology. For instance, issues surrounding positioning and feeding can be observed.

The data derived are often dependent on the skill of the provider. Therefore, choice of home care provider is crucial to ensure the most accurate and complete information. Whenever possible, a provider with a specialty in pediatrics should be used.

Summary

When dealing with in-home diagnostic testing, keep the following facts in mind:

- The most common in-home diagnostic testing includes apnea/bradycardia monitoring, ambulatory esophageal pH testing, and multichannel sleep testing. All are designed to detect disordered breathing.
- Apnea/bradycardia monitoring alerts the caregiver when an infant's respiratory effort falls below a prescribed standard.
- Gastroesophageal reflux is a common cause of disordered breathing. It is detected through ambulatory esophageal pH testing.
- Electrocardiogram, electroencephalogram, oral and nasal air flow, body position, and oxygen saturation are evaluated during multichannel sleep testing to provide as much information as possible about a patient's cardiorespiratory status.

Bibliography

Burstein L. Home care. In: Barnhart SL, Czervinske MP, eds. *Perinatal and Pediatric Respiratory Care.* Philadelphia, PA: W. B. Saunders Co; 1995:658-680

Cairo JM, Pilbeam SP. *Mosby's Respiratory Care Equipment.* 6th ed. St Louis, MO: Mosby; 1999

Johnson LF, Demeester TR. Twenty-four-hour pH monitoring of the distal esophagus. A quantitative measure of gastroesophageal reflux. *Am J Gastroenterol.* 1974;62:325-332

Meny R, Carroll JL. Sudden infant death syndrome and sleep disorders. In: Barnhart SL, Czervinske MP, eds. *Perinatal and Pediatric Respiratory Care.* Philadelphia, PA: W. B. Saunders Co; 1995:627-636

Richter JE, ed. *Ambulatory Esophageal pH Monitoring: Practical Approach and Clinical Applications.* New York, NY: Igaku-Shoin; 1991

Turner J, McDonald GJ, Larter NL. *Handbook of Adult and Pediatric Respiratory Home Care.* St Louis, MO: Mosby-Year Book; 1994

Chapter 20

Home Phototherapy – Equipment and Support

Robert J. Rose, MD

Introduction

Since the mid-1980s, devices that provide home phototherapy for hyperbilirubinemia have been available. Advantages of moving this technology into the home from the hospital include facilitating feeding schedules and maternal-infant bonding, convenience, and cost savings. Home phototherapy devices can be used successfully by most families. Good protocols keep the physician and other health professionals in the loop so tight control of an infant's progress is maintained.

Phototherapy Technology

Home phototherapy devices are similar to hospital units in that all provide blue-range light to an infant's skin to break down bilirubin. They are different, though, in several respects, including portability, safety features, light delivery techniques, light intensity, surface area, and treatment times.

▸ Portability

There is a trend toward greater portability and convenience of use. First generation devices weighed 40 pounds or more. Today, devices weigh 7 to 15 pounds and are carried easily.

▸ Safety Features

Eye Protection

Using eye patches has been standard in hospital units. There have been episodes of eye patches slipping off, sometimes over the infant's airway. The effect of patching an infant's eyes for several days is unknown. Current home phototherapy devices generally avoid eye patches. Fiber-optic devices only expose the trunk; other fluorescent devices use a baby face shield system.

Temperature Controls

The fluorescent device warms the baby chamber if it is less than 75°F and shuts off if it is more than 98°F. Fiber-optic devices allow for clothing or blankets.

Physical Safety

All devices are designed to fit into a crib, and some have various anti-tip design features.

▸ Light Delivery Techniques

Phototherapy devices use special blue fluorescent bulbs and reflection techniques to maximize the skin area being treated, or fiber-optic blankets that are applied to an infant's torso. The advantage of the fluorescent bulbs is high intensity, which allows intermittent therapy and shorter treatment times. An advantage of the fiber-optic devices is that the infant can be held and fed during treatment, albeit tethered to the light source.

▸ Light Intensity, Surface Area, and Treatment Times

The dosage of phototherapy can be defined as the light intensity multiplied by the skin surface area treated and by the time of skin exposure. Because bilirubin in the skin degrades rapidly when exposed to light, intermittent therapy, especially of high intensity, has been shown to be as effective as continuous therapy. Therefore, the time of light exposure appears to be less important than previously thought. Modern protocols now usually call for 10 to 16 hours under the light each day, allowing time out for feedings, cuddling, and sleep breaks for the caregivers.

For light intensity and skin surface area treated, a useful unit of measure is the phototherapy unit (PTU), which is light intensity at the baby's skin in $\mu W/cm^2/nm$ multiplied by the percentage of the total surface area exposed to the light therapy. Newer fluorescent and fiber-optic devices provide higher intensity light than older devices. Standard hospital devices provide 4 to 12 $\mu W/cm^2/nm$ while newer generation devices provide up to 60 $\mu W/cm^2/nm$. The skin area that is treated is as important as the intensity of the light. Fiber-optic devices generally treat less skin surface area than fluorescent devices. Treatment times therefore generally are longer for fiber-optic devices. Fluorescent units may provide the highest PTUs and the shortest treatment times (Table 20-1).

TABLE 20-1. Characteristics of Phototherapy Treatments

Type of Light	PTUs
Older fiber-optic	200
Other fluorescent	600
Newer fluorescent	1,100
Doublebank hospital	600
Newer fiber-optic	400
Newest fiber-optic	700
Newest fluorescent	2,200

Because bulb output degrades over time, photodosimeters are used with lower PTU devices to ensure an adequate (>4 $\mu W/cm^2/nm$) dose is being delivered. They are not needed for high-output (more than 1,000 PTU) devices as bulbs are replaced before they degrade 20%.

Daily serum bilirubin measurements are part of most home phototherapy protocols. Heel sticks and capillary blood samples are the standard of care. Accurate transcutaneous bilirubin monitoring devices now are available for home use.

Providers

Home phototherapy should be ordered and monitored by the attending physician. Home phototherapy services typically are provided by durable medical equipment (DME) dealers or home nursing services. Sometimes the DME dealer provides the equipment, while the visiting nurse provides the screening, education, and daily assessments. Less commonly, hospital-based or physician office-based home care services provide home phototherapy. Phototherapists provided through a DME dealer are likely to be respiratory therapists or nurses. Occasionally, other health professionals may be used.

▸ Clinician Considerations

Clinician concerns about home phototherapy generally fall in two categories, environmental safety and control of the treatment regimen.

Environmental Safety

Safety of the environment includes thermal and physical safety. Only infants who can maintain body temperature are selected for home phototherapy.

They are treated in a mildly warm environment, generally inside a crib —
an environment that is safe for most babies. Infant temperature should be
monitored regularly per protocol; rarely, a baby will develop hypothermia
and require hospitalization.

Control of the Treatment

Regimen control is ensured by using a clear and complete protocol that
keeps the clinician in the daily assessment and decision-making loop —
no different than hospital care. Having parents on the caregiver team may
reduce clinical expertise, but usually increases the motivation to succeed.
The key to achieving good results is good screening of parents.

Financial Considerations

▶ Price Comparisons – Hospital Versus Home

Because the clinician's evaluation and management fees are roughly the
same for hospital versus office care, and the daily bilirubin laboratory fees
are presumed to be the same, the price comparison between hospital and
home phototherapy depends on the hospital charges versus the equipment
rental and nurse visit costs of home care (Table 20-2).

TABLE 20-2. Price Comparison of Hospital and Home Phototherapy

Typical hospital daily charge = $1,000-$2,000 × 3 days average treatment = $3,000-$6,000 per
  infant treated

Typical home daily charge = $150-$300 × 3 days average treatment = $450-$900 per infant treated

The average savings of home vs hospital phototherapy is $2,550-$5,100 per infant.

▶ Reimbursement

Payment for home phototherapy is covered by virtually all private health
insurers offering all types of indemnity and managed care policies. The substantial savings compared to hospital costs are powerful motivation to provide
this coverage. Coverage by medical assistance programs varies from state to
state ranging from no coverage to full coverage.

Summary

The following is important information to know about home phototherapy:

- Home phototherapy equipment to treat hyperbilirubinemia has been available since the mid-1980s.
- Phototherapy equipment uses fluorescent bulbs or fiber-optic devices. Bulbs allow for shorter treatment times; fiber-optic devices allow an infant to be held and fed during treatment.
- Intermittent phototherapy has been shown to be as effective as continuous therapy. Modern protocols call for 10 to 16 hours of treatment per day.
- Home phototherapy should be ordered and monitored by the attending physician. Only infants who maintain body temperature can receive home phototherapy.

Bibliography

American Academy of Pediatrics, Provisional Committee for Quality Improvement and Subcommittee on Hyperbilirubinemia. Practice guideline: management of hyperbilirubinemia in the healthy term newborn. *Pediatrics*. 1994;94:558–565

Chapter 21

Assistive Technology in the Home Care Setting

Rani C. Kathirithamby, MD

Introduction

Early development of children is based heavily on gross motor and fine motor skills. Infants and children use these skills to explore and manipulate their environment. Inability to master the environment may lead to diminished socialization and delayed normal development. Assistive devices, when prescribed in a timely manner, can enhance the independence of children with chronic illnesses and disabilities and improve the quality of life.

Provision of assistive technology or durable medical equipment is best accomplished by following a multidisciplinary team approach. The team consists of a child's physician, parent caregiver, therapist (physical, occupational, or speech), teacher, social worker, and the vendor. Older children should be included when deciding on their assistive technology devices.

Prescribing Assistive Technology

When prescribing assistive technology, careful consideration must be given to many factors. The intended purpose of the device, biomedical principles, possible limitations of the device, and possible unwanted effects should be considered. Growth and development of the child also should be considered because many devices are costly and funding agencies may not allow replacement or adjustment of the equipment if it is outgrown too quickly. Devices should be easily integrated in day-to-day family life. Children with multiple or severe disabilities may require devices that interfere with the lifestyle of the family, meaning compromises may need to be made.

The natural course of the child's illness and the prognosis are important factors when considering assistive devices. This is important in progressive neuromuscular or degenerative disorders when the future functional and medical status may require frequent replacement or modification. Therefore, it is cost-effective to purchase devices that are adaptable to changes in medical and functional needs.

Durability of the device is important, especially when there are a number of moving parts and the device is used daily. It is vital to consider if repairs and replacement parts are easily accessible and installed so as not to interrupt the child's activities.

The physician and the team should be able to justify the medical necessity of the prescribed device so that the funding agency will approve the cost of the device and future repairs. When assistive devices are discussed with the family, it is advisable to show an actual sample to the child and family. If possible, the child should try the device to ensure it is comfortable. The parents should determine whether there is sufficient space in the home to accommodate the equipment.

Prior to the delivery of the device, the child and parents should receive adequate training and instructions on the use and care of the equipment. The parents should be able to make minor adjustments without having to call the vendor.

Types of Devices

Assistive devices can be categorized into the following basic groups:
1. Positioning devices
2. Mobility devices
3. Activities of daily living (ADL) devices
4. Recreation devices
5. Communication devices

Many devices fall into more than one category.

▶ Positioning Devices

This equipment, when used appropriately, promotes optimal posture and alignment of joints in children who have not achieved head or trunk control either because of muscle weakness or developmental delay. The devices prevent abnormal contractures and deformities and prevent decubiti formation by decreasing undue pressure on bony prominences. In addition, they can assist in ADLs such as feeding, bathing, toileting, homework, and play.

Positioning devices range from simple, inexpensive, and easy-to-use equipment to technologically advanced, expensive, and large devices.

Pillows, Wedges, and Inserts

Pillows traditionally have been used to keep children in optimal positions. In a child with hip abductor spasticity due to cerebral palsy or traumatic brain injury, scissoring of the hips can be minimized by placing a bolster pillow or an abduction pillow between the legs. This decreases the possibility of hip subluxation and helps personal hygiene. A rolled wash cloth can be placed in a fisted hand to prevent maceration of the skin on the palm due to sweat collecting in the palm. An infant with hydrocephalus and a large head can be positioned optimally to keep the head in midline with the help of a foam collar.

Foam wedges of various lengths and widths can be used to help children attain a supine or prone position or lie on their side. Foam arm and leg elevators can help reduce edema. Soft boots lined with fleece or sheepskin can be used to keep ankles in neutral alignment to prevent heel cord tightness and decubiti in a child who is confined to bed.

The Versa Foam pillow is a newly developed positioner made of styrene beads that can be molded into a firm support using a vacuum pump. This allows children to be placed in any position, which can be changed by remolding the beads.

Positioning Chairs

Children who are unable to maintain independent head control and sitting balance often lie in bed or sit in their wheelchair for ADLs or during socialization with the family. Positioning chairs offer an alternative means of optimal positioning at home and an opportunity to interact with the family during mealtime or other occasions (Figure 21-1). The complexity of the positioning chair depends on the functional status of the child and the amount of support and alignment needed. Children with good head and trunk control can sit in a simple wooden chair with seat and chest belts and foot rests. Children with decreased trunk control or tonal abnormalities require trunk supports, a chest harness, hip guides, armrests, and hip abductor pommels. Poor or absent head control requires headrests that are adjustable so the head and neck can be placed in the optimal position for feeding, to decrease abnormal postures, and for management of secretions. Most chairs

FIGURE 21-1. Positioning Chairs Offer an Alternative Means of Optimal Positioning at Home

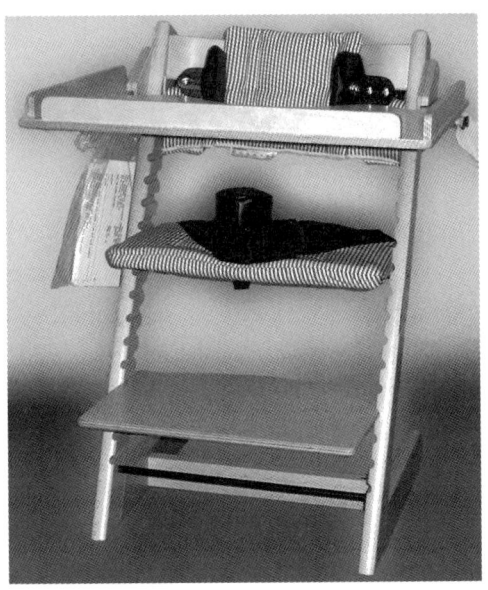

are equipped with wheels for mobility. The seats and back supports usually are upholstered and the belts and restraints are well padded to prevent skin irritation (Figure 21-2).

Standers

Standers are positioning devices that provide supported passive standing for children who are incapable of independent weight bearing. Standing sustains muscle strength, promotes stretching of tight muscles, and improves passive motion of lower limbs and head and trunk control. Standers can be used at home as part of a home exercise program. Many children use standers while they are doing homework or watching television.

There are three basic types of standers. The supine stander supports the child posteriorly and is capable of changing position from a horizontal to an upright position. The supine stander is indicated for children with absent or poor head and trunk control and/or increased extensor muscle tone. With the use of accessories such as head supports, lateral trunk supports,

FIGURE 21-2. The Seats and Back Supports of Positioning Chairs Usually Are Upholstered and the Belts and Restraints Are Well Padded

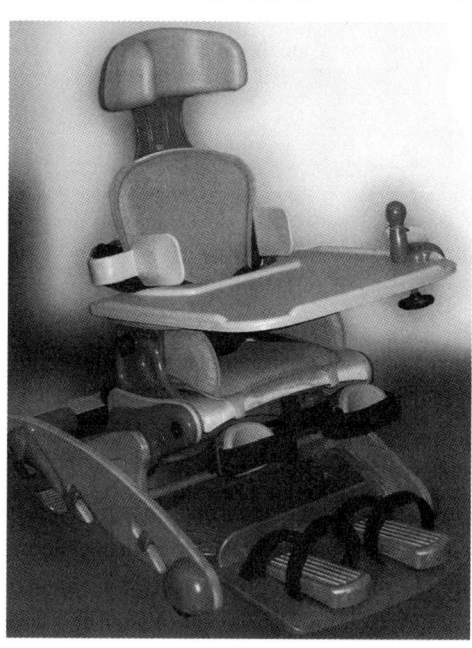

knee pads, and footrests, optimal alignment and weight bearing through the major joints is possible. Adding a tray allows children to use their hands to manipulate toys.

Prone standers are similar to supine standers, but they support the child anteriorly. They are not indicated for a child with poor head control. Prone standers have chin supports in addition to the accessories previously noted in the supine stander. Prone position enhances the extensor tone. Children are able to improve their trunk control and upper extremity weight bearing by using a prone stander.

An upright stander maintains children in an erect position through hip and knee supports. Upright standers have no head support and offer only a limited degree of trunk support. They can be used for weight bearing in children with spina bifida or low-level spinal cord injuries. (Children with high-level spinal cord injuries or with severe generalized muscle weakness benefit from a supine stander.)

Standers used for older or larger children should be equipped with hydraulic or manual lifts to assist the caregivers with positioning. When selecting a stander, the child's functional status accommodation for growth, the family's ability to use the device, space availability, and long-term goals for standing need to be considered carefully.

▸ Mobility Devices

Mobility aids can be categorized as follows:
- Ambulatory aids, which assist the children in standing and walking with support and safety
- Transfer aids, which help children and caregivers change the position from one surface to another
- Wheeled mobility aids, which assist children who are unable to walk, achieve mobility and independence

Ambulatory Aids

These devices are designed to help children improve balance and posture, provide support during walking, and decrease energy expenditure so they can explore their environment and achieve functional independence. The most common ambulatory aids are walkers, crutches, and canes.

Walkers

There are two types of walkers — forward or anterior and reverse or posterior. Forward walkers are the most traditional type; they promote trunk flexion. Forward walkers are not appropriate for a child with a tendency to stoop. Walkers with wheels are available, eliminating the need to lift the walker for forward progression and easy gliding. Reverse walkers facilitate more erect posture and therefore improve trunk extension.

Children with pronated posture of the forearms and wrists because of tonal abnormalities can benefit from the addition of upturned handles. Such handles will keep the forearms in greater supination and allow for a more erect posture. Platform troughs and handle attachments can be used to compensate for poor hand grip due to pain, weakness, or spasticity. Other accessories such as hand brakes, hip guides, swivel wheels, seats, baskets, and weights are available to customize the walker to meet the individual needs of the user. For children who are large and heavy and need more stability, heavy-duty walkers are available that are often wide, cannot be folded, and are difficult to maneuver through narrow spaces and doorways.

Crutches and Canes

Crutches can be used by children who have better trunk control. Two types, axillary and forearm, are commercially available. Axillary crutches are made of wood or aluminum and offer limited adaptability. Forearm crutches usually are made of metal and are lightweight. Forearm cuffs can be circumferential, half, or open. Handles vary in shape and size. Crutch tips of various sizes can be made of rubber or gel for stability and shock absorption. Tips made of studded cups that fit over the crutch tips facilitate walking in rain or snow. Crutches are available in a variety of bright colors and sizes and are easily adjustable to fit the height of any child. Types of canes available are straight canes, quadripod canes (four-prong), or hemi canes (combination of cane and walker); hemi canes have the widest base support.

Ambulatory aids should be checked and adjusted at regular intervals to accommodate for a child's growth. Prior to using ambulatory aids at home, children should be trained by a physical therapist. Adequate space should be available for walking. Parents and caregivers should be trained to assist and supervise as needed. The home environment should be barrier free and assessed for safety.

Transfer Aids

Transfer aids are used to assist children in changing their position on one surface, or transferring from one surface to another. A trapeze bar attached to a frame over a bed can assist a child in changing position from supine to sitting, or in side-to-side rolling transfers. A transfer board made of maple wood (8" × 24") can assist in sliding transfers from a bed to a chair. Sliding transfer can cause sheer stress and friction; a transfer board made of plastic on which a child glides laterally on a seat that rotates 360° decreases the risk of skin breakdown because of decreased friction.

There are larger and stronger transfer aids suitable for children with poor muscle strength who require total assistance in transfers. These are operated by the parents or the caregiver. The devices have heavy-duty canvass slings or supports that cradle the child and are operated manually or with power. Portable lifts are ideal for home use because they are lightweight and designed for narrow hallways and doorways.

Wheeled Mobility Devices

Wheeled mobility devices include wheelchairs, scooters, and strollers.

Wheelchairs

Wheelchairs come in a variety of sizes and shapes to meet the diverse needs of children with different levels of physical disabilities, cognitive limitations, and recreational interests.

Children with sufficient upper body strength to propel a wheelchair can use manual wheelchairs (Figure 21-3). Those who are unable to do so require a powered wheelchair. Children who have hemiparesis may be able to use a one-arm–driven manual wheelchair. There are various kinds of wheelchairs to suit the diverse interests of children. Rugged or outdoor wheelchairs are available for children who like camping and outdoor sports. Aerodynamic, three-wheeled chairs are used in wheelchair racing events. Lightweight sport chairs allow maximum independent mobility with minimum effort for everyday use or participation in group sport activities. Manual chairs with movable seats raise the user from a sitting to a standing position. Other types of manual wheelchairs include reclining wheelchairs for children who are unable to hold up and turn their head in an upright position, and tilt-in-space chairs for children who need changes in position during the day for various medical reasons. These chairs are usually propelled by parents or caregivers.

Proper selection of a wheelchair is essential for children to maximize their potential and to become independent in their environment.

Proper selection of a wheelchair is essential for children to maximize their potential and to become independent in their environment. When selecting a wheelchair, it is important to consider the following factors: the child's specific disability, level of function, medical interventions, prognosis for future function and cognitive ability, the family's ability to use the chair, and the family's willingness to integrate a child with a wheelchair into their daily life. The physician should consider funding sources prior to prescribing expensive and technologically advanced devices. Most of all, it is important to consider how the wheelchair will be used by the child and how much assistance it will provide. This should be done with the assistance of the multidisciplinary team, which must be involved in this process from beginning to end.

FIGURE 21-3. Children With Sufficient Upper Body Strength Can Use Manual Wheelchairs

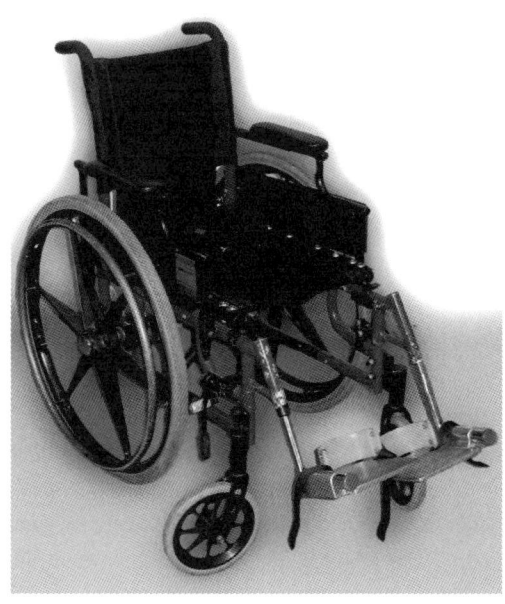

A powered wheelchair should be considered when the child's upper body strength or endurance is not sufficient to propel a manual chair effectively and independently. Children as young as 24 months can operate a powered mobility device safely. The child should be able to understand the concept of cause and effect, be able to follow one-step commands, have adequate visual skills to perceive child-size objects within a 10' radius, and have at least one reliable movement for activating a switch to operate the powered chair control. The movement must be one that the child can repeatedly stop and start at will, from a seated position. Because the powered chair can be driven with a variety of controls, a limitation in hand or arm control does not preclude powered mobility.

Powered and manual wheelchairs share the same basic components. Advances in technology have enabled powered wheelchairs to operate using joysticks, mouthsticks, jaw control, and sip-and-puff mechanisms. There are powered chairs that raise from a seated to a standing position, as well as elevate or lower the seat using a seat elevator. Children who are dependent on a ventilator can use the chairs for mobility. Wheelchair accessories allow ventilators to be mounted behind the seat of the chair.

Scooters

Three- or four-wheel scooters provide an alternate means of powered mobility. They are less expensive than other mobility devices, but they provide less alignment of the trunk and extremities. Positioning options are limited, as is the choice of child-size scooters. These scooters cannot be used when children need maximum trunk support.

Strollers

Young children who are unable to safely propel a wheelchair, or children with severe cognitive behavior or medical impairments that preclude them from propelling the wheelchair, may benefit from a stroller. There are a variety of strollers commercially available, ranging from simple lightweight strollers with small wheels, push handles, and restraints that can be used for younger children, to technologically complicated heavy strollers with multiple accessories. For children with multiple significant disabilities, there are complex seating systems with headrests, chest harnesses, lateral trunk supports, hip guides, foot rests, and armrests that can be adjusted to various angles. These seating systems are mounted on wheel bases and can be heavy and difficult to fold for transportation in a family vehicle. Many wheelchairs and strollers now are crash tested and have models equipped with accessories for transportation in school buses or ambulettes.

▸ Activities of Daily Living Devices

Activities of daily living devices help patients during feeding, grooming, bathing, and toileting. Occupational therapy evaluation determines the need for adapted equipment. Ongoing occupational therapy should be instituted to train the child in age-appropriate self-care activities. Adapted equipment should be tried out in the therapeutic setting to determine the child's ability to use the device and if there is a need for modifications before home use. Parents should be trained to follow through on home activities programs and to implement, assist, and supervise these activities.

Feeding

Children often have difficulty feeding themselves because of decreased muscle strength (muscle diseases), pain, limitations in range of motion (arthritis, burns, skeletal abnormalities), impaired motor coordination (cerebral palsy), or poor endurance (chronic illnesses). To improve the hand grip, built-up spoons or utensils with curved handles can be used. To improve the ability to scoop, spoons with shallow bowls and contours can be used. Plates and bowls can be stabilized by using nonskid mats. Shallow bowls can be used to facilitate the transfer of food. For children with significant weakness, mechanical or motorized feeders are available, which use switches that rotate plates, push food into spoons, and lift the spoon to the mouth level of the operator. The strength, coordination, and precision required to operate these devices are minimal. Other feeders use pulley systems to bring the arm to the mouth.

Grooming

Adapted equipment is available for brushing teeth, combing, cleaning after toileting, and dressing. Children need to be trained by an occupational therapist before they can use these devices successfully at home.

Bathing

Many devices are available to position children in bathtubs safely, including canvas bath chairs with belts, chest straps, and head supports. The chairs can be reclined or positioned upright, depending on the age and the functional status of the child. Caregivers can clean children easily without fear of the child falling into the water. The chairs may be positioned low in the bathtub with suction cups, or mounted on a frame at a higher level so that the caregivers can tend to the child without bending over. There are tub benches, bath seats, shower chairs, as well as tub rails and shower rails that can be used for older children with lesser disabilities. For children who are larger and heavy and require maximum assistance, there are hydraulic and powered bath lifts that raise and lower the child into the bathtub. Inflatable bathtubs are available for bathing children who are confined to the bed and cannot be moved.

Toileting

There are various models of potty-chairs and toilet seats available to help young children achieve continence of bladder and bowel. For children who require assistance when sitting, grab bars, toilet rails, seat belts, and footrests can be used to provide support and safety. There are complex toilet chairs for children who need maximum support, and commode chairs that can be placed by the bedside when bathroom doorways are too narrow to transfer the child to the toilet.

Car Seats

Car seats are important devices when considering the safety of children with chronic illnesses and disabilities. Car seats come in various sizes to accommodate children from infancy to youth. Some have appropriate positioning pads to support and align the head, trunk, and extremities; restraint systems; harnesses; and deep seat depths. Children who are in body casts or spica casts that limit the ability to change position can be placed in a Spelcast convertible seat. For children who are able to sit with support, an EZ-On Vest can be used. These can be used in both upright and horizontal positions in the back seat. See Chapter 22 for more detailed information on transportation of the child who is medically fragile.

Helmets

Helmets made of soft or hard materials, chin straps, face guards, and ear protectors can be used for children who have decreased balance, seizure disorders, are self-abusive, and exhibit self-stimulatory behavior to protect the head and face from injury. Parents sometimes have difficulty accepting custom-made helmets and often prefer to use bicycle helmets. For children who are liable to injure their face or ears, these may not be sufficient. Accurate measurements need to be taken to ensure the helmet fits properly.

▶ Recreational Devices

Children with disabilities and chronic illnesses need their toys to be adapted for easy manipulation. Adapted switches can be used to activate powered toys and educational games. Joysticks can be modified to help the grip when playing video and computer games. Mouth sticks or head pointers can be used to activate computer keyboards. For children with spina bifida who have weakness in lower extremities, carts are available so that the child can sit and propel using the upper extremities. Hand-operated bicycles and tricycles allow children to interact with nondisabled friends. Tricycles can be modified to include wide seats, head supports, foot sandals, seat backs, and chest belts. Scooters and powered cars can be modified so that the children can propel them with powered switches.

▶ Communication Devices

Communication behavior develops spontaneously in all children regardless of the severity and number of disabilities. These behaviors include gestures, eye gaze, and vocalizations to indicate satisfaction, dissatisfaction, and needs. Augmentative and alternative communication can be used to supplement children's diminished communication skills. They are indicated when a child's natural speech and language skills are not sufficient for communication purposes and academic learning. Children are evaluated by a speech and language pathologist, a psychologist, a teacher, and an occupational therapist to determine the most appropriate communication device for the child's disability. It is important that the device is available for home use so communication skills can be maintained at home and integrated into family life. Communication systems can be very costly and should be prescribed so that the devices have the capability to expand as the child's communication abilities expand.

Summary

When deciding whether to prescribe assistive technology, the following points should be made:

- Assistive devices can enhance the independence of children with chronic illnesses and disabilities and improve the quality of life.
- There are five basic types of assistive devices: positioning, mobility, ADL, recreation, and communication.
- A team that includes the physician, parent caregiver, therapist, teacher, social worker, and equipment vendor should be involved in making decisions about assistive technology. If the patient is old enough, he or she also should be involved.
- The physician and team should be able to justify the medical necessity of prescribed devices so that the funding agency will approve the cost of purchasing and maintaining the device.

Chapter 22

Transport of the Child Who Is Medically Fragile

Mhairi G. MacDonald, MBChB, FRCPE, DCH; Sharon Boyle-King, RNC, BSN, CCM; Rachel K. Lockwood, RNC, NNP; Linda Larson, MS, RN

Introduction

The transport of a child who is fragile and/or dependent on technology represents a period of increased vulnerability and risk for the patient. In addition to ensuring that the child is sufficiently stable to be discharged from the hospital to home, the safe transport of the child in both nonemergency and emergency circumstances must be carefully planned and conveyed to those caring for the child in the home setting as an integral component of the overall discharge plan.

The Transport Plan

An overview of transport options, the details of which will vary by state or county, is presented in Table 22-1. The importance of in-depth communication and information exchange between discharge-planning personnel and all community services that are involved in the care of the child in the home setting cannot be overemphasized. Such personnel not only include police and local emergency medical services (EMS), but others who might find themselves in key roles such as apartment managers and building attendants.

Major considerations for the development and communication of the transport plan are summarized in Table 22-2.

The Emergency Plan

The transport plan must be closely integrated with the child's overall emergency plan. The emergency plan is created by the child's treating physicians (including the local pediatrician) in close cooperation with parents and other home care providers. The plan must be available 24 hours a day. Guidelines for creating emergency plans have been developed by the

TABLE 22-1. Triage Guidelines for Pediatric Transport*

Triage Category[†]	Transport Options[‡]	Advantages	Disadvantages
Chronic, stable condition	Nonmedical (parent/caretaker escorts in family vehicle)	Low cost; readily available	Requires well-directed parents/caretakers who know how to trouble-shoot equipment and access emergency services. Allows for low likelihood of clinical instability. Vehicle may not accommodate special seats, prone frames, etc (Table 22-6).
	Public transport, taxi, modified van	Relatively low cost	May not carry car seats or other restraints appropriate for children. Family is responsible for care of the child en route.
	BLS ambulance or volunteer ambulance	Usually equipped with basic patient and passenger facilities and restraints	May not carry pediatric supplies, car seats, or appropriate-size stretchers with restraint belt. Implies ability to intervene if patient's condition deteriorates. Emergency medical technicians usually have little pediatric experience (approximately 100 hours of medical training) and volunteers usually have none.[§]
Acute illness; slowly progressive	ALS ambulance	Abilities of paramedics (1,500-2,000 hours of medical training) include administration of oxygen and nebulized medications, ALS, and airway skills (including endotracheal intubation)	Not all paramedics are skilled in pediatrics. Paramedics primarily are trained in extrication, intervention, and rapid transport, rather than monitoring, diagnosis, or prolonged transport.
	Critical care ambulance team	Presence of critical care nurse permits a higher level of assessment and intervention	Expertise in pediatric critical care is uncommon; risk of extrapolation of adult care principles to care of children is present.[§]

TABLE 22-1. Triage Guidelines for Pediatric Transport*, continued

Triage Category[†]	Transport Options[‡]	Advantages	Disadvantages
Acute illness; slowly progressive, continued	Specialized pediatric critical care transport service	Specialized pediatric assessment, monitoring, and diagnostic intervention skills. Medical supervision.	A relatively expensive and limited resource
Acute illness with potential for rapid deterioration of clinical condition and need for life-saving intervention	Specialized pediatric critical care transport service	See above	See above

*A minimum of one adult (excluding the driver) should travel with the child.

[†]No objective scoring system has been validated for use in pediatric transport. Local variation in transport patterns, geography, and distances traveled must be considered during triage.

[‡]Medicolegal implications of transport options must be recognized. The primary physician retains full responsibility for medical care of the child, whether he or she accompanies the patient on urgent/emergency transport, if transport is by private vehicle, taxi, or BLS or volunteer ambulance. BLS indicates basic life support; ALS indicates advanced life support.

[§]Family members are frequently prohibited from riding with the child in emergency circumstances.

Adapted from Table 3-1 of MacDonald MG, Ginzburg HM, eds. *Guidelines for Air and Ground Transport of Neonatal and Pediatric Patients.* 2nd ed. Elk Grove Village, IL: American Academy of Pediatrics; 1999:22-23

TABLE 22-2. Development and Communication of the Transport Plan

The plan should

- Be written prior to discharge of the child into the home care setting.
- Cover routine transport for outpatient appointments and family outings, as well as emergency transport.
- Be communicated on a need-to-know basis to personnel in the community likely to have a substantive role in transporting the child.
- Involve close collaboration between the discharge-planning coordinator at the hospital and those coordinating and providing home care.
- Be thoroughly communicated to the parents and other care providers prior to the child's discharge from hospital.
- Be based on in-depth knowledge of the capabilities of local EMS, specialized transport programs, and hospital services.
- Appropriately maintain confidentiality.

American Academy of Pediatrics (AAP) in collaboration with the American College of Emergency Physicians (ACEP) and are available in the policy statement "Emergency Preparedness for Children With Special Health Care Needs." (American Academy of Pediatrics, Committee on Pediatric Emergency Medicine. Emergency preparedness for children with special health care needs. *Pediatrics.* 1999;104) Major components of an emergency plan are listed in Table 22-3.

The Life Pack

An emergency travel bag or life pack must travel with the child at all times. The pack should contain all small equipment and supplies that might be needed during the time that the child is out of the home. Typical but not all-inclusive contents of the life pack include a bag-and-mask ventilator with appropriate-sized mask, spare tracheostomy tubes (if a tube of the same size cannot be replaced, one of the next smaller size should be carried; if neither spare tube can be replaced, a trimmed suction catheter can be used as a temporary airway), portable suction and a suction trap (eg, DeLee — if the suction equipment malfunctions), tracheostomy tube ties, an extra gastrostomy tube or foley catheter (if the child has a button that becomes displaced, a foley can be inserted to maintain patency of the stoma until

TABLE 22-3. Major Components of the Emergency Plan

- A method for identifying children who are at risk*
- Completion of a medical information data set (eg, the AAP/ACEP Emergency Information Form in the Appendix) by the child's physicians
- Education of family, caregivers, health care professionals, and school personnel (as appropriate) on use of the plan
- Regular updates of information
- Twenty-four hour access to the plan by authorized emergency health care personnel
- Maintenance of patient confidentiality

*Some EMS agencies are capable of placing this information in their 911 system; some hospitals have databases that can accommodate it. The not-for-profit MedicAlert Foundation has offered to act as a central repository for information on children with special needs. Adjuncts to such programs include window stickers identifying the homes of children who are medically fragile, and automatic information such as the location of a copy of the emergency plan within the home. The fine line between adequate communication and patient confidentiality must be maintained under all circumstances and involves parent/guardian informed consent.

the button can be replaced), saline bullets, and a unit dose of all medications needed during the time away from home, including prn/emergency medications. Extra time should be allowed for unexpected traffic and other obstacles when planning medications and feedings.

The life pack also should contain a copy of the patient's emergency information card or form. An emergency information form has been developed by the American Academy of Pediatrics in collaboration with ACEP (*see* Appendix). Essential data include the date of last update, patient's name, birth date, weight, parent/guardian's name, emergency contact information for the pediatrician, case manager, other health care personnel, and the predesignated primary emergency department. Clinical data should include major chronic illnesses and disabilities, baseline physical and mental status, baseline vital signs and laboratory results, immunization history, ventilator settings and baseline oxygen requirements, medication doses and schedules, and medication and/or food allergies. Also essential is insurance information and advance directive/modified code information (most states have a standard advanced directive form, and it is required that EMS honor the directive to withhold emergency lifesaving measures; the emergency data set can identify a need for a standard form). It also is valuable to place copies of recent, pertinent x-rays in the life pack.

Safety Equipment

The requirements for safety equipment within a transport vehicle vary with the specific needs of the child. The following are examples of basic safety equipment:

- Adapted car seats for children who have difficulty sitting (some have a detachable base that converts the seat into a stroller)
- Restraint vest for children requiring restraints in addition to seat belts
- Wheelchair tie-downs for children transported in a wheelchair

▶ Portable Equipment

Generic requirements for monitoring and other devices used during transport are listed in Table 22-4.

Backup equipment must always be available on transport in case of equipment failure so the child can be supported until arrival at home or the hospital (Table 22-5).

TABLE 22-4. Essential Features for Equipment Used in Pediatric Transport

- Portable (can be loaded by two people)
- Lightweight
- Durable (able to withstand 4g deceleration forces)
- Easily maintained
- Portable power (twice the expected transport time as minimum)
- Alternating current/direct current capable (whenever possible, use converters to conserve power)
- Produces no electromagnetic interference
- Resistant to electromagnetic interference
- Displays physiologic data clearly in digital and wave form
- Audible and visible alarms
- Securable
- Compatible with all other equipment
- Meets all federal, state, and Federal Aviation Administration codes, including hazardous material regulations
- Able to withstand altitude, temperature changes, and vibration
- Able to fit through standard doors

Adapted from Table 9-1 of MacDonald MG, Ginzburg HM, eds. *Guidelines for Air and Ground Transport of Neonatal and Pediatric Patients.* 2nd ed. Elk Grove Village, IL: American Academy of Pediatrics; 1999:106

TABLE 22-5. Examples of Backup Procedures/Equipment for Transport

Portable Equipment	Backup
Ventilator	Bag-and-mask ventilator
Suction machine	Suction trap (eg, DeLee)
Feeding pump	Adjust clamp on feeding tubing and use gravity
Nebulizer	Multidose inhaler; oxygen at high flow
Oxygen	No substitute; always have an extra tank available
Battery*	A backup battery; an alternating current/direct current adapter can be plugged into the cigarette lighter in a car

*The length of battery charge and average life of the battery need to be known for each piece of equipment. Information also should be available about whether the equipment will run on an external battery. Emergency vehicles should be fitted with alternating current inverters and, ideally, a shore line with multiple outlets into which equipment can be plugged during transport.

The Transport Vehicle

The appropriate vehicle in which to transport a child who is medically fragile will vary with the circumstances of the transport (ie, emergency versus nonemergency), clinical stability, size and mobility of the child, and size and quantity of the special equipment required.

For nonemergency transport, the choice of family vehicle requires keeping the considerations listed in Table 22-6 (see also Table 22-1) in mind.

▶ Personnel

In addition to the driver, the child who is medically fragile should be accompanied during transport by, at minimum, one adult with the required expertise. The need for additional personnel is based on the clinical stability of the child, the need for ongoing assessment and/or the potential requirement for immediate intervention (eg, airway management), and the frequency of scheduled interventions (Table 22-1).

Long-Distance/Vacation Transportation

When planning a long-distance trip, it is essential that the accessibility of the destination facility, other than a hospital or clinic, be assessed in advance. It is important to check that entrances and exits (eg, fire exits), in addition to

TABLE 22-6. Selection Considerations for the Optimal Family Vehicle*

For the small or larger child who can self-transfer or has independent mobility, consider the following:

- The chassis should be sufficiently low to allow self-transfer from a wheelchair and to facilitate the transfer of necessary medical equipment.
- There should be four doors.
- There must be sufficient space for optimal positioning of the child, at least one adult in addition to the driver, and the necessary medical equipment.
- Additional space should be available for a folded wheelchair and/or walker, if needed.

For the larger child who is dependent on a wheelchair or cannot self-transfer, consider the following:

- A van usually is required.[†]
- Frequently required vehicle modifications include elevation of the roof to increase headroom, a lift to transfer the chair and patient into the van, and safety restraints on the floor of the van to keep the chair in place.

*Vehicles should be fitted with handicap license plates; a car phone is optimal.

[†]An adapted van may be beyond family resources. Third-party payers may reimburse for van transport provided by a private company to medical appointments. In many states, funding for van transportation to medical appointments is provided, on advance notice, by Medicaid. Supplemental Security Income (SSI) funds can be used for public transportation and toward the purchase of adapted vans. Public health departments frequently provide transportation for routine medical appointments (eg, hemodialysis). Most states also have programs based on the Individuals with Disabilities Act that provide transportation to schools and special education programs. Additional sources include Lions & Rotary Clubs, charitable foundations (eg, Ryan White), and church groups (which often assist families with fundraising activities such as raffles).

the main entrance, are accessible to the child and that oxygen use will not represent a hazard. The child's pediatrician should be involved in planning the trip, including the choice of vehicle, and should be aware of the intended route. If traveling with oxygen, planned stops along the way may be required to refill oxygen tanks; equipment supply issues en route and at the destination should be discussed in advance with the company supplying the child's home equipment. The child may require additional oxygen at certain altitudes.

If traveling by bus or train, the service should be contacted to discuss the child's needs prior to the trip. The vehicle should have a lift ramp if the child is dependent on a wheelchair and too heavy to carry, and there must be an adequate nonsmoking area. Most bus companies will allow portable oxygen, but may not allow additional oxygen tanks; stops may have to be arranged to refill oxygen tanks. Most railroads will allow medical equipment, including oxygen, and may allow hookup of equipment to the train's electrical supply.

Airlines should be contacted to discuss the child's needs prior to making a reservation. Most airlines will accommodate those who are dependent on a wheelchair. Cabins are only partially pressurized, so even if a child does not regularly use oxygen, it may be required while in flight. Most airlines will not allow oxygen to be brought onto the plane; the airline will supply oxygen during the flight, but oxygen availability at the destination or during layovers is the responsibility of the care providers. There is a charge for oxygen used during a flight, and a written physician's order may be required. The home medical equipment company should be able to assist the family in locating the necessary equipment suppliers for oxygen and other needs.

If nursing care is required, options should be discussed with the nursing agency and third-party payer. The parents should be supplied with the name and location of a suitable hospital in the destination vicinity and along the intended route of travel. Ideally, there should be physician-to-physician communication about the child's clinical status and needs.

Other Considerations

Prior to initial hospital discharge, it may be valuable to run a mock 911 call with parents/guardians and home health care providers. Select EMS personnel should be employed as needed for special equipment and other transport requirements.

Summary

As is the case for other aspects of home care for the child who is medically fragile, the keys to safe transport are meticulous preplanning; optimal communication between the hospital, the child's pediatrician, and community services to develop a safety network; in-depth knowledge of appropriate services available; and effective instruction of parents and other care providers.

Bibliography

Ahmann E. *Home Care for the High-Risk Infant: A Family-Centered Approach*. 2nd ed. Gaithersburg, MD: Aspen Publishers; 1996

American Academy of Pediatrics, Committee on Pediatric Emergency Medicine. Emergency preparedness for children with special health care needs. *Pediatrics*. 1999;104:e53. Available at: http://www.pediatrics.org/cgi/content/full/104/4/e53. Accessed September 18, 2001

Joint Task Force for the Management of Children with Special Health Care Needs. *Supervisor's Guide for Transporting Children with Special Health Needs.* Baltimore: Maryland State Dept of Education; 1991. Publication MdHR923384

MacDonald MG, Ginzburg HM, eds. *Guidelines for Air and Ground Transport of Neonatal and Pediatric Patients.* 2nd ed. Elk Grove Village, IL; American Academy of Pediatrics; 1999

Seidel JS, Knapp JF, eds. *Childhood Emergencies in the Office, Hospital, and Community: Organizing Systems of Care.* Elk Grove Village, IL: American Academy of Pediatrics; 2000

PART THREE

Disease-Management Programs

Chapter 23

Case Management of Children With Special Health Care Needs

Carol Marsiglia, RN, BSN, CCM; Karen Ann Lichtenstein, MA; Sharon Boyle-King, RNC, BSN, CCM; Barbara McCord, MS

Introduction

This chapter presents community case management on behalf of children who require technology and have complex medical needs. Case management will be presented within a conceptual framework best described as child and family centered. Planning for home care considers the needs of the child and the capacities of the family in a holistic manner. Professionals from diverse disciplines and the family members, who are responsible for the nurturing and care of the child, form a partnership with health promotion of the child and family as the focal point. This perspective explains why the term that is used throughout this section is "care" management as opposed to "case" management.

In the recent past, children dependent on technology typically remained in hospitals for many months and sometimes years, often beginning their lives in the pediatric intensive care unit. The medical concerns were related to prematurity, congenital anomalies, genetic or chromosomal disorders, neurological or nutritional complexities, trauma, or other childhood syndromes. These children required technology such as a ventilator, tube feedings, or specialized parenteral infusion to support their daily needs. Many of the children required frequent skilled assessments of their body systems to determine what intervention should be delivered to maintain homeostasis and medical stability.

Care management is indicated for those children dependent on technology or who have complex medical needs and require significant support and coordination of multiple systems, services, and providers. All children should have a medical home where care is accessible, family-centered, continuous, comprehensive, coordinated, compassionate, and culturally competent. The need for care management can be determined through a screening tool used to identify potential risks. Table 23-1 is an example of a community-based screening tool. If multiple indicators are identified as risks, care management is indicated and the process begins.

Process

Children who require technology or other assistance to carry out typical daily functions need specialized services to enable participation in routine childhood activities. Careful, deliberate planning methods promote a smooth transition from hospital to home. The complex nature of these specialized needs requires extensive coordination of medical and therapeutic services, community resources, and financial planning. Additionally, a frequently over-looked or assumed factor is the presence of a parent (primary caregiver) and at least one backup caregiver with the desire and ability to care for the child at home.

Home care coordination addresses these needs through a four-phase process: assessment, planning, implementation, and evaluation. The care manager facilitates the family's role as an active participant in each phase of this process (Table 23-2).

Assessment

The assessment phase begins at the time the child is hospitalized. During this phase, a site visit to the home or environment where the child's care will be provided is essential. This site visit may be referred to as a predischarge home visit and scheduled in conjunction with the parent or primary caregiver. The predischarge home visit ideally is done by a care manager, but it may be performed by a hospital discharge planner, social worker, nursing provider, medical equipment company representative, or other discipline trained to identify existing and potential supports, resources, and obstacles to care. The predischarge home visit should occur 1 to 2 weeks before the targeted date of discharge from hospital to home, depending on the complexity of the child's requisite technology. Adequate time allows the family to make plans for any necessary accommodations in the home environment prior to the child's discharge from the hospital. For example, an older child may require more intensive home modifications related to

TABLE 23-1. The Coordinating Center Care Management
Risk Assessment

Risk Factors	Indicators	Comments
Housing/ Environmental	• Potential for loss of housing • No permanent housing conditions • Barriers to accessibility • Home is crowded (>4 people sleeping in room) • Requires basic necessities (eg, household goods, beds, dishes, etc) • Non-habitable home • Safety issues (specify) • Utilities at risk for turnoff • Telephone not accessible	Requires on-site environ-mental assessment Requires change of address Other concerns
Health Behavior	• No primary care physician identified • Child requires routine immunizations • Inappropriate or frequent use of emergency room (>3 visits in 6 months) • Requires specialty physician care and follow-up • Requires transportation to medical appointments • Consistent missed medical appointments • Requires education/family planning services • Requires disease management education • Requires dietary education and information • Not taking prescribed medication • Requires home care services • Requires education about growth and development • Requires information/education about physician follow-up/notification	
Psychosocial	• No backup caregiver available • Primary caregiver is a minor • Primary caregiver is age 65 or older • Primary caregiver is single parent • Primary caregiver has health issues that affect care giving • Primary caregiver cares for other people with disabilities in the home • Primary caregiver has cognitive delay/mental illness • Home has more than two other children age 10 or younger • Primary caregiver is known substance abuser • Client is actively followed by child protective services • Client is at risk for parental neglect/abuse • Caregiver requests support group	

TABLE 23-1. The Coordinating Center Care Management Risk Assessment, continued

Risk Factors	Indicators	Comments
Psychosocial, continued	• Caregiver is illiterate • Caregiver requires respite • Communication barrier • Cultural mores affect client's care • Client/caregiver has insufficient income to meet routine needs	
Home Health	• Client requires nutritional supplement • Client requires in-home nursing care • Client requires total assistance with activities of daily living • Client requests change in service providers • Client requires durable/disposable equipment and supplies • Client requires specimen collection in home • Client requires reinforcement of teaching or skilled intervention • Client requires a monitoring device in the home • Client requires frequent (eg, weekly) monitoring of weight • Client is not following prescribed plan	
Developmental/ Rehabilitation	• Client has or is at risk for developmental delay • Client requires rehabilitation services • Client requires educational services • Client has school health services needs during the school day • Client requires assistance in attending class (ie, nursing care)	

Used with permission from The Coordinating Center.

accessibility, whereas any child with technology such as ventilator dependency will require a review of items such as electrical capacity and other safety concerns.

A predischarge home visit includes environmental and needs assessments to determine if the home environment will support the necessary care of the child with technology. When the environment will not support the care of the child, the goal is to identify accommodations that are necessary to support the child's needs. The environmental assessment may include considerations for space and location of the child's room or living space, accessibility inside and outside of the home, provision of adequate electricity and lighting, functioning utilities and telephone services, and basic safety considerations essential for any child (Table 23-3).

Completing a needs assessment will assist the family and care providers in prioritizing issues that may require resolution before the child comes home. The family should identify willing and available caregivers as well as a trained

TABLE 23-2. The Coordinating Center Process for Planning Home Care for Children With Complex Medical Needs

Assessment	Expected Outcomes
• Predischarge home visit • Environment • Family needs	• Satisfactory environmental assessment • Functioning utilities • Plan for accessibility to the home • Prioritization of family needs related to care of child dependent on technology

Planning
• Meet with multidisciplinary team prior to discharge.
• Develop plan of care.
• Identify any need for nursing or related services.
• Identify goals for medical management, nursing services if applicable, and other services identified on the plan of care.
• Identify funding for plan.
• Develop a plan for physician notification and emergency protocol.
• Identify anticipated date for home care to begin.
	Expected Outcomes
	• Comprehensive, individualized plan of care documenting needs of child
	• Medical, nursing, therapy, and home care goals identified
	• Completed emergency protocol
	• Referrals to community agencies made
	• Funder determines services it will fund on plan of care
	• By date of discharge
	   ~ Equipment and supplies delivered to the home or hospital
	   ~ Documented training of caregiver and backup caregiver
	   ~ Stable or predictable medical status with no acute changes in status
	   ~ Pharmacy items available
	   ~ Nursing schedule available with reasonable staffing for 2 weeks

Implementation • Schedule on-site visits as indicated. • Monitor plan of care to ensure services are being provided as anticipated. • Identify and locate resources and plan as needs indicate.	**Expected Outcomes** • Coordination pathway identifies outcomes of ongoing care management. • Ultimate goal is family as care manager (*see* coordination pathway components and outcomes in Table 23-7).
Evaluation • Schedule regular plan of care review meetings with the home care multidisciplinary team and physician. • Update current medical status and review outcomes of home care. • Identify goals for medical management, home care, and other services listed on the plan of care. Make changes as necessary. • Update physician notification and emergency plan.	**Expected Outcomes** • Review plan of care at review meetings. • Review status of medical, nursing, therapy, and home care goals. • Identify new goals for medical, nursing, therapy, and home care goals. • Review emergency protocol for changes.

Used with permission from The Coordinating Center.

TABLE 23-3. The Coordinating Center Environmental Assessment Tool

Name: **Address:**

Date:

Neighborhood
- Access to transportation.
- Access to emergency services.
- Handicapped parking space.
- Identify other issues or concerns.

Access
- Exterior ramping/lift.
- Entry door/adequate width.
- Interior passage doors/adequate width.
- Interior stairs to child's room.
- Toilet and bathing facilities accessible.
- Identify other issues or concerns.

Utilities
- Functioning heat.
- Functioning plumbing.
- City water/sewage.
- Well and septic tank.
- Access to laundry facilities.
- Functioning electrical service.
- Likelihood of loss of service.
- Refrigerator.
- Identify other issues or concerns.

Allergens
- Smoking in home
- Dogs, cats, or other pets
- Pests (rodents, bugs)
- Pesticide use
- Clutter
- Trash accumulation
- Molds or mildews
- Fireplace

Safety Features
- Functioning smoke detectors.
- Filled fire extinguisher.
- Fire escape plan.
- Child safety precautions (covered outlets, safety gates).
- Space heaters.
- Flashlight.
- Easily identifiable building (house numbered/light).
- "No smoking" signs if oxygen in use.
- Medication storage.
- Identify other issues.

Child's Area
- Bed/crib
- Adequate area for child's needs
- Space for equipment
- Supply storage convenient to child and caregivers
- Adequate lighting
- Electrical outlets (adequately spaced for child's needs)
- Power strip
- Grounded outlets (three prong)
- Telephone convenient for caregiver
- Room shared with other siblings or adults
- Communication center (calendar, clock with second hand, bulletin board)
- Access to family living area

Used with permission from The Coordinating Center.

backup caregiver prior to discharge. This is essential for a successful home care plan.

Inclusion of family from the start promotes partnership between the family and the professionals. Need is based on an individual's judgment of the discrepancy between actual states or conditions and what is considered normative, desired, or valued from the help seeker's, and not the help giver's, perspective. Thus it is imperative the care manager recognize the potentially overwhelming position of the family when planning care for the child with extraordinary medical needs. See Table 23-4 for sample needs-assessment questions.

Planning

It is prudent to identify and convene a multidisciplinary team and meet prior to the anticipated discharge date. Members of the team include the parent or legal guardian, physician, care manager, therapists, social worker, hospital discharge planner, representatives from the home care nursing agency and equipment company, and school nurse. The multidisciplinary team is not limited to this list of people; anyone involved in the care of the child may be included. A meeting provides a forum where all the participants in the team hear the same information and have the opportunity to pose questions and clarify information. This is important to optimize outcomes and avoid unnecessary phone calls and potential miscommunication. The purpose of the meeting is to review current medical needs and develop a plan for home care. The meeting should last no longer than 2 hours and can be conducted effectively in less time with a skilled facilitator and preparation in advance by team members. It is important to identify clear goals for home care and the purposes for home care services.

Goals for home care should be consistent with concepts of normalization, promotion of health and well-being of the child and family, and participation in family and community life. Goals may reflect medical outcomes (eg, weaning of mechanical ventilation or decannulation). Nursing goals relate to education for caregivers or to the provision of care so that caregivers can sleep or work. Goals also relate to specific home care services such as

TABLE 23-4. The Coordinating Center Family Needs-Assessment Questions

Family Structure/Roles

- Do you want to care for your child at home?
- Are you aware of alternatives to home care?
- Are you willing and available to provide your child's care at home?
- Can you identify another person to act as a backup caregiver for your child?
- Are there others (friends/family members) who can assist you with your child with special needs, your other children, or your family obligations?

Medical Management

- Have you completed hospital training in your child's care?
- Has your child's backup caregiver completed the training? If not, what is left to learn?
- Do you have transportation to medical appointments?
- Do you need help in selecting a nursing agency or medical equipment company?
- Do you have a pharmacy that makes deliveries?

Nutrition

- How is your child fed?
- If formula, will you need help to buy or locate the formula?
- Have you applied for the Special Supplemental Nutrition Program for Women, Infants, and Children (WIC)?
- Does your child have a need for diapers that is greater than the norm?

Education

- Will your child be attending school?
- Do you know which school your child will attend?
- Has your child been referred to the Infant and Toddler program (for ages 0-3) or the early intervention program?
- Do you have a current educational plan for special services?
- Do you have a contact person in the school program?
- Will your child need adaptive equipment at home, child care, or school? Does your child currently have a wheelchair?

Parenting/Child Care

- Do you work outside of the home? Do you go to school?
- Do you think your child will require skilled nursing care or other home health care providers?
- What is your plan if home health nurses are not provided?
- Have you considered medical day care or adaptive child care? What resources are available to offset the costs?
- What is your plan to care for your child if the nurse is absent or shifts are not staffed?
- Have you planned child care for your other children?

TABLE 23-4. The Coordinating Center Family Needs-Assessment Questions, continued

Financial Resources

- Does your child have medical insurance?
- Do you need more information about or referrals to the Department of Social Services, WIC, Supplemental Security Income, food stamps or local food banks, housing, or respite care?
- Can you access everyday supplies for your child such as a crib, clothing, and toys?
- Will you need resources to help with budgeting?

Community Resources

- Are you involved with any helping agencies or people, especially those you would like to include in the planning process?
- Do you or other family members belong to a church, social groups, clubs, or associations?
- Would you like to talk to another parent who has a child with special needs?
- Would you like a referral to a support group?

Family Life

- Do you see your child's homecoming as making a significant change in your lifestyle?
- Do you have concerns about your other children?
- What are your short-term and long-term goals for your child with technology needs?
- What do you see as your family needs at this time?
- Do you understand the role of the care manager?
- Do you have any questions or other concerns that have not been addressed?

Used with permission from The Coordinating Center.

occupational, physical, or speech therapy. The plan of care serves as a template for implementation of services. It is a document that identifies all services the child requires, including professional services such as skilled nursing care; home health aide services; physical, occupational, or speech therapy; educational services; medications; medical equipment; medical supplies; therapeutic adaptive equipment; physician visits; outpatient services; anticipated laboratory work; testing for diagnostic or monitoring purposes; and nutrition. The plan of care also may include a cost analysis of services (Table 23-5).

Avoid planning home care around hospital routines. Again, this is an opportunity to respect family preferences. Of course, frequency of medical interventions at home should be requested based on need for intervention but not directed by hospital routine. Acute versus chronic nature of needs also should be considered when identifying goals.

TABLE 23-5. Basic Components of the Plan of Care

Component	Examples of Required Entries
Nursing interventions	Level of care, hours of care, provider name and phone number
Medications (include PRN)	Medication, route, dosage, frequency
Nutrition and special diets	Nutritional formulas, supplements, feeding assistance
Rehabilitative	Developmental/speech therapy, physical therapy, occupational therapy, vision services, child life, etc
Education	Level of education, school, home tutoring
Durable equipment	Medical, therapeutic, and adaptive equipment
Supplies	Medical supplies, amount, frequency
Clinics	All community physicians/clinics, frequency of visits
Technology services	Diagnostic tests, x-rays, laboratory tests
Planned hospitalizations	Elective surgeries or hospitalizations

▸ Level of Nursing Services

Nursing is often a requested component of care for children who are dependent on technology at home. There is inconsistency in the recommendation of frequency and level of nursing services throughout the health care system. Data from participants on a Medicaid waiver program indicate that nursing service is one of the most costly components in caring for children who are dependent on technology at home. It is essential that these services are prescribed and used in situations where there is a clear indication for need. There is much discussion about need, amount, and frequency of nursing services. With no clear guidelines to determine the number of nursing care hours, decisions should be based on justifiable factors. Consistency in recommending the number of nursing care hours for home settings may assist in the development of universal standards. Upon initial discharge from the hospital, the level of nursing support usually is more intensive to assist the family and child with the transition to home. Nursing support should be weaned to a maintenance level within 1 week in most circumstances to prevent family dependency on unnecessary nursing support, and reviewed regularly by the multidisciplinary team. The care manager reviews nursing notes and the plan of care regularly to determine the effectiveness of and need for this service. Considerations for nursing care include a variety of issues summarized in the following questions:

- Who is available to care for the child?
- Are parents working and is it reasonable for the family to make adjustments in lifestyle?
- Does the child require an awake caregiver (at night while family sleeps) to maintain safety?
- Does the child require nursing in school?
- Does the child attend school where a nurse is on staff?
- Are medical day care or inclusive child care an option?
- How long has the child been cared for at home with the technology?
- What other social factors support the need for skilled nursing?
- Is nursing the appropriate service to meet the needs?
- Are there circumstances when increases are indicated (eg, birth or death in family, other sibling hospitalized)?
- Is typical child care with a trained provider adequate?
- What are the criteria for weaning?

▶ Funding Home Care

When planning for home care, it is important to select services based on the needs of the child, rather than on allowed benefits. Identifying funding for the items listed on the plan of care should be the responsibility of the care manager or discharge planner. Identifying funding for items not covered by private insurance or public medical assistance must be a part of this process. The emphasis on cost of care from third-party payers and limited insurance benefit packages may create incentives that are unethical for planning optimal care. Again, the family can take an active role by working with the care manager to pursue leads for potential funding. It is wise to include a representative from the insurance company or payer source on the multidisciplinary team to answer questions related to allowed benefits.

When planning for home care, it is important to select services based on the needs of the child, rather than on allowed benefits.

Family contribution is not an unreasonable concept, but it is important to understand the overwhelming costs incurred for a child dependent on technology. Some indirect costs include increased use of electricity, telephone service, over-the-counter items not covered by insurance, co-payments for services and prescriptions, and adaptations to the home environment. Options for funding a costly home care plan include third-party insurers,

Medical Assistance (Title XIX), State Maternal Child Health Programs (Title V), state waivers, local health departments, departments of social services, developmental disabilities administrations, private foundations, charitable organizations, and other community-based advocacy organizations. Locating funding for such complex plans demands creativity.

Community involvement with funding promotes a successful home care plan. A plan for physician notification and emergency protocol should be developed at the discharge planning meeting (Table 23-6). The emergency plan includes parameters for physician notification as well as specific descriptions of what constitutes an emergency for each child. This is an opportunity to address an end-of-life plan when appropriate. It also is helpful for the family to have a copy of the discharge summary and the plan of care to carry in an emergency supply bag, so that if the child must be taken to an emergency room, a brief description of status, medical needs, and contacts can be used to provide historical information.

Implementation

After the plan is developed, the implementation phase begins. Once the child is discharged to the home, community care management is essential in preventing rehospitalization as well as fostering a typical home environment. An inherent danger in bringing a child requiring technology home is the re-creation of an intensive care setting. Therefore, a challenge in implementing the home care plan is maintaining the home and community as the normal environment for the child.

The purpose of community care management is to integrate the child into the home and community safely and effectively while encouraging family independence relative to managing the child's care. Community care management is most effective when the family assumes appropriate care management roles, using a designated care manager for authorization and resource information. Making regular contact through home visits and the telephone accomplishes this goal. As the family becomes more independent and confident about coordinating their child's complex needs, the need for intensive professional care management lessens. However, it is important for a family to have access to care management services as medical and

TABLE 23-6. Sample Form for Physician Notification and Emergency Protocol, Developed by The Coordinating Center

Physician Notification and Emergency Protocol

In the event of

	Greater than	Less than
Heart rate		
Respiratory rate		
Temperature		
Blood pressure		
Emesis (vomiting)	more than _____ /24-hour period	
Stools (diarrhea)	more than _____ /24-hour period	
Weight gain	more than _____ /24-hour period	
Weight loss	more than _____ /24-hour period	

Please call _____ at _____ (phone)

Emergency Protocol Plan

- *What interventions are to be performed?*

- *Name and number to notify in emergency (physician, rescue squad).*

Emergency Transport Plan

Indicate name, address, and phone of local hospital nearest to home and nearest to school (for stabilization/emergency treatment).

Individualized Considerations

Indicate

- *What constitutes an emergency?*

_____   _____
Client Name   Physician Signature/Date

Used with permission from The Coordinating Center.

social situations change, as this may disrupt the balance within the home and ultimately affect the child's health management.

A best-practice model developed and practiced by The Coordinating Center in Maryland has identified eight essential components to effective community care management for children (Table 23-7). The Coordinating Center uses a Coordination Pathway to map care management intervention and monitor family-centered outcomes. As the family accomplishes the outcomes, they achieve the skills necessary to provide care management.

Evaluation

The last phase of the care management process is evaluation. The care manager reviews the goals and plan of care at each site visit with the family. Regardless of the site visit schedule, a review of the plan should be accomplished at minimum on a monthly basis. As site visits decrease in frequency, the plan evaluation can be done over the telephone. This evaluation includes a review of goals and services listed on the plan of care and should assess the need for new services and alternative funding sources.

Evaluation of the plan of care services can be done effectively through a multidisciplinary team meeting. The child with a high level of technology needs and intensive services may require a systematic review of the plan with the multidisciplinary team 3 months after discharge. In addition to reviewing the components of the plan of care (Table 23-4), this meeting includes a medical update by the family and physician, an update of the emergency protocol, special transportation issues, a review of current goals, and identification of new goals. It also provides an opportunity for equipment company representatives and nursing providers to participate in the child's treatment plans. The team determines the frequency of subsequent meetings based on intensity of services and stability of the home care plan. If a hospitalization occurs that requires adjustments to the plan of care, it is advisable to convene an additional meeting to ensure that any new needs have been identified and addressed.

In addition to the expected family-directed care management outcomes listed in Table 23-7, care management can improve quality of care and access to services. Combined, these outcomes ultimately contribute to reduced health care spending.

TABLE 23-7. The Coordinating Center Coordination Pathway Components and Outcomes

Components of Care Management	Care Management Outcomes
Medical Management	• Communication among primary and specialty physicians facilitated. • Criteria for medical stability established and optimal wellness maintained. • Goals for medical management established and reviewed as appropriate. • Physician notification and emergency protocol updated including notification of local emergency medical services system.
Plan of Care	• Plan of care developed by team and reviewed at designated intervals. • Cost of plan established. • Review of plan and use of services monthly or at designated interval.
Family as Care Manager	• Primary and backup caregiver are identified and trained. • Caregiver can identify and use medical equipment and supplies safely and efficiently. • Caregiver can access medications and understands purpose and regimen. • Caregiver can identify and access primary/specialty physicians as recommended. • Caregiver can identify and access all service providers and describe their role (eg, nursing and durable medical equipment). • Caregiver initiates reorder of supplies and develops system for monthly reorder. • Caregiver participates in development and implementation of education and/or rehabilitation plan. • Caregiver recognizes the role of the care manager and implements care management tasks as negotiated. • Caregiver participates in multidisciplinary team to review plan of care and develop home care goals. • Family is independent in coordinating care of the child and does not require ongoing professional care manager.
Nursing	• Copy of current physician orders obtained and distributed to appropriate team members. • Preauthorization in place for nursing services. • Nursing schedule in place. • Caregiver anticipates changes in authorization and develops alternate child care as needed.
Education and Rehabilitation	• Referrals to early intervention programs, educational system, or community rehab program initiated. • Education and/or rehabilitation goals identified. • Therapeutic and adaptive equipment needs addressed by multidisciplinary team. • Caregiver participates in educational meetings to develop and review long-term and short-term goals and services.

TABLE 23-7. The Coordinating Center Coordination Pathway
Components and Outcomes, continued

Components of Care Management	Care-Management Outcomes
Physical Environment	• Maintain safe environment for child's care. • Maintain utilities and phone service. • Maintain functional equipment and supplies in home. • Medical equipment in the home will be safe and accessible.
Community Resources	• Identify community resources presently used. • Identify other resources as indicated. • Caregiver initiates contact with relevant community agencies independently to access new supports.
Community Inclusion	• Plan for accessibility outside of home. • Travel transportation plan established for physician, educational services, and other desired destinations. • Special parking permits or license plates obtained. • Adaptive car seating/safety restraints obtained. • Wheelchair/adapted stroller obtained, if necessary. • Portable medical equipment available and charged.

Used with permission from The Coordinating Center.

Summary

The following should be included when discussing care management for
a child with high-technology needs:
- Care management plays a significant role in planning for care of the child
  dependent on technology. A proactive approach using care management
  to locate, coordinate, and monitor services for children with complex
  needs will improve quality of life and ensure optimal medical and
  psychosocial outcomes for home and community inclusion.
- Care management must continue to explore innovative ways to meet
  the needs of this complex population. Creative care-management interventions include investigation of the use of service animals, telemedicine,
  and the identification of other unconventional resources.
- Participation by care managers in advocacy groups and in the legislative
  and health policy arena can help shape standards and improve services
  available to families and children dependent on technology.

Bibliography

Bond N, Phillips P, Rollins JA. Family-centered care at home for families with children who are technology dependent. *Pediatr Nurs.* 1994;20:123-130

Leeka AB. Ethical delivery of specialized care beyond hospital walls. *Caring.* 1995;14:18-20, 22

Marsiglia C, Boyle S. *The Coordination Pathway.* Millersville, MD: The Coordinating Center; 1999

Chapter 24

Care of Low Birth Weight Infants in the Home

Judy Bernbaum, MD; JoAnn D'Agostino, RN, MSN, CPNP; Marsha Gerdes, PhD; Deborah Calvert, MSW, LSW

Infant Mortality and Changes in Neonatal Care

Low birth weight is a major factor affecting infant survival. However, improvements in neonatal care have had a significant effect on infant mortality. The rate of prematurity has remained relatively stable over several decades — approximately 7% of all live births are infants weighing less than 2,500 g and approximately 1.5% are infants weighing less than 1,500 g. In 1961, mortality for infants weighing 1,001 to 1,500 g was 50%. In the past decade mortality rate substantially decreased to less than 10% for infants of the same birth weight.

The outcome for infants with birth weights less than or equal to 1,500 g generally is favorable, with most studies showing 60% to 80% developing normally. However, the lower the gestational age and birth weight, the greater the risk for sequelae after discharge.

In addition, the presence of any neurologic insult or prolonged illness places the infant at further risk for adverse medical and neurodevelopmental sequelae. Infants most at risk include those with the following characteristics:

- Birth weight less than or equal to 1,500 g
- Small for gestational age (SGA) with symmetric SGA being most at risk
- Perinatal asphyxia
- Prolonged mechanical ventilation
- Central nervous system abnormalities
- Hyperbilirubinemia at a level requiring an exchange transfusion
- Chronic lung disease
- Perinatal infections
- Genetic or metabolic disorders

Preparation for Discharge of the Infant at High Risk

Because of the potential for ongoing problems after discharge, preparing an infant at high risk for discharge from the hospital begins with a thorough assessment of all aspects of the infant's care needs. The goal is to ensure a smooth transition from hospital to home with minimal disruption in the level of care. The process begins shortly after the infant's admission and is updated periodically over the course of the hospital stay. Table 24-1 lists the factors that should be assessed to determine the feasibility of discharge.

TABLE 24-1. Factors to Consider Prior to Discharge

- Infant's medical stability
- Adequate nutrition for optimal growth
- Maintenance of body temperature in an open crib
- Child's care at a level that is manageable at home
- Caregiver capable and comfortable with infant's care
- Community resources identified
- Insurance coverage identified and sufficient to cover infant's post-hospitalization needs
- Primary care and subspecialty providers identified and comfortable with provision of infant's care

As more infants with low birth weight enter the pediatric population, primary care providers must become confident in managing their unique medical conditions and developmental progress and recognizing early signs of neurologic disorders. Primary care providers play a major role in the identification of problems early. The primary care provider's role in discharge planning depends on the level of involvement in an infant's neonatal care. Neonatal intensive care in a tertiary care unit is directed by a neonatologist who generally will not be involved with providing primary care after discharge. The transition from the tertiary care setting to the community has the greatest potential for breakdown in communication. Therefore, it is important that there be good communication throughout the infant's hospital course and that the events of the entire hospitalization are reviewed just before the infant's discharge.

Most preterm infants spend time after discharge recovering from the neonatal intensive care unit (NICU) experience. Many are left with little in the way of residual problems. Others, however, leave the nursery with continuing health problems and need treatment for weeks or months, which often affects many aspects of their growth and development. Although they still require well-child care, many have needs that are far from routine. Special attention must be given to the following areas:

▶ Growth

The pattern of growth following discharge is a valuable indicator of an infant's well-being, particularly during the first 2 years of life. Aberrant growth may reflect a variety of disorders including inadequate caloric intake, chronic illness, feeding difficulties, abnormalities in gastrointestinal motility, or social or emotional difficulties. Although these factors can affect all infants discharged from nurseries, the preterm infant is particularly vulnerable to such problems. It is important to monitor nutritional intake closely and to interpret growth rates with a complete understanding of the infant's past history, current problems, and expectations for growth.

Many factors affect the growth of a preterm infant, including gestational age, birth weight, severity of neonatal illness, caloric intake, ongoing illnesses, environmental factors in the home, and heredity. Caloric requirements for a healthy, preterm infant generally exceed those of a normal term infant, especially during rapid catch-up growth. Chronic illnesses, such as broncho-pulmonary dysplasia, that increase caloric expenditure add to an infant's daily requirements. Malabsorption after necrotizing enterocolitis and chronic emesis from gastroesophageal reflux may impair growth because of increased losses. In contrast, decreased intake may be caused by fatigue, hypoxemia, oral motor dysfunction, or esophagitis from gastroesophageal reflux. Neurologic complications such as intraventricular hemorrhage or periventricular leukomalacia also may affect motor skills, which can result in feeding problems. Finally, infants with intrauterine growth retardation caused by congenital infections, chromosomal abnormalities, or other syndromes may never achieve optimal growth.

Patterns of Growth

When evaluating the growth of a low birth weight infant, the gestational age should be taken into consideration. Growth parameters should be plotted on preterm growth charts according to the infant's adjusted age until 2½ years. Various patterns of growth emerge from different groups of patients.

Healthy, low birth weight, appropriate for gestational age (AGA) infants generally experience catch-up growth during the first 2 years of life with maximal growth rates between 36 and 44 weeks' postconception. Little catch-up growth occurs beyond a chronological age of 3 years. More than 80% of preterm infants who were AGA at birth will achieve normal growth reflecting the family's genetic makeup. Head circumference usually is the first parameter that demonstrates catch-up growth and commonly will fall at a higher percentile than weight or length during the first several months after discharge. Increases in weight commonly are followed by linear growth increases within several months. Because rapid head growth may represent the onset of post-hemorrhagic hydrocephalus, caution should be used when interpreting rapid head growth as catch-up growth in the preterm infant who has suffered a grade III or IV intraventricular hemorrhage. An imaging study may be necessary if the infant's history or symptoms suggest increasing intraventricular pressure. In contrast, a head circumference that measures more than three standard deviations below the mean often is associated with significant developmental disabilities. Head growth at 8 months of age is one of the best predictors of eventual growth and neuro-development. Slowing of head growth at 5 to 6 months of age is an ominous sign.

It is important to evaluate an infant's growth velocity for weight and length.

It is important to evaluate an infant's growth velocity for weight and length. Some infants will grow at a slow but progressive rate during this period. However, a low weight for length or a decline in all growth parameters suggests inadequate nutritional intake and may warrant further investigation. If a preterm infant's weight significantly exceeds length in percentiles, the possibility of overfeeding should be discussed with the family. Ironically, obesity may occur in a previously underweight preterm infant because of compensatory overfeeding or in an infant whose medical problems have resolved but whose diet remains high in calories.

Growth of the SGA infant is influenced strongly by the etiology of the intrauterine growth retardation. Most premature SGA infants have gradual improvement of height over the first 2 years of life, but severely SGA infants have the highest incidence of no catch-up growth by age 2. Symmetric SGA infants with head circumference at birth similar in percentile to birth weight are less likely to demonstrate catch-up growth than are SGA infants whose head circumference at the time of birth exceeds the percentiles for length and weight. As with AGA infants, head circumference normally is the first parameter to demonstrate catch-up, followed by weight and then by length.

Because of the wide range of growth that is considered within the normal range for preterm infants during the first several years of life, it is best to analyze trends rather than make assumptions based on single measurements. When abnormalities are noted in growth trends, investigation into the infant's nutritional status during hospitalization, the results of cranial sonography studies, and the status of continuing illnesses should be undertaken to identify a possible cause.

▸ Nutritional Requirements

Traditionally, although somewhat controversial, the goal for preterm infants is to achieve a growth rate approximating the expected fetal growth rate at the same postconceptional age. Because weight gain is suboptimal during acute illness, all efforts should be made to promote catch-up growth once the medical condition is stable. The nutritional needs of the preterm infant during the first few months of life exceed those of a term infant and may persist for the first year of life. Caloric requirements for adequate growth vary. Healthy preterm infants generally require 110 to 130 kcal/kg/day but some infants with chronic disease may require up to 150 or more kcal/kg/day. Caloric intake should be increased as tolerated until weight gain is satisfactory.

Special considerations should be given to the following situations:

Infant Discharged on Breast Milk

Because of prolonged illness, delayed initiation of breastfeeding, or low milk supply because of maternal stress and mechanical expression of milk, infants may not be fully breastfed by the time of discharge. The primary care provider will then be responsible for providing guidance on how to safely progress to full breastfeedings, monitoring for signs of dehydration and adequate growth. Additional supplements (Table 24-2) may be necessary and can be provided through breast milk fortification offered by bottle or use of supplemental nursing systems.

TABLE 24-2. Common Caloric Supplements

Supplement	kcal/mL	Properties
Vegetable oil	9	Inexpensive; must blend into formula
Medium-chain Triglycerides oil	7.6	Expensive; must blend into formula
Microlipids	4.5	Expensive; can be difficult to obtain (order through pharmacy and some home agencies)
Dry baby cereal	10 kcal/T	Readily available; inexpensive; may help with gastroesophageal reflux
Polycose glucose Polymers	2 (liquid) 3.8 kcal/g (powder)	Well-tolerated; order through pharmacy

Adapted from Bernbaum. *A Practical Guide to the Office Management of the Preterm Infant.* Columbus, OH: Ross Publications; 2000.

Note: Caloric supplements dilute the nutrient density of a formula. Preterm infants who require supplementation generally need additional nutrients as well as calories. For this reason, using a nutrient-dense formula or concentrating the formula (to 24 cal/fl oz) may be preferred to adding a caloric supplement.

Infant Discharged on Formula

As a result of rapid growth rates experienced after initial hospital discharge, preterm infants often require higher caloric intake for optimal growth. Formulas specially designed to meet the special nutrient and caloric needs of the growing premature infant after discharge are available. These typically are formulated to provide 22 kcal/oz. In general, these formulas are appropriate for the first 9 months of chronologic (postnatal) age. If additional calories are required because of inadequate growth, formula can be concentrated or nutritional supplements can be added (Table 24-3).

Infant Discharged on Supplemental Tube Feedings

Because supplemental tube feedings are an additional stress to families of infants at high risk, careful consideration should be given to determine when this is necessary (Table 24-3). Infants who typically require post-discharge supplemental tube feedings include those with significant neurological impairment, feeding dysfunction, chronic lung disease, or infants who have plateaued in their progression to oral feedings despite meeting all other criteria for discharge. The primary care provider frequently is responsible for monitoring weight gain, adjusting nutrient intake to meet caloric requirements, adjusting feeding schedules to encourage oral feeding readiness, and monitoring for conditions that may impede oral feeding such

TABLE 24-3. Issues in Home Enteral Feedings in Infants

- Feedings may be given orally throughout the day and by tube at night (either bolus or at a continuous rate). This should be considered as long as the infant has progressed in feeding skills such that at least one half of the required daily volume of feedings is being taken by mouth.

- If continuous feedings are given through the night, stop them at least 2 hours before the infant awakens to allow enough time for hunger cues to develop by the first morning feeding. Gradually decrease amounts given at night to support increased appetite during the day.

- If the nasogastric tube results in increased gagging or interferes with oral feedings, consider removing the tube during the day.

- If the infant has what seems to be a blunted appetite for oral feedings, the volume of feedings given by tube may be excessive or scheduled too closely together. Adjust feeding volumes and schedules to allow hunger cues to develop.

- If oral intake is close to being adequate, tube feedings may be discontinued for a trial period. Weight and urine/stool output should be monitored closely during this time. A temporary plateau or modest decline in weight ($\leq 5\%$) may be acceptable for a week or two only if the infant is otherwise healthy and well nourished and maintains adequate hydration status.

- Once adequate weight gain is established with oral feedings alone, gradually decrease the excess concentration of feedings and/or discontinue supplements.

- If the feeding tube has been surgically placed, maintenance of adequate oral feedings over a 1-month period usually is required before removal of the feeding tube is considered.

as gastroesophageal reflux or hypoxia. Timely referral to a feeding specialist should be encouraged to promote oral feedings.

As the infant's oral skills progress and feeding volumes approach adequacy, tube feedings can gradually be decreased and eventually discontinued. The weaning process can be accomplished in a variety of ways and should be individualized based on the infant's and family's needs and circumstances.

▶ Gastroesophageal Reflux

Most infants regurgitate small amounts of feedings, usually because of physiologic immaturity. If health and growth are not affected, regurgitation is not considered a significant problem. It usually is managed with modest changes in feeding, handling, and positioning. Gastroesophageal reflux is a common cause of regurgitation affecting up to 50% of all newborns; it is even more common in preterm infants. It may be considered pathologic, requiring more aggressive intervention if it is associated with growth failure, feeding aversion, esophagitis, or respiratory compromise including apnea, reactive airways disease, or aspiration pneumonia. In these situations, pharmacologic interventions are often required.

▶ Immunizations

Preterm infants should receive the same immunizations as term infants on similar schedules without correcting for prematurity. The American Academy of Pediatrics Committee on Infectious Diseases recommends that full doses of diphtheria and tetanus toxoids and acellular pertussis (DTaP), *Haemophilus influenzae* type b (Hib), pneumococcal conjugate vaccine, inactivated polio, and measles–mumps–rubella (MMR) vaccines be administered to prematurely born infants at the appropriate *postnatal (chronologic) age*. For the DTaP vaccine, the pertussis component should not be withheld because of prematurity or underlying chronic disease (Table 24-4).

Hepatitis B vaccine should be withheld until the infant weighs more than 2 kg and can be initiated prior to hospital discharge if the preparation is free of thimerosal. Otherwise, delay administration until 2 months of age.

Special consideration should be given to the following:

Influenza Vaccine

Infants with chronic pulmonary disease or cardiac disease with pulmonary vascular congestion are at high risk for developing serious illnesses if infected with an influenza virus. To protect vulnerable infants, immunization with the influenza vaccine is indicated for household contacts, including siblings, primary caretakers, and home care nurses, as well as hospital personnel. For infants 6 months (chronologic age) or older, two doses of split-virus vaccine should be given 1 month apart between October and December followed by one annual dose. Adults and older siblings with natural immunity or who have received previous immunizations need only one yearly dose (Table 24-5).

Respiratory Syncytial Virus

The preterm infant is particularly at risk for the development of serious sequelae from respiratory syncytial virus (RSV) disease. It is the most common and serious infection in these infants and may result in the need for bronchodilator therapy, reinstitution of supplemental oxygen, rehospitalization, and, at times, ventilator support. Although a vaccine to protect against RSV disease still is unavailable, passive immunity can be provided in the form of a monoclonal antibody preparation (Synagis) or an immune globulin

TABLE 24-4. Recommended Childhood Immunization Schedule

Recommended Childhood Immunization Schedule
United States, 2002

	range of recommended ages					catch-up vaccination				preadolescent assessment		
Age ▶ **Vaccine ▼**	Birth	1 mo	2 mos	4 mos	6 mos	12 mos	15 mos	18 mos	24 mos	4-6 yrs	11-12 yrs	13-18 yrs
Hepatitis B[1]	Hep B #1 only if mother HBsAg(-)										Hep B series	
		Hep B #2			Hep B #3							
Diphtheria, Tetanus, Pertussis[2]			DTaP	DTaP	DTaP		DTaP			DTaP	Td	
Haemophilus influenzae type b[3]			Hib	Hib	Hib	Hib						
Inactivated Polio[4]			IPV	IPV		IPV				IPV		
Measles, Mumps, Rubella[5]						MMR #1				MMR #2	MMR #2	
Varicella[6]						Varicella					Varicella	
Pneumococcal[7]			PCV	PCV	PCV	PCV			PCV	PPV		
Hepatitis A[8]		Vaccines below this line are for selected populations								Hepatitis A series		
Influenza[9]						Influenza (yearly)						

This schedule indicates the recommended ages for routine administration of currently licensed childhood vaccines, as of December 1, 2001, for children through age 18 years. Any dose not given at the recommended age should be given at any subsequent visit when indicated and feasible. ▓▓▓ Indicates age groups that warrant special effort to administer those vaccines not previously given. Additional vaccines may be licensed and recommended during the year. Licensed combination vaccines may be used whenever any components of the combination are indicated and the vaccine's other components are not contraindicated. Providers should consult the manufacturers' package inserts for detailed recommendations.

Approved by the Advisory Committee on Immunization Practices (www.cdc.gov/nip/acip), the American Academy of Pediatrics (www.aap.org), and the American Academy of Family Physicians (www.aafp.org).

1. **Hepatitis B vaccine (Hep B).** All infants should receive the first dose of hepatitis B vaccine soon after birth and before hospital discharge; the first dose may also be given by age 2 months if the infant's mother is HBsAg-negative. Only monovalent hepatitis B vaccine can be used for the birth dose. Monovalent or combination vaccine containing Hep B may be used to complete the series; 4 doses of vaccine may be administered if combination vaccine is used. The second dose should be given at least 4 weeks after the first dose, except for Hib-containing vaccine which cannot be administered before age 6 weeks. The third dose should be given at least 16 weeks after the first dose and at least 8 weeks after the second dose. The last dose in the vaccination series (third or fourth dose) should not be administered before age 6 months.
   Infants born to HBsAg-positive mothers should receive hepatitis B vaccine and 0.5 mL hepatitis B immune globulin (HBIG) within 12 hours of birth at separate sites. The second dose is recommended at age 1-2 months and the vaccination series should be completed (third or fourth dose) at age 6 months.
   Infants born to mothers whose HBsAg status is unknown should receive the first dose of the hepatitis B vaccine series within 12 hours of birth. Maternal blood should be drawn at the time of delivery to determine the mother's HBsAg status; if the HBsAg test is positive, the infant should receive HBIG as soon as possible (no later than age 1 week).

2. **Diphtheria and tetanus toxoids and acellular pertussis vaccine (DTaP).** The fourth dose of DTaP may be administered as early as age 12 months, provided 6 months have elapsed since the third dose and the child is unlikely to return at age 15-18 months. **Tetanus and diphtheria toxoids (Td)** is recommended at age 11-12 years if at least 5 years have elapsed since the last dose of tetanus and diphtheria toxoid-containing vaccine. Subsequent routine Td boosters are recommended every 10 years.

3. ***Haemophilus influenzae* type b (Hib) conjugate vaccine.** Three Hib conjugate vaccines are licensed for infant use. If PRP-OMP (PedvaxHIB® or ComVax® [Merck]) is administered at ages 2 and 4 months, a dose at age 6 months is not required. DTaP/Hib combination products should not be used for primary immunization in infants at ages 2, 4 or 6 months, but can be used as boosters following any Hib vaccine.

4. **Inactivated polio vaccine (IPV).** An all-IPV schedule is recommended for routine childhood polio vaccination in the United States. All children should receive 4 doses of IPV at ages 2 months, 4 months, 6-18 months, and 4-6 years.

5. **Measles, mumps, and rubella vaccine (MMR).** The second dose of MMR is recommended routinely at age 4-6 years but may be administered during any visit, provided at least 4 weeks have elapsed since the first dose and that both doses are administered beginning at or after age 12 months. Those who have not previously received the second dose should complete the schedule by the 11-12 year old visit.

6. **Varicella vaccine.** Varicella vaccine is recommended at any visit at or after age 12 months for susceptible children, ie, those who lack a reliable history of chickenpox. Susceptible persons aged ≥13 years should receive 2 doses, given at least 4 weeks apart.

7. **Pneumococcal vaccine.** The heptavalent **pneumococcal conjugate vaccine (PCV)** is recommended for all children age 23 months. It is also recommended for certain children age 24-59 months. **Pneumococcal polysaccharide vaccine (PPV)** is recommended in addition to PCV for certain high-risk groups. See *MMWR* 2000;49(RR-9);1-35.

8. **Hepatitis A vaccine.** Hepatitis A vaccine is recommended for use in selected states and regions, and for certain high-risk groups; consult your local public health authority. See *MMWR* 1999;48(RR-12);1-37.

9. **Influenza vaccine.** Influenza vaccine is recommended annually for children age ≥6 months with certain risk factors (including but not limited to asthma, cardiac disease, sickle cell disease, HIV, diabetes; see *MMWR* 2001;50(RR-4);1-44), and can be administered to all others wishing to obtain immunity. Children aged ≤12 years should receive vaccine in a dosage appropriate for their age (0.25 mL if age 6-35 months or 0.5 mL if aged ≥3 years). Children aged ≤8 years who are receiving influenza vaccine for the first time should receive 2 doses separated by at least 4 weeks.

For additional information about vaccines, vaccine supply, and contraindications for immunization, please visit the National Immunization Program Web site at www.cdc.gov/nip or call the National Immunization Hotline at 800/232-2522 (English) or 800/232-0233 (Spanish).

This immunization schedule is updated annually. Please access the current schedule at http://www.aap.org/family/parents/immunize.htm.

TABLE 24-5. Recommended Doses of Split-Virus Influenza Vaccine*

0.25 mL	(6 to 35 months)
0.50 mL	(3 years and greater)

*Dosages are those recommended in recent years. Product circular should be reviewed yearly to determine the appropriate dosage.

intravenous (IGIV) specially formulated to provide a high titer of anti-RSV antibodies (RespiGam).

Either palivizumab or RSV-IGIV should be administered monthly beginning at the onset of the RSV season and terminated at the end of the RSV season. (The season generally runs from October through April, but varies regionally.) Indications for palivizumab and for RSV-IGIV appear in Tables 24-6 and 24-7.

Retinopathy of Prematurity and Other Visual Problems

Retinopathy of prematurity (ROP) is a disorder that interrupts the normal vascularization of the developing retina. It occurs primarily in infants at 32 weeks' gestation or younger. The lower the gestational age, the higher the incidence of ROP, with a 40% incidence among those infants at 28 weeks or younger increasing to a 70% incidence for those at 24 weeks' gestation or younger. Most cases of ROP resolve spontaneously, but even with complete resolution, scarring of the retina may occur. The initial examination should not take place before 4 to 6 weeks' chronologic age because a vitreous haze may interfere with visualization of the retina and the yield for identifying ROP is low. The initial examination should be at 7 to 9 weeks of age to catch the peak period during which ROP occurs. A schedule of follow-up visits is based on the initial findings. All infants with immature fundi or any stage of ROP require close monitoring until the eyes have matured or the ROP has completely resolved. Thereafter, follow-up to assess for refractive errors should be at 1 year of age and before kindergarten, or earlier if there are clinical signs.

Sequelae of ROP depends largely on the extent of retinal scarring. As many as 80% of stage 3 ROP cases resolve spontaneously without significant scarring, but there may be subtle retinal changes resulting in refractive errors, strabismus, or amblyopia. Early identification of a child with a visual disability

TABLE 24-6. Use of Palivizumab (Synagis)

Recommendations

1. Palivizumab or RSV-IGIV Prophylaxis should be considered for infants and children younger than 2 years of age with CLD who have required medical therapy for their CLD within 6 months before the anticipated RSV season. Palivizumab is preferred for most high-risk children because of its ease of administration, safety, and effectiveness. Patients with more severe CLD may benefit from prophylaxis for two RSV seasons, especially those who require medical therapy. Decisions regarding individual patients may need additional consultation from neonatologists, intensivists, or pulmonologists. There are limited data on the efficacy of palivizumab during the second year of age; risk of severe RSV disease exists for children with CLD who require medical therapy. Although those with less severe underlying disease may receive some benefit for the second season, immunoprophylaxis may not be necessary.

2. Infants born at 32 weeks of gestation or earlier without CLD or who do not meet the criteria in recommendation 1 also may benefit from RSV prophylaxis. In these Infants, major risk factors to consider are gestational age and chronologic age at the start of the RSV season. Infants born at 28 weeks of gestation or earlier may benefit from prophylaxis up to 12 months of age. Infants born at 29 to 32 weeks of gestation may benefit most from prophylaxis up to 6 months of age. Decisions regarding duration of prophylaxis should be individualized, according to the duration of the RSV season. Practitioners may wish to use RSV rehospitalization data from their own region to assist in the decision-making process.

3. Given the large number of patients born between 32 to 35 weeks and the cost of the drug, the use of palivizumab in this population should be reserved for those infants with additional risk factors until more data are available.

4. Palivizumab and RSV-IGIV are not licensed by the FDA for patients with CHD. Available data indicate that RSV-IGIV is contraindicated in patients with cyanotic CHD. However, patients with CLD, who are premature, or both, who meet the criteria in recommendations 1 and 2 and who also have asymptomatic acyanotic CHD (eg, patent ductus arteriosus or ventricular septal defect) may benefit from prophylaxis.

5. Palivizumab or RSV-IGIV prophylaxis has not been evaluated in randomized trials in immunocompromised children. Although specific recommendations for immunocompromised patients cannot be made, children with severe immunodeficiencies (eg, severe combined immunodeficiency or severe acquired immunodeficiency syndrome) may benefit from prophylaxis. If these infants and children are receiving standard immune globulin intravenous (IGIV) monthly, physicians may consider substituting RSV-IGIV during the RSV season.

6. RSV prophylaxis should be initiated at the onset of the RSV season and terminated at the end of the RSV season. In most areas of the United States, the usual time for the beginning of RSV outbreaks is October to December, and termination is March to May, but regional differences occur. The onset of RSV infection occurs earlier in southern states than in northern states. Practitioners should contact their health departments and/or diagnostic virology laboratories in their geographic areas to determine the optimal time to begin administration.

7. RSV is known to be transmitted in the hospital setting and to cause serious disease in high-risk infants. In high-risk hospitalized infants, the major means to prevent RSV disease is strict observance of infection control practices, including the use of rapid means to identify and cohort RSV-infected infants. If an RSV outbreak is documented in a high-risk unit (eg, pediatric intensive care unit), primary emphasis should be placed on proper infection control practices. The need for and efficacy of prophylaxis in these situations has not been evaluated.

8. The guidelines for modification of immunizations after RSV-IGIV have not changed. Palivizumab does not interfere with the response to vaccines.

Reprinted from American Academy of Pediatrics, Committee on Infectious Diseases and Committee on Fetus and Newborn. Prevention of respiratory syncytial virus infections: indications for the use of palivizumab and update on the use of RSV-IGIV. *Pediatrics.* 1998;102:1211-1216

TABLE 24-7. Use of RSV-IGIV (RespiGam)

Respiratory syncytial virus (RSV)-immune globulin intravenous (IGIV) provides additional protection against other respiratory viral illnesses and should be considered in certain selected infants at high risk. However, it requires intravenous access, large volumes (15 mL/kg) of fluid, and several hours to administer – all on a monthly basis.

Consider RSV-IGIV for

1. Infants receiving replacement IGIV (secondary to underlying immune deficiency or human immunodeficiency virus infection).

2. Infants with severe chronic lung disease who are bronchodilator, oxygen, or ventilator dependent and who are likely to develop severe sequelae from any viral respiratory-related illness, not only RSV.

The RSV-IGIV is contraindicated in children with cyanotic congenital heart disease.

is essential to provide the child and family with services available on county and state levels for children who are visually impaired.

Hearing Problems

The incidence of sensorineural hearing loss in preterm infants generally is reported to be between 1% and 3%. Several factors place these infants at particular risk for hearing loss, including birth weight less than 1,500 g, hypoxia, hyperbilirubinemia, prolonged mechanical ventilation, perinatal asphyxia, meningitis, and ototoxic drugs. Passing an initial hearing screening does not preclude the possibility of acquired hearing loss. Absent or abnormal responses to auditory stimulation, delays in speech development, poor articulation, or inattentiveness should raise the suspicion of hearing loss and lead to a more thorough evaluation. All infants who fail an initial hearing screening should be referred to an audiologist for further testing and intervention.

Neuromuscular Disorders

Abnormalities in muscle tone and reflexes during the first year of life are common, and have been reported in up to 70% of infants weighing less than 1,500 g. The most common abnormality seen is hypertonicity affecting the shoulder girdle, trunk, and/or lower extremities. Tone usually increases over the first few months, peaks at 3 to 6 months, then gradually resolves. Tone should be completely normalized by 18 months of age. Tone abnormalities, albeit transient, can negatively affect the acquisition or quality of motor milestones. Referral to intervention services should be initiated to help ameliorate the impact of these tonal abnormalities. Persistent abnormalities beyond 18 months' adjusted age associated with a delay in acquisition or quality of gross motor skills may be consistent with the diagnosis of cerebral palsy. The incidence of cerebral palsy has been reported in up to 6% of the preterm population, with the most common type being spastic diplegia. Consistent physical and/or occupational therapy services should be considered strongly in a child with the diagnosis of cerebral palsy to promote progression of skills and minimize orthopedic deformities such as contractures or subluxation. Referral to an orthopedist should be considered to monitor for hip dislocation and/or scoliosis.

Developmental Problems

Developmental surveillance of preterm infants takes on greater importance because these children are more likely to experience mild to moderate developmental problems. In addition, parents often are more anxious about their infant's progress. The diagnosis of disabilities in a low birth weight infant is a process that continues through the early years of life. The timing of diagnosis varies because of the variable learning rate during the preschool years, the difficulty of predicting learning, the strong influence of environment, and the learning experiences.

▶ Risk Factors for Developmental Disabilities

In addition to prematurity, there are other medical and environmental factors that place a child at risk for developmental disabilities. An important process in screening and diagnosing disabilities is the review of the child's history for factors that increase their individual risk (Table 24-8).

TABLE 24-8. Biologic and Environmental Risk Factors for Developmental Disabilities

Biologic Factors	Environmental Factors
• Extremely low birth weight	• Poverty
• Grade III or IV intraventricular hemorrhage	• Low parental educational level
• Periventricular leukomalacia with cystic changes	• Pattern of illicit drug use in the environment
• Prolonged bronchopulmonary dysplasia or any chronic illness	• Maternal depression or maternal mental illness
• Birth asphyxia	

▸ Mental Retardation

The incidence of mental retardation (IQ less than 70) is reported to be between 4% and 5% in the preterm population. Unless severe, diagnosis is often delayed until 4 years of age because developmental tests that correlate with school outcome cannot be used in the early years. Mental retardation is defined as

- Having significantly below-average intellectual functioning as measured by an individually administered, culturally fair IQ test
- Having deficits in adaptive and self-help behavior, with onset before 18 years of age

Mental retardation often is assumed to refer to only the most severe types of impairments. The anxiety of parents of a low birth weight infant who are informed of the possibility of mental retardation affecting their infant can be minimized by describing the four subtypes of mental retardation (Table 24-9).

The diagnosis of mental retardation generally is not applied to the infant and preschool population because many delays may be transient. It is possible that a deficit in a single area of a child's development can give the appearance of a global delay. Recovery from illness or environmental deprivation can also ameliorate early delays. It is appropriate to use the term *developmental delay* in the preschool population.

▸ Minor Disabilities

A high percentage of children born with low birth weight have intellectual outcomes that fall into the "slow learner" or "borderline" range of intelligence. These are children who are able to achieve the major developmental milestones within the normal range. However, their achievement in language and conceptual thinking lags slightly behind their age mates. In school, these children are at risk for lags in academic learning, but they may not qualify for services or be identified because of the mild degree of the lags. Unfortunately, this is an often unrecognized group who can benefit from services. Parents should be counseled to be aware of subtle learning lags and to offer support to their children. Teaching in a comfortable, supportive environment; learning through multiple teaching methods; and opportunities for practice are important.

TABLE 24-9. Four Subtypes of Mental Retardation

Category	Developmental Course	Educational Intervention	Expected Educational Outcome	Expected Life Skills Outcome
Mild MR*: IQ level= 50 to 70	• Slow attainment of milestones • Language within preschool years	• Varying degrees of inclusion in typical classes with special, individualized instruction	• Achievement at approximately the 6th-grade level	• Independent to semi-independent living
Moderate MR: IQ level= 35 to 55	• Slow attainment of milestones • Language within preschool years	• Special, individualized instruction with varying degrees of inclusion • Vocational instruction	• Achievement at early elementary school level	• Limited independent living • Sheltered workshops
Severe MR: IQ level= 20 to 40	• Language (often limited) develops during school years • Significant delays in acquisition of developmental milestones	• Special, individualized instruction • Emphasis on self-help, adaptive skills, and communication	• Pre-academic	• No independent living • Self-care (personal hygiene) can be expected
Profound MR	• Co-morbidities are frequent and include sensory deficits and cerebral palsy	• Special, individualized instruction and care; self-care; and sensory awareness	• Pre-academic	• No independent living • Variable levels of self-care

*MR = mental retardation.

▶ Learning Disabilities

It has become increasingly apparent that children born with low birth weight often experience significant functional learning impairments at school age. Learning problems affect the ability of a low birth weight child to comprehend math, reading, and other academic subjects. Related learning problems affect 11% to 45% of the preterm population.

These learning problems, best described as *learning deficits* or *learning disabilities,* are found in children with average intelligence and normal sensory acuity. Learning disabilities cannot be diagnosed before the child enters school.

▶ Available Resources

Educational intervention is available for children with learning disabilities in all public school districts. The process of obtaining these services is described in the public law PL94-142, the Individuals with Disabilities Education Act, which provides the framework for

- A process of identification
- A description of learning disabilities
- Provision of services in the least restrictive setting possible

It is important to offer support to the child and family and suggest alternative approaches if academic frustrations develop.

▶ Developmental Interventions for Young Children

Early intervention programs have proven valuable for children with special needs or who are disadvantaged. The intervention must be designed to meet the individual needs of each child. The goals of the program are to maximize the individual child's potential, improve family well-being, and ready the child for the least restrictive setting at school age. The intervention should include services in which the family is an important member of the inter-disciplinary team and helps prioritize goals for the child.

The characteristics of a well-designed early intervention program include the ability to maximize the child's potential, use of an individualized program, and presence of an appropriately trained staff. Positive outcomes of early intervention can be found in the improved developmental progress in the child and support for families. Referrals should be made when there are delays in development, atypical or unusual developmental characteristics, or parental concerns.

Legislation

Federal legislation provides for early intervention services for all children from birth to 3 years of age who demonstrate developmental delays or have a diagnosis that places them at risk for delays. These services are available in all states; however, each state determines its own definition of developmental delay and the appropriate services that should be provided. Generally, services should be family focused, multidisciplinary in service, and provided in the child's natural environment.

Family Adjustment

The stresses on families of preterm infants during hospitalization are overt and dramatic. For families of preterm infants who require attention at home, the stress continues to be significant after discharge. Because of these home care needs, the family centers their attention on the child and normal activities may become difficult. As a result, siblings often feel neglected. Not only has a new baby come home, but the baby demands extra attention. The stress of caring for a child with a medical condition also can strain the parents' relationship. Financial stress often adds to marital problems. It is often necessary for one parent to stay home and not work because of the medical needs of the child. Inadequate insurance coverage along with additional expenses all contribute to increased conflict for families. Exacerbating the situation is the sense of isolation felt by families caring for a child with a chronic illness at home.

The effect on these families after discharge is described in the following three phases (the severity and timing vary among families):

1. **Euphoria.** Euphoria occurs during the first few weeks after discharge. Parents experience the thrill of having their child home. They finally feel like parents.

2. **Despair.** The parent's support system from the NICU is gone and families and friends in the community are often unable to understand what the family is going through. Exhaustion may prevail. Parents may realize that their child is much sicker and at higher risk for developmental problems than they thought.

3. **Acceptance.** Parents start to integrate the child with complex medical needs into their lives. By accepting their child and the attendant life style, the family is able to resume a more normal life.

▶ Vulnerable Child Syndrome

Despite a child's recovery from illness, some parents continue to experience anxiety because they perceive their child as fragile, vulnerable, and having special needs. This behavior by the parents can adversely affect the child's behavior and negatively affect the child's normal acquisition of develop-

mental skills. The parents' perception of a child's vulnerability persists for
the following reasons:

1. A history of infertility, miscarriages, stillbirth, or intrauterine demise.
2. Questions about the infant's survival that preoccupied the parents'
   emotions during hospitalization linger after discharge.
3. Parents may lack confidence in their parenting ability. This may be
   because of an interruption in the normal development of parenting
   skills as a result of prolonged hospitalization or persistent feelings that
   the hospital staff is more competent at caregiving.
4. Concern over problems with the child's future development often
   leads to parental feelings that the child perpetually remains sick, is
   different from other children, and warrants special status in the family.
   This can result in the inability to distinguish minor health problems
   from serious problems, causing parents to overuse medical services.

Parent-child behavior problems frequently result in feeding and/or sleeping problems. Another problem is difficulty in separation from parents. The
mother, in particular, may think that she is the only one capable of providing
care. Families also may overindulge their child and have difficulty in setting
age-appropriate disciplinary limits, interfering with normal development.
The child becomes dependent, demanding, and out of control; the child,
not the parent, is running the household.

What can be done to prevent vulnerable child syndrome?

1. Parents of preterm infants need more time with their primary
   care physician because of the anxiety over the medical status of
   the preterm child.
2. It is important to establish rapport with the family, being sensitive
   to the family's needs and providing support.
3. Families need to feel comfortable in expressing fears and concerns.
4. Families should be encouraged to normalize the caregiving of their
   preterm infant and daily activities as they are able, which is critical
   in the development of a healthy parent-child relationship.
5. Encourage families to be firm and establish disciplinary limits and
   schedules. Give them permission to set limits and be in control.
6. Educate parents about adjusted age for preterm infants. Communicate
   that developmental delays are common and, in most cases, temporary.

7. It is important that infants with developmental delay be enrolled in early intervention programs as soon as possible. The intervention program promotes developmental progress and provides an opportunity for parental involvement and support.
8. Parents should be encouraged to join community support groups or to seek counseling.
9. Recognize parents' concerns and provide a careful explanation and continued clarification of the infant's true health status. This can alleviate unnecessary concerns and promote more effective use of the primary care physician.

Summary

Caring for low birth weight infants is challenging. The following should be included in any home care program:

- Care of the preterm infant after discharge is a challenge for the pediatric home care team. All premature infants should be monitored through infancy, preschool, and school years because of common medical, neurological, and developmental concerns inherent in this population of children.
- Medical providers need to identify the preterm infants who are at greatest risk for ongoing problems so that those children can be closely monitored for the development of later sequelae.
- Infants who are at risk should be referred to early intervention programs and families should be given support through the pediatrician and community resources.

Bibliography

American Academy of Pediatrics. *2000 Red Book: Report of the Committee on Infectious Diseases.* Pickering LK, ed. 25th ed. Elk Grove Village, IL: American Academy of Pediatrics; 2000

American Academy of Pediatrics, Committee on Infectious Diseases and Committee on Fetus and Newborn. Prevention of respiratory syncytial virus infections: indication for the use of palivizumab and update on the use of RSV-IGIV. *Pediatrics.* 1998;102:1211-1216

American Academy of Pediatrics, Committee on Nutrition. Nutritional needs of preterm infants. In: Kleinman RE, ed. *Pediatric Nutrition Handbook.* 4th ed. Elk Grove Village, IL: American Academy of Pediatrics; 1998:55-87

American Psychiatric Association. *Diagnostic and Statistical Manual of Mental Disorders.* 4th ed. Washington, DC: American Psychiatric Association; 1994

Bernbaum. *A Practical Guide to the Office Management of the Preterm Infant.* Columbus, OH: Ross Publications; 2000

Casey PH, Kraemer HC, Bernbaum J, Yogman MW, Sells JC. Growth status and growth rates of a varied sample of low birth weight, preterm infants: a longitudinal cohort from birth to three years of age. *J Pediatr.* 1991;119:599-605

Hokken-Koelega AC, De Ridder MA, Lemmen RJ, Den Hartog H, De Muinck Keizer-Schrama SM, Drop SL. Children born small for gestational age: do they catch up? *Pediatr Res.* 1995;38:267-271

Hussain N, Clive J, Bhandari V. Current incidence of retinopathy of prematurity, 1989-1997. *Pediatrics.* 1999;104:e26. Available at: http://www.pediatrics.org/cgi/content/full/104/3/e26. Accessed October 5, 2001

Marino AJ, Assing E, Carbone MT, Hiatt IM, Hegyi T, Graff M. The incidence of gastroesophageal reflux in preterm infants. *J Perinatol.* 1995;15:369-371

Chapter 25

Short-bowel Syndrome and Enteral Feedings

Gilberto R. Pereira, MD; Beth Leonberg, MS, RD, CSP

Introduction

Short-bowel syndrome (SBS) is defined as the malabsorption that follows substantial congenital shortening or postnatal resection of the small or large intestine. It is a chronic condition that requires parenteral nutrition and specialized enteral feedings for several months or a few years after birth. Consequently, the treatment of this condition has great implications for the home health care of affected infants. This chapter reviews the etiology of SBS, the pathophysiology of SBS, the process of intestinal adaptation that follows surgical resection, the methods of enteral feeding, the types of enteral feeding, the medical and surgical therapies required by infants with SBS, and the clinical and laboratory parameters used for patient monitoring.

Etiology of Short-bowel Syndrome

A significant number of patients with SBS (20% to 50%) acquire this condition soon after birth, most commonly after the surgical treatment of necrotizing enterocolitis. Other etiologies include multiple intestinal atresias (12% to 31%), midgut volvulus (6% to 12%), extensive aganglionosis (6% to 12%), and omphalocele or gastroschisis (8% to 12%). The site and the length of the intestinal resection have the greatest effects on the clinical manifestation and treatment of SBS. Table 25-1 summarizes the different sites of enzyme secretion and nutrient absorption along the gastrointestinal tract.

Pathophysiology of Short-bowel Syndrome

Loss of the stomach results in decreased secretion of pepsin and intrinsic factor, impairing protein digestion and vitamin B_{12} absorption. The absorption of medium-chain triglycerides (MCTs) by the stomach is impaired but often compensated by the absorption of MCTs in the jejunum and ileum. The response of the stomach to massive intestinal loss is hypergas-

TABLE 25-1. Sites of Secretion and Absorption Along the Gastrointestinal Tract

Sites	Secretion	Absorption
Stomach	Gastric lipase Hydrogen chloride, pepsin Intrinsic factor	Medium-chain triglycerides
Duodenum	Pancreatic trypsin Lipase, amylase	Iron, calcium, magnesium, folate, glucose Water-soluble vitamins Bicarbonate
Jejunum	Secretin Cholecystokinin Disaccharidases: lactase, sucrase, and maltase	Amino acids, fats Zinc, phosphorus, bile acids Conjugated bile salts
Ileum	Enteroglucagon Peptide YY	Vitamins B_{12}, A, D, E, K Intrinsic factor, cholesterol
Colon	Potassium, bicarbonate	Chloride, sodium, water, oxalate Short-chain fatty acids

trinemia, which results in gastric hypersecretion in approximately 50% of patients with SBS. This hypergastrinemia is secondary to the loss of the normal feedback that shuts down gastric secretion in response to an increase in acid load in the small intestine. Hyperacidity can lead to peptic ulcer disease, esophagitis, and impairments in intraluminal micelle formation, stomach protein digestion, and pancreatic lipase activation.

The duodenum and the jejunum have a greater capacity for nutrient absorption than the ileum, being the primary sites for absorption of iron, calcium, magnesium, folate, glucose, and water-soluble vitamins. Loss of the duodenum and jejunum results in severe mineral and nutrient deficiencies, steatorrhea, and cholestasis.

The ileum is the primary site for the absorption of bile acids, conjugated bile salts, vitamin B_{12}, zinc, and fat-soluble vitamins. Loss of the ileum can result in vitamin deficiencies, steatorrhea, diarrhea, and fat malabsorption. The ileum also is the site for the production of peptide YY, a gastrointestinal hormone that delays gastrointestinal transit time in response to the presence of fat in the small intestine. Resection of the ileum eliminates this adaptive response. The ileocecal valve regulates the flow of enteric contents from the ileum to the colon, slowing down gastrointestinal transit time and improving fluid and nutrient absorption. While the presence of the ileocecal valve no longer is considered critical for the survival of patients with SBS, its resection adversely affects the process of intestinal adaptation and prolongs weaning off parenteral nutrition.

The colon, especially its ascending part, is the primary site for the absorption of water and sodium and for the excretion of potassium and bicarbonate. Loss of the colon can lead to hypovolemia, dehydration, and electrolyte abnormalities. Carbohydrates that were malabsorbed can adversely affect colonic function by the small intestine. This can result in an increased osmotic load to the colon, causing fluid and electrolyte losses.

Intestinal Adaptation

The process of physiologic adaptation is a response that occurs after massive intestinal resection. The remaining gut surface area progressively increases over time by means of mucosal hyperplasia, deepening of the crypts, lengthening of the villi, increments in hormone production and enzyme synthesis, and by delay in gastrointestinal transit time. The intestinal adaptation process is slow and, in some patients, might take as long as 2 to 3 years. In infants who acquired SBS during the neonatal period, no further intestinal adaptation is seen after the age of 3 years. Factors known to enhance the process of intestinal adaptation include the administration of intraluminal nutrients; the presence of endogenous secretions, principally pancreaticobiliary; and circulating gut hormones such as enteroglucagon.

Several clinical factors have been associated with improvements in the outcome of patients with SBS. The length of the residual small bowel after initial surgery and the preservation of the ileocecal valve have the strongest correlations with the length of time necessary to achieve complete intestinal adaptation and weaning off parenteral nutrition. Other factors include the site of intestinal resection (ileum has greater adaptation potential than jejunum), the gestational age of the infant (premature infants have greater intestinal growth potential than full-term infants), and the adequacy of the parenteral nutrition support to maintain growth and to replace nutrient losses. Conversely, the occurrence of bacterial overgrowth and associated enterocolitis has been reported to impair the adaptation process by prolonging the course of parenteral nutrition. A recent study showed that it is possible to estimate the duration of parenteral nutrition on patients with SBS early in the newborn period. This estimation can be made by an equation that takes into account the length of the residual small bowel after initial surgery and the daily energy intake tolerated by the administration of enteral feedings.

Methods of Enteral Feeding

It is essential that enteral feedings be introduced to the patient with SBS as early as possible to promote gut adaptation and to minimize the risk of developing liver disease. During transition from parenteral nutrition support and up to the time that the child is able to support appropriate growth through oral intake, enteral feedings by tube represent the primary source of nutrition support. Nasogastric tubes are most often used to initiate enteral feedings. If nasogastric feedings are well tolerated and the anticipated duration of supplemental feedings is short (3 to 6 months), the nasogastric tube may continue to be used until supplemental feedings are no longer needed.

If reflux, delayed gastric emptying, or frequent emesis occurs, tolerance to feedings may be improved by placing the tip of the tube just past the pylorus in the duodenum. Using a naso-duodenal feeding tube with a weighted tip helps keep the tube in the small bowel; placement should be checked with an x-ray before feeds are initiated. Placing the tube too far into the small bowel must be avoided to prevent rapid transit of feedings through the bowel, which may cause an increase in malabsorption and in stool output.

Oral feeding should be maintained simultaneously with tube feedings to promote normal development of feeding skills. If oral feeding skills are not achieved during the first year, especially during the critical period of 9 to 12 months, feeding aversion often develops. The treatment of this condition requires intensive behavioral and oral motor therapy. For the child with very short bowel associated with oral motor delay or feeding aversion, transition to full oral feeding may take months or years to achieve. For this child, placement of a gastrostomy tube is indicated at initial surgery or after several months of nasogastric feedings. Because of previous surgery to the bowel, percutaneous endoscopic gastrostomy tubes often are contraindicated, requiring a surgically placed gastrostomy tube. Once an established track for the tube is achieved, skin-level gastrostomy devices such as the button can be placed. These devices are invisible below clothing and help the child to feel more comfortable in child care or school settings.

▶ Continuous Feedings

Enteral feedings typically are initiated as a continuous infusion administered by electric pump. Continuous administration of enteral feedings may promote better tolerance and absorption than bolus feedings. For those patients with severe SBS who require home parenteral nutrition support, tube feedings and parenteral feedings often are given simultaneously overnight. Nighttime administration of continuous feedings allows for maximization of oral feedings during the day. The rate of administration of continuous feedings should be based on the age and size of the infant or child. Feedings are initiated slowly and advanced as tolerated to the volume estimated to meet calorie needs for growth and development. Once tolerated, feeding rates may be advanced further to shorten the infusion period and to minimize the length of time the child remains attached to the pump.

▶ Bolus Feedings

Alternatively, feedings may be delivered as boluses, either by gravity or by pump, over short infusion periods. This type of feeding often is less tolerated by patients with SBS because it may result in a dumping syndrome or in osmotic diarrhea. However, bolus feedings may be appropriate and better tolerated later in the course of SBS, when gut adaptation has progressed but the child still is unable to take adequate calories orally. A combination of bolus and continuous feedings can be used to maximize absorption and promote a more normal feeding schedule. It is extremely important to choose a schedule and method of administration that meet the family's lifestyle and the child's developmental needs.

Types of Enteral Feeding

Choosing an enteral feeding formula for the child with SBS requires careful consideration of multiple factors, including the child's age, site and extent of resection, and degree of malabsorption present. There is controversy over the necessity of using formulas with modified protein, fat, or carbohydrate content. However, standard cow's milk or soy-based infant and pediatric formulas generally are not well absorbed or tolerated by patients in the early stages of intestinal adaptation. Standard formulas may be used later in the course of treatment after adaptation has occurred, but the need for calories to support normal growth and development cannot be met by oral intake alone. Table 25-2 provides guidelines for distinguishing the types of formulas available for patients with SBS and their indications for use.

Human milk (breast milk) or infant formulas are indicated for at least the first year of life and may be used for longer periods, depending on tolerance and nutrient requirements. Pediatric formulas are designed for children from 1 to 10 years of age but may be used for older children and adolescents. Adult formulas often are the best choice for older children and adolescents, but they should be carefully evaluated to determine whether nutrient needs are being met in the smaller volumes administered to provide the calorie needs of the child.

Though there is some controversy about whether they are required, elemental formulas typically are used at initiation of enteral feedings. These formulas contain protein in the form of synthetic-free amino acids to maximize absorption and minimize allergic response. In addition, they contain a greater percentage of fat calories than MCTs. Medium-chain triglycerides are beneficial for patients with fat malabsorption because they are absorbed more readily than long chain fats. Elemental formulas are lactose free and contain glucose and glucose polymers as carbohydrate sources.

Oral feedings should be introduced when appropriate for the chronological and developmental age of the child.

Formulas derived from hydrolyzed cow's milk protein may be well tolerated in infants and children with resections of isolated segments of the bowel or in transition from an elemental diet to one containing intact nutrients. These formulas contain proteins of low molecular weight that are readily absorbed. Short-chain peptides have been shown to be beneficial in promoting intestinal adaptation following resection. Like elemental formulas, hydrolyzed protein and peptide-based formulas are relatively low in fat, contain MCT oil, and are lactose free.

Oral feedings should be introduced when appropriate for the chronological and developmental age of the child. Complex carbohydrates such as cereal and vegetables generally are well tolerated. Simple sugars such as sucrose or fructose may cause osmotic diarrhea and should be avoided; most

TABLE 25-2. Composition of Enteral Formulas for Patients With Short-bowel Syndrome

Category	Features	Available Products		Composition		
				% Carbohydrates	% Protein	% Fat
Free amino acid, fat modified, lactose free	Composed entirely of synthetic free amino acids with no intact protein.	Infant:	Neocate® (SHS North America)	47% corn syrup solids	12% free amino acids	41% safflower, coconut, and soy oils
	Contains increased medium-chain triglycerides (MCT).	Pediatric:	Neocate One Plus® (SHS North America)	58% corn syrup solids	10% free amino acids	32% MCT, coconut, canola, and safflower oils
			Elecare® (Ross)	43% corn syrup solids	12% free amino acids	43% high-oleic safflower, soy, and fractionated coconut oils
			Vivonex Pediatric® (Sandoz)	63% maltodextrin and modified starch	12% free amino acids	25% MCT and soy oil
Protein hydrolysate, fat modified, lactose free	Composed of short-chain peptides derived from hydrolyzed protein.	Infant:	Pregestimil® (Mead Johnson)	41% corn syrup solids, modified corn starch, and dextrose	11% casein hydrolysate	48% MCT, corn, soy and safflower oils
			Alimentum® (Ross)	41% sucrose and modified tapioca starch	11% casein hydrolysate	48% MCT, safflower, and soy oils
		Pediatric:	Peptamen Jr.® (Nestle)	55% maltodextrin and starch	12% hydrolyzed whey	33% MCT, soy and canola oils, lecithin

TABLE 25-2. Composition of Enteral Formulas for Patients With Short-bowel Syndrome, continued

Category	Features	Available Products		% Carbohydrates	Composition % Protein	% Fat
Polymeric	Composed of intact and complex macronutrients. Balanced in fat, carbo-hydrate, and protein to mimic an oral diet consumed ad libitum.	Infant:	Cow's milk and soy-based formulas	40%-44% lactose, maltodextrins, sucrose, or corn syrup solids	8%-12% cow's milk, whey, or soy proteins	46%-49% palm olein, coconut, sunflower, or soy oils
		Pediatric:	Pediasure® (Ross)	44% hydrolyzed corn starch and sucrose	12% casein, whey	44% safflower, corn and soy oils, lecithin
			Kindercal® (Mead Johnson)	50% maltodextrin and sucrose	13% calcium and sodium caseinate, milk protein concentrate	37% canola, MCT, corn, and high oleic sunflower oils
			Nutren Jr.® (Nestle)	51% maltodextrin and sucrose	12% isolated casein and whey proteins	37% soy, MCT, and canola oils

patients tolerate juice poorly. Lactose-containing or high-fat foods generally are not well tolerated and should be avoided initially. While some of these intolerances may improve as adaptation occurs, it is not unusual for lactose intolerance and fat malabsorption to persist throughout childhood, necessitating long-term avoidance of high-fat foods and use of lactose-reduced milk products.

Medical Therapy

During the acute phase of SBS, medical management should focus on the adequate provision of parenteral calories and nutrients to maintain positive nitrogen balance, to promote growth, and to stabilize fluid and electrolyte status. During the chronic phase of SBS the medical management should focus on the advancement of enteral feedings and on the treatment of medical complications associated with SBS and the chronic use of parenteral nutrition.

▸ Hyperacidity

Hyperacidity occurs transiently during the first few months after small bowel resection. Untreated, this condition may lead to peptic ulcer disease, esophagitis, and impairment in protein and fat digestion. Gastric hypersecretion is treated effectively with hydrogen antagonists that can be administered intravenously until enteral feedings are well tolerated.

▸ Hypermotility

Hypermotility commonly is seen after intestinal resection and includes shortening in gastric emptying time and in total gastrointestinal transit time. The continuous administration of enteral feedings over a 24-hour period appears to be better tolerated than bolus feedings on patients with this complication. Hypermotility may need to be treated with antiperistaltic agents such as codeine and loperamide hydrochloride, which have been shown to alleviate persistent diarrhea.

▸ Fat Malabsorption

Fat malabsorption can result from the occurrence of bile acid insufficiency. Following ileal resection, bile acids may enter the large intestine, causing irritation of the colon and eliminating bile acids in diarrheal stools. This condition may be improved significantly by treatment with bile acid-binding agents such as cholestyramine. Conversely, bile acids may enter the colon and be de-conjugated by colonic bacteria and rapidly reabsorbed. Under these circumstances the administration of bile acid-binding agents may decrease further the bile salt pool and aggravate fat malabsorption.

▸ Vitamin B$_{12}$ Deficiency

Vitamin B$_{12}$ deficiency can occur on patients who underwent severe ileal resections after the discontinuation of parenteral nutrition. This deficiency results from poor enteral absorption of the vitamin and it is clinically manifested by the development of macrocytic anemia. Treatment includes the intramuscular or subcutaneous administration of vitamin B$_{12}$ at initial doses of 100 μg/day for 10 to 15 days and maintenance doses of 60 μg monthly.

▸ Bacterial Overgrowth

Bacterial overgrowth and associated enterocolitis are known to adversely affect the outcome of infants with SBS. These complications are recognized by the detection of an elevated number of bacteria in jejunal aspirate or adhered to the mucosal surface of biopsy specimens, by elevated plasma lactate concentration, and by the abnormal breath hydrogen excretion after the use of glucose substrate. Treatment of bacterial overgrowth and associated enterocolitis is the administration of antibiotics (neomycin, gentamicin, cephalexin, metronidazole, trimethoprim-sulfamethoxazole) alone or in combination with sulfasalazine and prednisone for periods of 1 to 2 weeks. The selection of these drugs is based on the results of bacterial culture and antibiotic sensitivity.

▸ Complications

Metabolic and septic complications of parenteral nutrition are common for patients with SBS. They include catheter-related sepsis (54%), hepato-biliary dysfunction (40%), anemia (50%), osteopenia (6%), and endocarditis (4%). The high rate of line sepsis on patients with SBS probably represents translocation of enteric bacteria into the blood stream. The administration of antibiotics through the central line for 7 to 10 days is effective therapy for most patients. Removal of the central line is recommended for patients with *Candida* sepsis and for those in whom bacteremia persists despite antibiotic therapy. Parenteral nutrition-associated liver disease can be progressive and lead to liver failure, which accounts for 42% to 56% of the mortality in patients with SBS. The etiology of parenteral nutrition-associated liver disease is multifactorial and probably related to prematurity, immature liver function, lack of enteral alimentation, formation of toxic bile salts, and repeated episodes of sepsis. The medical management of this condition includes the following measures:

- The progressive advancement of enteral feedings and weaning of parenteral nutrition solutions while maintaining adequate nutritional intake for growth
- The administration of cyclical parenteral nutrition over 12 to 16 hours, instead of 24-hour periods
- The administration of medications such as phenobarbital to improve cholestasis and chenodeoxycholic acid (Ursodiol) to promote excretion of bile salts
- The supplementation of liposoluble vitamins A, D, E, and K to prevent deficiency status

Osteopenia

Osteopenia is seen commonly on premature infants with SBS receiving long-term parenteral nutrition. In severe cases, pathological fractures may occur on ribs and long bones in association with minimal trauma. The etiology of osteopenia is multifactorial, in most cases occurring because of an inadequate intake of calcium and phosphorus in parenteral nutrition solutions. Other causes of osteopenia include deficiency of vitamin D secondary to fat malabsorption, inadequate conversion of vitamin D to active metabolites secondary to liver disease, and increased calciuria secondary to chronic use of diuretics. The treatment of osteopenia includes high daily intakes of calcium (250 mg/kg/day), phosphorus (125 mg/kg/day), and vitamin D (400 to 1,000 IU/day), and the discontinuation of calciuric diuretics. While improvement occurs with increasing age, the bone mineral content of patients with SBS is lower than that of controls up to the age of 6 to 7 years.

Essential Amino Acids

Glutamine presently is considered a conditionally essential amino acid for premature and stressed full-term infants. Glutamine is present in human milk and infant formulas but absent from parenteral nutrition solutions. The supplementation of glutamine to enteral feedings and to parenteral nutrition solutions has been evaluated by a small number of controlled studies in babies with very low birth weight. The results of these studies were beneficial and included decreased tissue catabolism; enhanced gluconeogenesis; improved feeding tolerance; lower incidence of sepsis; and shorter duration of parenteral nutrition, mechanical ventilation, and hospitalization. In addition, this supplementation produced no notable side effects. The supplementation of glutamine to one child with SBS resulted in improvement in intestinal absorption. Further studies are needed to determine whether glutamine should be routinely supplemented to infants with SBS.

Surgical Therapy

Conservative intestinal resection during the initial surgery is strongly recommended to spare small sections of viable intestine and to minimize the severity of SBS. Patients with SBS who become dependent on parenteral nutrition because of slow intestinal adaptation or hypermotility may benefit from palliative surgical procedures to slow down intestinal motility or to increase intestinal absorption capacity. The insertion of 2.5- to 4-cm segments of ileum on a reversed peristaltic manner and the isoperistaltic interposition of a colonic segment into the proximal small bowel may decrease intestinal transit time and facilitate the absorption of water, electrolytes, and nutrients. Dilated bowel segments with ineffective peristalsis can be halved in diameter and doubled in length, while keeping the same mesenteric blood supply (Bianchi procedure). Experimental lengthening of the jejunum is preferable compared to that of the ileum.

Liver and bowel transplantation have been performed in a limited number of patients with severe SBS complicated by irreversible liver failure. These patients have a stormy postoperative course, a high rate of medical complications, prolonged hospitalizations, and a limited survival rate. Small-bowel transplantation for patients with severe SBS has been more successful when performed prior to the onset of end-stage liver disease. However, this procedure has been done only in a very small number of patients and long-term course presently is unknown. With the development of techniques that lower the risk of rejection and infection complications, bowel transplantation may become a viable therapy for patients with SBS in the future. Patients with SBS who might benefit from intestinal transplantation include those at risk of developing liver failure secondary to prolonged courses of parenteral nutrition.

Monitoring

The child's primary doctor should provide routine pediatric care, while the management of dietary, medical, and surgical interventions is best accomplished by a multidisciplinary team including a gastroenterologist, surgeon, dietitian, and nurse. Serial visits with the team should be scheduled to follow up with the patient for the management of malabsorption, administration of tube feedings, advancement of feedings, the assessment of growth, and laboratory monitoring.

▶ Growth

Advancement of enteral feedings is made based on symptoms of intolerance and malabsorption, including emesis, stool frequency, and stool consistency. While patients on parenteral nutrition alone grow well on regimens that provide expected calorie needs for age and gender, those with severe malabsorption on enteral feedings may require up to double their estimated calorie needs to grow at normal rates. Feeding regimens should be adjusted to promote weight gain and linear growth at expected rates for age. Because bowel growth corresponds to the overall linear growth of the child, maximizing nutrition support will result in more rapid adaptation of the bowel and ultimately more rapid transition from parenteral to enteral nutrition. Nutrition support should be weaned gradually to ensure that growth is not compromised during the period of adaptation.

Growth may be compromised by the inability to consume adequate calories in the face of malabsorption and should be monitored by serial measurements of weight, length, and head circumference plotted on the appropriate growth chart. Arm anthropometry, including mid-arm circumference and triceps skinfold (which can be measured by a trained pediatric dietitian) may reflect fat and muscle stores more accurately than the assessment of weight for length alone.

▶ Bone Density

Dual energy x-ray absorptiometry may be useful for the monitoring of bone density and body mass (lean versus fat). Infants and children with SBS are at risk for decreased bone density because they often receive inadequate intakes of calcium and phosphorus while on parenteral nutrition and later malabsorb vitamin D, calcium, and phosphorus while enterally fed. The inability to absorb adequate total calories may lead to depleted fat and muscle stores.

▶ Diet

The diets of children with SBS may be limited by their poor tolerance to certain kinds of foods, especially lactose-containing dairy products, high-fat foods, and hyperosmolar liquids. A pediatric dietitian should routinely monitor the child's dietary intake by analysis of dietary recalls or 3-day diet records. These techniques allow for the identification of nutrients at risk in the child's diet and the need for possible supplementation. For infants and young children maintained on tube feedings for prolonged periods of time, assessment of oral feeding skills also should be made routinely to ensure proper development or to treat preexisting feeding disorders.

▶ Laboratory

Laboratory monitoring is essential to evaluate the patient's response to dietary interventions and the need for nutritional supplementation and to assess effectiveness of medical and surgical therapies. The site of intestinal resection is a useful guide in determining specific nutrient deficiencies that the patient may be at risk of developing (Table 25-1). Subclinical nutrient deficiencies have been noted in children several years after discontinuation of specialized nutrition support, emphasizing the importance of ongoing monitoring. Table 25-3 displays the recommended guidelines for anthropometric, dietary, and laboratory monitoring of children with SBS receiving enteral feedings at home.

TABLE 25-3. Parameters for Monitoring Children With Short-bowel Syndrome

1. Weight, length, and head circumference	
0–1 year of age	At each visit or every 2-4 weeks
1–3 years of age	At each visit or every 1-3 months
3 years of age or older (weight and height only)	At each visit or every 4-6 months
2. Arm muscle and arm fat area	Every 3-6 months
3. Dual energy x-ray absorptiometry	Every 6-12 months
4. Dietary adequacy	Every 6-12 months
5. Feeding-related development	At each visit
Critical period at 9–12 months Referral to feeding specialist if indicated	
6. Laboratory measurements	
Chemistry panel (fluid balance, glucose, calcium, phosphorous, albumin, total protein, triglycerides, cholesterol, bilirubin, aspartate transaminase, γ-glutamyl transferase, alkaline phosphatase)	Every 1-2 months
Carbon dioxide breath test	As indicated by symptoms of small-bowel bacterial overgrowth
Serum magnesium, zinc	Every 6 months
Complete blood count, red blood cell indices	Every 6-12 months
Iron studies (serum iron, ferritin % saturation)	Every 6-12 months
Plasma vitamin A, 25-hydroxy vitamin D, and vitamin E levels	Every 6-12 months
Serum vitamin B12 levels	Every 6-12 months
Serum folate levels	Every 6-12 months
Serum copper and manganese (patients with hepatic cholestasis)	Every 6-12 months

Summary

The following are critical facts to remember:

- Short-bowel syndrome is a chronic condition that requires parenteral nutrition and specialized enteral feedings for a period of time after birth. Consequently, the treatment of SBS has great implications for home health care.
- It is essential that enteral feedings be introduced as early as possible to promote gut adaptation and to minimize the risk of liver disease.

- Nasogastric tubes are used most often to initiate enteral feedings. The feedings typically are initiated as a continuous infusion administered by electric pump. Feedings also may be delivered as boluses.
- Oral feedings should be maintained simultaneously with tube feedings to promote normal development of feeding skills.
- A variety of medical therapies are used to treat the complications of SBS and the problems associated with the chronic use of parenteral nutrition.
- Surgical therapy is used to spare small sections of viable intestine and to minimize the severity of SBS.
- Monitoring a child with SBS requires the primary physician as well as a multidisciplinary team that includes a gastroenterologist, surgeon, dietitian, and nurse.

Bibliography

Allen SJ, Pierro A, Cope L, et al. Glutamine-supplemented parenteral nutrition in a child with short bowel syndrome. *J Pediatr Gastroenterol Nutr.* 1993;17:329-332

Anagnostopoulos D, Valioulis J, Sfougaris D, Maliaropolous N, Spyridakis J. Morbidity and mortality of short bowel syndrome in infancy and childhood. *Eur J Pediatr Surg.* 1991;1:273-276

Bianchi A, Lendon M, Ward ID. A reassessment of surgical techniques for neomucosal growth. *Pediatr Surg Int.* 1992;7:41-46

Bristol JB, Williamson RCN. Mechanisms of intestinal adaptation. *Pediatr Surg Int.* 1988;3:233-241

Clark JH. Management of short bowel syndrome in the high-risk infant. *Clin Perinatol.* 1984;11:189-197

Cooper A, Floyd TF, Ross AJ III, Bishop HC, Templeton JM Jr, Ziegler MM. Morbidity and mortality of short-bowel syndrome acquired in infancy: an update. *J Pediatr Surg.* 1984;19:711-718

Dellert SF, Farrell MK, Specker BL, Heubi JE. Bone mineral content in children with short bowel syndrome after discontinuation of parenteral nutrition. *J Pediatr.* 1998;132:516-519

Dorney SF, Ament ME, Berquist WE, Vargas JH, Hassall E. Improved survival in very short small bowel of infancy with use of long-term parenteral nutrition. *J Pediatr.* 1985;107:521-525

Dowling RH. Small bowel adaptation and its regulation. *Scand J Gastroenterol.* 1982;74(suppl):53-74

Galea MH, Holliday H, Carachi R, Kapila L. Short-bowel syndrome: a collective review. *J Pediatr Surg.* 1992;27:592-596

Georgeson KE, Breaux CW Jr. Outcome and intestinal adaptation in neonatal short-bowel syndrome. *J Pediatr Surg.* 1992;27:344-350

Goulet O, Maurage C, Revillon Y, et al. Extensive small intestinal resection in newborn infants. *Arch Fr Pediatr.* 1990;47:415-420

Goulet OJ, Revillon Y, Jan D, et al. Neonatal short bowel syndrome. *J Pediatr.* 1991;119:18-23

Grosfeld JL, Rescorla FJ, West KW. Short bowel syndrome in infancy and childhood. Analysis of survival in 60 patients. *Am J Surg.* 1986;151:41-46

Illingworth RS, Lister J. The critical or sensitive period, with special reference to certain feeding problems in infants and children. *J Pediatr.* 1964;65:839-848

Kaufman SS, Loseke CA, Lupo JV, et al. Influence of bacterial overgrowth and intestinal inflammation on duration of parenteral nutrition in children with short bowel syndrome. *J Pediatr.* 1997;131:356-361

Lacey JM, Crouch JB, Benfell K, et al. The effects of glutamine-supplemented parenteral nutrition in premature infants. *JPEN J Parenter Enteral Nutr.* 1996;20:74-80

Langnas AN, Shaw BW Jr, Antonson DL, et al. Preliminary experience with intestinal transplantation in infants and children. *Pediatrics.* 1996;97:443-448

Leonberg BL, Chuang E, Eicher P, Tershakovec AM, Leonard L, Stallings VA. Long-term growth and development in children after home parenteral nutrition. *J Pediatr.* 1998;132:461-466

Matsuo Y, Nezu R, Kubota A, et al. Massive small bowel resection in neonates — is weaning from parenteral nutrition the final goal? *Surg Today.* 1992;22:40-45

Neu J, Roig JC, Meetze WH, et al. Enteral glutamine supplementation for very low birth weight infants decreases morbidity. *J Pediatr.* 1997;131:691-699

Perdum PP III, Kirby DF. Short-bowel syndrome: a review of the role of nutrition support. *JPEN J Parenter Enteral Nutr.* 1991;15:93-101

Ricketts RR, Jerles ML. Neonatal necrotizing enterocolitis: experience with 100 consecutive surgical patients. *World J Surg.* 1990;14:600-605

Roig JC, Meetze WH, Auestad N, et al. Enteral glutamine supplementation for the very low birthweight infant: plasma amino acid concentrations. *J Nutr.* 1996;126(suppl4):1115S–1120S

Sondheimer JM, Cadnapaphornchai M, Sontag M, Zerbe GO. Predicting the duration of dependence on parenteral nutrition after neonatal intestinal resection. *J Pediatr.* 1998;132:80-84

Todo S, Reyes J, Furukawa H, et al. Outcome analysis of 71 clinical intestinal transplantations. *Ann Surg.* 1995;222:270-282

Treem WR. Short bowel syndrome. In: Wyllie R, Hyams JS, eds. *Pediatric Gastrointestinal Disease: Pathophysiology, Diagnosis, Management.* Philadelphia, PA: W.B. Saunders Co; 1993:573-603

Vanderhoof JA, Langnas AN, Pinch LW, Thompson JS, Kaufman SS. Short bowel syndrome. *J Pediatr Gastroenterol Nutr.* 1992;14:359-370

Weber TR, Tracy T Jr, Connors RH. Short-bowel syndrome in children. Quality of life in an era of improved survival. *Arch Surg.* 1991;126:841-846

Chapter 26

Care of Children With Human Immunodeficiency Virus Infection

Richard Rutstein, MD; Constance Cleary, RN; Denise E. Ramsden, RN

Introduction

By the end of 1998, more than 8,500 cases of pediatric acquired immunodeficiency syndrome (AIDS) had been reported to the Centers for Disease Control and Prevention. This number only included children with an advanced stage of human immunodeficiency virus (HIV) infection; a much larger number of children living with earlier stages of HIV infection exist. More than 95% of new pediatric HIV cases in children younger than 13 years of age are perinatally acquired. It is estimated that the sero-prevalence of HIV infection in pregnant women in the United States is 1.5 per 1,000 women, which equals approximately 6,000 exposed neonates born each year. In the United States, where breastfeeding by women with HIV is discouraged, the peri-natal transmission rate (in the absence of perinatal therapy) is approximately 20%.

In the early 1990s, a multisite National Institutes of Health-sponsored trial demonstrated the efficacy of perinatal antiretroviral therapy (in this case, zidovudine [AZT] monotherapy) in decreasing the perinatal transmission rate from 22% to 8%. Most recently, with the use of potent multidrug antiretroviral therapy and elective cesarean sections, the rate of perinatal transmission in many centers is less than 3%. This translates into hundreds of pediatric HIV infections prevented annually.

For children who are infected, the standard of care is for multidrug regimens, which are known as highly active antiretroviral therapy (HAART). These three- or four-drug regimens generally are from two or more classes of anti-retroviral agents. State-of-the-art treatment recommendations are available online and are continuously updated. Laboratory monitoring of patients with HIV requires a complete blood count, chemistry profile, CD4 count, and assay of viral replication (using ribonucleic acid [RNA] quantification assays, or "viral load") every 3 months, at a minimum.

For children with CD4 counts low for their adjusted age, prophylaxis against common

289

opportunistic infections (trimethoprim/sulfamethoxazole for *Pneumocystis carinii* pneumonia, azithromycin for disseminated Mycobacterium avium complex) is also required. With the use of new antiretroviral therapies and prophylaxis against opportunistic infections, both morbidity and mortality have significantly decreased. Hospitalization and mortality rates have plummeted, and the median survival for children with HIV is now into the teenage years.

With the new therapies, however, come new problems. Medication regimens are complex and burdensome. All regimens require at least twice-daily dosing, and some agents are given three times a day. In addition, many of the medications come only as tablets or capsules; others are available in liquid or powder, but many infants and children find the taste intolerable. Therefore, younger children, incapable of swallowing pills or capsules, have limited treatment options.

To maximize and sustain drug effectiveness, patients must comply with a complex medication schedule consistently and indefinitely at this point. Because of the rapid development of drug resistance, compliance with the medication schedule must be nearly complete to maximize virologic suppression. Results of multisite studies indicate that anything less than 80% to 90% compliance with the medication schedule is associated with early drug failure, as measured by increasing viral load and decreasing CD4 counts. Unfortunately, at least 30% to 40% of families report having missed more than 20% of doses the previous week. Most children are dependent on their caregivers to help maintain their medication schedules. Caregivers may have multiple psychosocial issues that may influence their ability to consistently administer medications. Many are infected with HIV themselves and have difficulty adhering to their own medication regimen. For some, substance abuse remains an active issue. The caregivers' knowledge of HIV issues, as well as cultural and religious beliefs, are all factors that affect their ability to care for the child and comply with a complex medication schedule.

Among the population of children with HIV, there is a high incidence of developmental disabilities. These range from catastrophic progressive encephalopathy, to static encephalopathy, as well as specific learning disabili-

> *To maximize and sustain drug effectiveness, patients must comply with a complex medication schedule consistently and indefinitely at this point.*

ties and attention-deficit/hyperactivity disorder. Prior to the use of HAART, up to 25% of children with HIV developed progressive encephalopathy. An additional 25% will have significant developmental issues requiring special educational services.

It is believed that as many as 20% of new adult infections are acquired in adolescence. In addition, the population of children with perinatally acquired HIV continues to age, with many entering adolescence. Adolescence is a time of behavioral unrest, and classically includes noncompliance with medications and risky behaviors. With HIV infection, the importance of these behaviors is magnified.

Referral to Home Care

Patients with HIV enter the home care system through various avenues, with a wide array of presenting symptoms and needs. Home care units may receive the initial referral at the time of birth/discharge from the maternity unit. Alternatively, referral may occur at the time of family crisis or acute illness in the child or parents. Critical to assisting the family is a working knowledge of HIV, including recent recommendations on home care, education, and therapeutic options. It also is critical to ensure that families are linked to specialized HIV treatment centers for ongoing HIV-related care. In many areas, there are several social support agencies funded to provide case management services to families affected by HIV. The most common reasons for referral are the need for respiratory medications (primarily aerosolized pentamidine), nutritional support, medication review/ compliance, follow-up, and developmental therapies.

Many families referred to home care are subsequently linked to multiple service providers. These providers must strive to minimize the fragmentation of care, and mechanisms must be in place to facilitate communication between the medical treatment team and home care providers. When possible, interagency team meetings serve to optimize family treatment plans, decrease redundancy in services, and facilitate open discussions of the emotional burden of caring for children with chronic or fatal illnesses.

Providing ongoing HIV-related education is key to keeping all agency personnel current within this rapidly changing field. Education efforts must include issues related to patient confidentiality, as well as employee exposure to infected body fluids.

Home Care Therapies for Children With Human Immunodeficiency Virus Infection

Home care agencies may be called on to provide routine nursing care along with respiratory therapy and developmental therapies. Case management services are also frequently required. Staff should be well educated in the care and treatment of persons with HIV and should be chosen for their nonjudgmental, compassionate nature and sensitivity to cultural issues. Specific indications for home care involvement with clients with HIV may include the following:

▸ **Nutritional Support**

Disorders of growth, particularly failure to thrive and/or the HIV-related wasting syndrome, are exceedingly common in infants and children with HIV. Even with the advent of more aggressive and effective antiretroviral treatment regimens, nutritional support is key to optimizing the quality of life. Morbidity and mortality increase in the presence of significant malnutrition. Therapies include early implementation of caloric supplementation by the oral route and, when needed, provision of enteral feedings via nasogastric or gastrostomy tubes. Home care staff may be called on to monitor nutritional status through frequent assessments of the patient's weight and review of caloric intake. In addition, home care staff may provide family education and initiate or supervise enteral feedings.

▸ **Respiratory and Intravenous Therapies**

Home care agencies may be called on to deliver monthly aerosolized pentamidine (for prophylaxis against *Pneumocystis carinii* pneumonia) or bronchodilator therapy. In patients with HIV who are in the late stages of the disease and have chronic lung disease, home oxygen supplementation and monitoring of respiratory status may be needed. Home intravenous (IV) therapy may be indicated to complete courses of therapy for pneumonia or opportunistic infections. Some patients also may receive monthly infusions of IV gamma globulin as prophylaxis against recurrent bacterial infections. Patients with cytomegalovirus retinitis or colitis may require lifetime daily IV therapy with antiviral agents.

▶ Medication Review, Education, and Compliance Monitoring

It has become clear that the major hurdle in the treatment of patients with HIV is adherence to complex medication schedules. As noted, most patients are treated with at least three agents in combination, requiring a total of six or more doses of medicines per day. For patients able to take capsule or tablet formulations, total daily pill counts frequently exceed 20. It is also clear that viral resistance invariably develops when patients are unable to comply with at least 90% of weekly doses.

Intervention strategies to enhance compliance vary with each patient and family. Home visits are essential to developing individual treatment plans. Interventions may include weekly calendars with prizes for taking all of a day's or week's doses, or weekly pillboxes, as well as beepers or watches with alarms set at the time of medicine taking. At times, recruiting additional family members to help monitor medicine-taking behavior is an important intervention. Many of the medications have specific and different dietary restrictions. Helping the family develop a realistic medication schedule with allowances for dietary restrictions is a major part of adherence interventions. There also are multiple behavioral issues related to the poor taste of the liquid formulations and difficulty swallowing multiple large pills or capsules. Teaching younger patients swallowing techniques may allow conversion to the pill or capsule and improve compliance. It is imperative to stress adult supervision of all doses, even for patients in the early teenage years.

▶ Developmental Therapies

Home-based developmental therapies may be appropriate for younger children. Up to 25% of infected children will develop progressive encephalopathy (though the incidence is less now with advanced therapy) and an additional 25% of children have static encephalopathy, or a significant learning disability requiring special school resources. All children with HIV should be considered at risk for developmental problems and have at least yearly developmental and psychometric testing. They should be referred at diagnosis to early intervention programs for monitoring of developmental progression and in-home services as needed.

▸ Pain Control/Hospice Care

Patients with late-stage HIV infection may be referred to specialized home care programs for hospice care and/or pain control. The same guiding principles exist for patients with HIV as for patients with other diseases (such as cancer) referred for hospice services.

Additional Considerations for Effective Home Care

▸ Disclosure of Diagnosis and Confidentiality

The HIV infection differs from other chronic or life-threatening illnesses of childhood in that the issue of disclosure of the diagnosis is a difficult one. For many families, the diagnosis of HIV infection is a closely guarded secret. In some, the parents may not have disclosed this to anyone, including other family members. Families are understandably anxious about disclosure, fearing the unwarranted stigma and prejudice of others. Adults are still at risk for losing their jobs and standing in religious and social groups should their HIV status be disclosed. In some cases, the family has not disclosed the diagnosis to all of their health and home care providers. Agency workers must be very circumspect when discussing the diagnosis with other family members and health care providers, insurance, and educational agencies. At times, this means caring for a child in the presence of family members who do not know the diagnosis. Most state laws forbid disclosure between providers without specific written consent from the patient or the guardian. HIV-specific information should never be included on school or child care health forms.

One of the most difficult issues facing families is the timing of disclosure of the diagnosis to the child or adolescent with the infection. Many parents are understandably worried that the child will indiscriminately disclose the diagnosis to friends, teachers, or other family members. In addition, disclosure may force the adult to come to terms with his or her own illness and the emotional distress related to transmission of the illness to the child.

Unlike cancer or cystic fibrosis, the child and family with HIV is still at risk for social ostracism. Most children respond with a matter-of-fact attitude and less anxiety than expected. Many children have had an idea of the true diagnosis for years prior to parental disclosure and are relieved to have an open dialogue. It must be emphasized that the issue of disclosure is a time-based process and can only be understood within the context of the family and their social environment. Disclosure to a child without the parents' consent is not allowed. Each family dynamic in this situation is unique and must be respected.

▶ Occupational Exposure

There are many illnesses that home care workers are exposed to, including bacterial infections (eg, the patient is recovering from meningitis), tuberculosis, and other blood-borne infections (most notably, hepatitis B and C), but a key cause of staff anxiety involves exposure to HIV. Transmission of HIV via occupational exposure occurs in approximately 1 out of every 300 episodes of parenteral exposure, and in no more than 1 in 1,000 mucous membrane exposures.

Despite continued public concern, it is clear that HIV is not transmitted by casual contact. Ongoing prospective studies have not documented any seroconversion among family members despite shared utensils, sleeping areas, and bathrooms. Of the handful of suspected cases of horizontal transmission of HIV, all are believed to have occurred from inapparent exposure to blood or blood-containing body fluids. Biting has never been proven to transmit virus. There have been two reports claiming potential transmission via this route, but they could not be confirmed. American Academy of Pediatrics guidelines suggest that gloves are not necessary in routine day-to-day care, such as feeding and diaper changes, unless there is visible blood contaminating the specimen.

All home care agencies should have well-understood and well-disseminated policies on occupational exposures to potentially infectious material. Procedures must be developed to ensure rapid counseling, baseline testing of the employee, testing of the patient (if warranted), and administration of postexposure prophylaxis if indicated. Updated recommendations are available from the Centers for Disease Control and Prevention.

Summary

For infants and children with HIV, the following guidelines should
be followed:

- The standard of care for children infected with HIV is multidrug
  regimens (HAART).
- To maximize and sustain drug effectiveness, patients and caregivers
  must comply with a complex medication schedule.
- The most common reasons why children infected with HIV are referred
  to home care are their need for respiratory medication, nutritional support,
  medication review/compliance follow-up, and developmental therapies.
- Patients with late-stage HIV may be referred to home care for hospice
  care and/or pain control.
- Exposure to HIV may cause anxiety among caregivers, so home
  care agencies should have clear policies on occupational exposure
  to potentially infectious material. American Academy of Pediatrics
  guidelines suggest that gloves are not necessary in routine care unless
  there is visible blood.

Bibliography

American Academy of Pediatrics, Committee on Pediatric AIDS and Committee on Infectious
Diseases. Issues related to human immunodeficiency virus transmission in schools, child care, medical settings, the home, and community. *Pediatrics.* 1999;104:318-324

Centers for Disease Control and Prevention. 1995 revised guidelines for prophylaxis against
Pneumocystis carinii pneumonia for children infected with or perinatally exposed to human immunodeficiency virus. *MMWR Morb Mortal Wkly Rep.* 1995;44:1-11

Kovacs A, Xu J, Rasheed S, et al. Comparison of a rapid nonisotopic polymerase chain reaction
assay with four commonly used methods for the early diagnosis of human immunodeficiency
virus type 1 infection in neonates and children. *Pediatr Infect Dis J.* 1995;14:948-954

Shearer WT, Quinn TC, LaRussa P, et al. Viral load and disease progression in infants infected with
human immunodeficiency virus type 1. Women and Infants Transmission Study Group. *N Engl J
Med.* 1997;336:1337-1342

Simonds RJ, Chanock S. Medical issues related to caring for human immunodeficiency virus-
infected children in and out of the home. *Pediatr Infect Dis J.* 1993;12:845-852

Working Group on Antiretroviral Therapy and Medical Management of HIV-Infected Children.
Guidelines for the use of antiretroviral agents in pediatric HIV infection. HIV/AIDS Treatment
Information Service. US Department of Health and Human Services. Available at:
http://www.hivatis.org. Accessed August 6, 2001

Chapter 27

Comprehensive Home Care Program for the Socially High-Risk Infant

Tove S. Rosen, MD; Jennifer Rosen, JD, MSW

Introduction

Socially high-risk infants face a multitude of needs simultaneously, making them extremely vulnerable and increasing their chances of falling through the cracks and becoming lost in the system. The term "socially high-risk infants" encompasses those children who are born into the cycle of poverty. These children receive the poorest medical care, are at the highest risk of school failure and drop out, and frequently find themselves in situations of unemployment, drug addiction, and crime. Many socially high-risk infants are born to single parents and are often dependent on governmental assistance to meet the basic needs of food, shelter, and medical care.

Unfortunately, socially high-risk infants are often trapped in an unending cycle of poverty. They may be born into families whose members faced similar conditions of poverty growing up and have been unable to break the cycle. Many of these infants are born to women addicted to drugs of abuse and/or alcohol. They also include infants born to women who experienced abuse in the past or domestic violence in the present, or who experienced some form of mental illness. Because of this cycle, many parents of socially high-risk infants have poor support networks, limited coping skills, and poor parenting skills. They may feel isolated, alone, and unable to access the resources, social services, or support they need. They may be stressed, depressed, and have low self-esteem.

The rate of premature birth is higher in the socially high-risk infant population and is secondary to poor nutrition, minimal or no prenatal care, and drug abuse. Newborns exposed to drugs in utero may be more irritable and difficult to care for. These infants also have been reported to have difficulties with attention and self-regulating behaviors. This may be taxing on the caregiver, stressing limited resources and

coping skills, especially when the caregiver does not understand the source
of the irritability and/or has not received adequate parental role modeling.
Poor development has been described in infants and children born and raised
by women who are stressed, depressed, and have limited social support. In
all of these groups, caregivers fail to provide adequate consistency, structure,
and discipline for their children.

Comprehensive Home Care Program

A comprehensive home care program (CHCP) using a team-driven, family-
based approach to treatment is an alternative method for providing care and
services to socially high-risk children and their families. Comprehensive
home care programs use a holistic approach to intervention; they address
the multitude of needs that children and their families face simultaneously
rather than use a single-problem approach. The program teams start where
the family is; they help the family access necessary resources and services
and work with parents to develop their self-confidence, self-reliance, and
self-determination, in addition to teaching caregivers concrete skills such
as parenting. Comprehensive home care programs work in the home and
community so that extended family, friends, and community members
become better integrated into the family's informal support network. By
using a home-based system for delivery of care, CHCPs teach families to
live successfully in their communities with the stressors that are part of daily
life. Too often, treatment programs remove parents and/or children from a
difficult situation, give them services they need such as parenting skills and
drug treatment in a vacuum, and place them back into the same situation
without assisting in the reintegration process. The CHCPs aim to teach
parents and children how to function within the community and within
their current life context so that they learn the community's strengths,
resources, and limitations.

The Comprehensive Home Care Team

Initially, each CHCP team is composed of formal supports, including a
pediatrician, nurse, social worker, and community worker, in addition to
the family members. Each professional on the team has been included to
offer an area of expertise essential to the successful functioning of the team

as a whole. The pediatrician, who provides medical expertise and services, also coordinates and supervises the work of the team. Each CHCP team has a nurse with expertise in child care, development, parenting, and health issues. The social worker is included because of expertise in family dynamics, intervention techniques, and knowledge of and ability to access resources. Finally, the community worker serves as a volunteer mentor and model for the family and is a constant presence in the community on whom the family members may rely. Ideally, the community worker is a member of the particular community of which the family is a part, and is of a similar race/ethnic background as the family.

Each professional on the team has been included to offer an area of expertise essential to the successful functioning of the team as a whole.

All professional team members have received extensive training and experience with socially high-risk families, including the community worker who must complete 40 hours of training prior to being assigned to a CHCP team. Over time, the composition of the CHCP team should change to become less professionally focused and more family and community focused. The CHCP team hopes to accomplish this by actively linking the family members with community resources, involving the family in community activities, and helping the family to develop a network of informal supports, including extended family and friends, in addition to teaching the family to function independent from formal supports as much as possible.

The Comprehensive Home Care Program Process

Ideally, the CHCP team makes contact with the mother and begins the CHCP process when she first becomes pregnant. Pregnancy and early postpartum are the most vulnerable times for intervention. This is an unrealistic expectation initially, because word about the program must be spread and relationships with community services, resources, and active community members must be developed for people to even know that the program exists so that referrals are made. If there is no contact with the mother until she gives birth, contact should be made with her while she and the baby are still in the hospital, or as soon after release as possible, to introduce the program and encourage the family to participate.

The most important task, once the initial contact is made, is to establish a solid working relationship between the parent/family and the professional members of the CHCP team. This may take time and a great deal of effort on the part of the professional team members. Many parents do not ask for help because of pride, poor knowledge of what help is available, disorganization on the part of the family, fear of potential consequences of asking for help (ie, fear of the child welfare system becoming involved), or fear of being labeled a failure. It is essential for the professional team members to be nonjudgmental, kind, and sympathetic in their interactions with the family. While the establishment of communication may be difficult, kindness and persistence will eventually prevail.

▶ Family Assessment

Once a family agrees to participate, it undergoes an initial comprehensive assessment that includes demographic information, psychosocial history, medical health history, and family strengths/needs assessment. These assessments will be administered in questionnaire format. Demographic information includes information on education, housing, finances, employment history, and criminal history. The psychosocial history includes a home study; educational history (including any learning disabilities or special needs); mental health history and treatment; drug/alcohol abuse and treatment; any history of abuse, neglect, or domestic violence; as well as information on family dynamics and interactions. The mother's attitude toward pregnancy, and relationship with the father of her child, her own parents, and her support network should be explored. The caregiver's parenting skills and her interaction with her child should be observed carefully. Careful attention also should be paid to her coping abilities and techniques for problem solving and discipline. The health history includes the general medical background of the family as well as information on the mother's pregnancies and the medical care of her children, if any, including immunization records and growth and development measures. While the initial evaluations are taking place, the social worker and community worker assess community resources to determine what services and resources currently exist in the community in which the family lives.

Certain formal assessment instruments are administered to determine the extent of symptomatology and for purposes of measuring improvement and follow-up. The caregiver is administered scales of depression, stress, and self-esteem. Developmental assessments (eg, the Bayley Scales of Infant Development), will be used to measure the developmental milestones and progress of the child. The home environment will be evaluated using the Home Observation for Measurement of the Environment (HOME) Inventory. The initial assessment process may have to occur over time as communication and trust develop between professional team members and the family.

▶ Developing an Individualized Family Care Plan

Following the assessment process, the CHCP team meets to develop an individualized family care plan. The plan's goals and objectives build on family strengths and priorities, and the family actively participates in determining these goals. The plan is family centered rather than child centered, so that the CHCP team meets all of the needs facing the family rather than just the particular child's needs. At all times, the professionals on the team take care to avoid making judgments and applying their own beliefs and values. Instead, they look to the cultural traditions, beliefs, and values of the individual family.

▶ The Social Worker's Role

The social worker is the primary liaison between the other professional team members, and the family and is responsible for supervising the community worker. The social worker, nurse, and community worker meet with the family three times per week for the first 6 months. Each visit will be carefully documented and include the time spent with the family, the content of the meeting, and the quality, productivity, and progress of the activity.

The social worker uses the meeting time to assess and help improve the caregiver's interactions with the children, family, friends, and others in the community. The social worker teaches the caregiver coping skills and strategies for problem solving related to interaction with the children and the father of the children, financial issues, and any issues relating to abuse. A mother with a history of drug abuse should be referred to an appropriate treatment program. To encourage her attendance and completion of the program, child care should be provided. The social worker is available to provide crisis intervention services for the family and teach the family how to access those services and other resources in the community, such as entitlement programs, food stamps, and medical care. The social worker may assist the caregiver with educational and employment needs. The social worker provides direction and helps the family become more organized and function better as a unit.

▶ The Nurse's Role

The nurse works on parenting and child care skills with the caregiver to improve the caregiver's ability to successfully meet the needs of the children and to stimulate them properly so that they are developmentally on target. Some of the caregivers have a great deal of difficulty parenting because of their own depression, drug abuse, or lack of knowledge of proper parenting. Caregivers of infants exposed to drugs are taught that the irritable, difficult baby is not exhibiting hostility toward them, but is exhibiting symptoms resulting from the drug exposure. The nurse will teach the caregiver how to provide comforting, responsive, and consistent care to the child. The caregiver will learn to play with and talk to the infant, what toys are age appropriate, and techniques of proper stimulation. The nurse will teach the caregiver about what to expect developmentally from the child at different ages. The nurse also will instruct the caregiver in proper nutrition, signs of illness, and safety measures to follow in the home.

▶ The Community Worker's Role

The community worker is a constant presence with the family and attends meetings with the social worker, nurse, and family. Initially, the community worker's primary role is to mentor the family and provide suggestions to improve the link between the family and professional members of the CHCP team. The community worker also serves as a role model for the family in areas of child care, parenting skills, and maneuvering in the community to access resources under the supervision of the social worker and nurse.

As the child gets older, the frequency of the visits by the nurse and social worker decreases. They will visit the home one to two times per week when the child is between 6 and 12 months old (provided the family is ready for this and the team agrees that this is an appropriate step), then only every other week for years 2 and 3. As the nurse and social worker reduce the direct time they spend with the family, the community worker assumes more responsibility for assisting, monitoring, and modeling for the family. As this occurs, the community worker becomes the primary liaison between the family and other professional members of the team. When the family's involvement in the program nears its end, appropriate referrals will be made to Head Start or other intervention programs as needed.

Monitoring the Comprehensive Home Care Program

One important component of the home care program is monitoring its progress and efficacy. The entire CHCP team will meet at 3-month intervals for the first year and then every 6 months thereafter. The team members will report on the progress of the family and discuss any relevant issues. These meetings are an important time for each team member to express satisfaction or dissatisfaction with the family plan, goals, and progress. If difficulties are encountered and goals are not being met, new strategies will be introduced, discussed, and implemented. The meetings are flexible and may occur more frequently if the family so requires. Additionally, several of the instruments administered in the initial assessment process, such as the maternal scales, mother-child interaction, and evaluation of the home environment, will be re-administered at certain dates to monitor the family's progress and the efficacy of the program. Neuro-developmental assessments should be done to evaluate the outcome of the child.

Summary

Holistic home-based and community-based care using a flexible team approach is an alternative intervention for socially high-risk infants and their families. The CHCP model presents a framework to build on when developing a system of care. With highly trained professionals working intensively from the outset with the children and family in the home and the community, CHCP surrounds the family with a formal support system with the goal to work with the family to build on the family members' strengths. The professional members of the team phase out over time at a pace that is consistent and appropriate for the family as necessary child-rearing skills are gained and necessary services are received. An informal support network is developed so that at the end of the average 3-year period, the family has developed self-confidence, self-determination, and essential skills for living fulfilling and constructive lives in the community. The need for this type of intervention exists and, if implemented, CHCPs will serve to benefit the lives and well-being of socially high-risk children and their families.

Bibliography

Ahmann E. The family and home care: common challenges and resources. In: Ahmann E, ed. *Home Care for the High-Risk Infant: A Family Centered Approach.* 2nd ed. Gaithersburg, MD: Aspen Publishers Inc; 1996:17-23

Anderson M, Elk R, Andres RL. Social, ethical and practical aspects of perinatal substance use. *J Subst Abuse Treat.* 1997;14:481-486

Black MM, Dubowitz H, Hutcheson J, Berenson-Howard J, Starr RH Jr. A randomized clinical trial of home intervention for children with failure to thrive. *Pediatrics.* 1995;95:807-814

Bradley R, Caldwell B. Using the HOME inventory to assess the family environment. *Pediatr Nurs.* 1988;14:97-102

Burchinal M, Lee M, Ramey C. Type of day-care and preschool intellectual development in disadvantaged children. *Child Dev.* 1989;60:128-137

Campbell FA, Ramey CT. Effects of early intervention on intellectual and academic achievement: a follow-up study of children from low-income families. *Child Dev.* 1994;65:684-698

Eisenberg L. Experience, brain, and behavior: the importance of a head start. *Pediatrics.* 1999;103:1031-1035

Escalona SK. Babies at double hazard: early development of infants at biologic and social risk. *Pediatrics.* 1982;70:670-676

Fiks KB, Johnson HL, Rosen TS. Methadone-maintained mothers: 3-year follow-up of parental functioning. *Int J Addict.* 1985;20:651-660

Johnson HL, Glassman MB, Fiks KB, Rosen TS. Resilient children: individual differences developmental outcome of children born to drug abusers. *J Genet Psychol.* 1990;151:523-539

Johnson HL, Nusbaum BJ, Bejarano A, Rosen TS. An ecological approach to development in children of prenatal drug exposure. *Am J Orthopsychiatry.* 1999;69:448-456

Johnson HL, Rosen TS. Mother-infant interaction in multirisk population. *Am J Orthopsychiatry.* 1990;60:281-288

Johnson JL, Leff M. Children of substance abusers: overview of research findings. *Pediatrics.* 1999;103(suppl):1085-1099

Mayer JB, Meshel R. An early intervention program for high-risk children in a health care setting. *Soc Work Health Care.* 1981;7:35-43

Ramey CT, Ramey SL. Early intervention and early experience. *Am Psychol.* 1998;53:109-120

Ramey CT, Ramey SL. Which children benefit the most from early intervention? *Pediatrics.* 1994;94(suppl):1064-1066

Wallace JM Jr. The social ecology of addiction: race, risk, and resilience. *Pediatrics.* 1999;103(suppl):1122-1127

Werner MJ, Joffe A, Graham AV. Screening, early identification, and office-based intervention with children and youth living in substance-abusing families. *Pediatrics.* 1999;103(suppl):1099-1112

Chapter 28

Care of Children Requiring Home Mechanical Ventilation

Stephanie Storgion, MD

Introduction

The improved survival of infants and older children with chronic illnesses of a pulmonary or neuromuscular nature has resulted in many children requiring some type of home ventilation. Home ventilation has become more common in the past 10 to 20 years among children who are dependent on long-term ventilation because of the development of ventilating equipment for out-of-hospital use. The move to outpatient management of children with complex technological needs should not be endorsed simply as a managed care initiative, but embraced as a strategy of caring for the child and family with the goal of integrating the child as completely as possible into the daily routine of the family. The child, along with the family, should be the main focus of the care plan, with the primary care pediatrician providing a medical home with the assistance of a pediatric pulmonologist and other subspecialists.

Once an infant or child has shown an inability to maintain ventilation, efforts should be focused on incorporating the ventilator into daily life like any medication, rather than on trying to wean the child off ventilatory support. Dealing with the more usual aspects of a child's life can enable the child, family, and medical team to begin to focus on long-term care, especially on discharge planning to an out-of-hospital environment such as the home. The transition to the home should not change the home into an extension of the intensive care unit, but truly should allow for the child and family to function in a relatively routine lifestyle.

Transitioning to Home Care

The transition to home care should begin as soon as it is apparent that the child will need long-term mechanical ventilatory support, which usually occurs in the neonatal or pediatric intensive care unit. This can be implemented effectively by a medical discharge planning team who will evaluate the situation and determine whether the patient is able to progress from the *acutely* critical to the more *chronically* critical phase of their illness. Accurate prognostication is complex and must take into account the underlying disease causing the need for chronic ventilation, the implications of care on quality of life, and the appropriateness of care for the patient. Once these issues have been addressed and the decision is made to proceed with continued support, informed choices about types of equipment and invasive procedures can be made.

▶ Case Management

Making complicated decisions in an informed fashion is facilitated by using a team approach to case management. The family, often divorced from the care of the child who is acutely critically ill, must be brought back into the fold to be actively involved in the care of the child and empowered with skills to advocate in the short- and long-term on the child's behalf. The primary physicians involved with the care of the child include critical care specialists, pulmonologists, and other subspecialists. Identifying a primary care pediatrician must be accomplished as early as possible so that the physician is actively involved in the discharge planning process. Medical social workers with a keen interest in the child who is medically complex are essential to successful discharge of these children. Social workers must have knowledge of how the local children services system works and have links to payer case managers and home health agencies, often in several different regions or states depending on the location of the hospital. Third-party payers must be encouraged to assign case managers to facilitate the discharge planning process by thorough coordination of care. Hospital-based providers of nursing and respiratory care must work with home-based providers and members of the discharge planning team to ensure that family training is completed in a coordinated fashion. In addition, pediatric-based dieticians, occupational and physical therapists, speech pathologists, and educators must be involved in the case management process to optimize services provided to the child after discharge. Weekly conferences with all the members of the discharge planning team help to keep the focus on transitioning the child to the home while continuing to meet the medical needs of the child and the educational and psychosocial needs of the family.

Medical Stability for Home Ventilation

Determining medical stability prior to discharging the patient increases the success of home therapy by decreasing potential complications and reducing return admissions. Each patient should have stable ventilator settings on the home equipment for at least 2 weeks prior to discharge. The patient should have no adverse events during this time and should need no major manipulations in any therapies. Infants must weigh at least 6 kg because home ventilation equipment cannot safely deliver tidal volumes small enough for infants weighing less. Children also need to have a well-established weight gain for at least 4 weeks prior to discharge.

Long-term Ventilation

The initial commitment to long-term ventilation should occur only after the goals of the therapy have been clearly defined and discussed with the family. If the child is old enough to understand the implications of the therapy, he or she must be brought into the conversation and have an active role in the decision-making process. The use of long-term ventilation should focus on the benefit that can be achieved for the child (eg, allowing for lung repair and growth). Patients with progressive neuromuscular diseases eventually progress to permanent respiratory failure. While the family may choose long-term ventilation, the option to discontinue support if the underlying neuromuscular dysfunction is no longer tolerable must be clearly defined. The goal of home ventilation for a child who is terminally ill is to provide ventilatory support and alleviate suffering so that the child can die peacefully at home. Although the logistics of providing hospice care to patients dependent on a ventilator may seem daunting, the positive experience for the patient and family is well worth the effort. A difficult decision must be made when providing long-term ventilation to children who are severely brain injured and exist in a persistent vegetative state. Medical providers and parents must determine the benefits to the child, and the family should be provided with the option to discontinue ventilatory support. Long-term ventilation is not a cure for an illness, but is a palliative intervention.

Predischarge Education

A program for predischarge education for the family should be developed for every child prior to discharge. Such a program requires a dedicated staff of medical professionals within and outside of the hospital. Families need to be trained in all aspects of the child's care, from the workings and trouble-shooting of the ventilator to developmental exercises. Before any training can begin, primary family caregivers need to be identified and recruited into the care schedule of the child. If a family cannot commit to the care of the child outside the hospital, efforts need to focus on securing a foster care home for a child who is medically fragile. For various reasons, a family may not be able to provide a safe environment as long as the child is on a ventilator, but can provide a safe home once the child has been weaned off support. At least two caregivers living in the home need to be fully trained in all aspects of the child's care. Consistent techniques need to be taught and family members need to demonstrate the various techniques. Cardio-pulmonary resuscitation (CPR) needs to be mastered and demonstrated. Prior to discharge, the primary family caregivers need to stay and provide all the care for the child for at least a 48-hour period to ensure that they are prepared for discharge. Some programs have the luxury of a step-down facility that simulates a home environment prior to discharge. More of these types of facilities would be of great value to families, but financial implications have prevented widespread development.

Preparing the Home

Prior to discharge, the home to which the child is to be discharged must be physically inspected by skilled personnel (eg, a respiratory therapist from a durable medical equipment company). The room in which the child is to sleep must be large enough to accommodate all needed equipment and personnel. There must be adequate space in the home to store equipment, and throughout the home for the child in a wheelchair. Utilities, including a phone, must be in place, working, and able to support the extra demands of the equipment. Often, a simple power strip can increase the number and types of outlets needed. Utility companies should be notified that there is a child on a ventilator in the home to shorten the time it takes to return service in the event of an outage.

Many of these children come from multifamily homes and the number of people living in the home should be taken into consideration. Some families may be able to apply for improved housing with assistance, such as federal housing grants, because of the needs of the child who is dependent on technology. By working closely with local, state, and federal government agencies, housing needs can be met in an expeditious manner.

Care in the Home

Once the child is home, the cost of care usually is less than in the hospital; however, the amount of work for the family or other caregivers increases significantly. Twenty-four hour home nursing care should be provided for the child who is dependent on a ventilator for at least 1 full week initially, decreasing over time as the patient stabilizes at home and the family becomes more accustomed to the routine of caring for the child. Skilled nursing care should only be decreased in frequency by the physician managing the child's ventilatory support in conjunction with the family. Unfilled caregiving shifts must be taken into consideration when decreasing nursing coverage. Plans for respite care should be made before discharge. At least two family members or friends should be fully trained in the care of the child. Other respite care alternatives include extended care facilities or nursing homes for children, medical day care, or rehospitalization. By working with the family, medical caregivers and third-party payers can create a workable plan of care.

Airway Management

Tracheostomies are needed for long-term ventilatory support to provide more permanent airway access. Some patients who require extended ventilatory support may eventually have the tracheostomy tube removed when they prove they no longer need the assistance of a ventilator. Exceptions are those patients with neurologic dysfunction or with an abnormal upper airway (eg, severe subglottic stenosis, paralyzed vocal cord) that cannot be repaired satisfactorily with current surgical techniques.

Advanced surgical techniques and improved materials have allowed for the safe placement of tracheostomy tubes in small patients (ie, those weighing less than 2 kg). The type and size of the tracheostomy tube chosen is dependent on the patient and the underlying need for an artificial airway. Softer, more pliable tubes can be used for those children who do not require stenting of the airway. New tight-to-shaft cuffed tubes that are filled with water provide a safer cuffed tube with decreased risk of tissue injury than previously available. Some companies make customized tubes for patients.

▶ Tracheostomy Care

The care of children at home with tracheostomies is safe if family education is comprehensive and individualized for each child. Education should include suctioning and changing the tracheostomy tube, humidification, and the routine care and cleaning of the tubes and equipment. Pediatric CPR should be taught to the parents and modified for a child with an artificial airway. Caregivers should be given scenarios focusing on airway compromise requiring removal of the tube and the use of bag-and-mask ventilation while blocking the ostomy opening. Family caregivers need to have the chance to change the tracheostomy tube and repeatedly demonstrate their ability in all tracheostomy care techniques. Equipment for ambulatory and home care of the child with a tracheostomy tube should include a self-inflating resuscitation bag, replacement tracheostomy tubes, replacement ties, suction catheters, gloves, and stationary and portable suction machines. In addition, it is essential that infants and young children with tracheostomy tubes have cardiopulmonary monitoring when sleeping or unattended, whether they are spontaneously breathing or on mechanical ventilatory support. In a study of infants with tracheostomy tubes, deaths occurred in 11% of the patients, with most being related to not using the prescribed apnea monitor. At least two caregivers should be trained, in addition to home nurses, to provide all the care for the child.

When a child no longer requires a tracheostomy, removal of a tracheostomy tube usually is done in a stepwise fashion by sequentially decreasing the size of the tracheostomy tube. The child usually is admitted to the hospital overnight when the tracheostomy is finally removed to ensure that the airway is protected throughout all phases of sleep and wakeful states. Some children have irreversible upper airway obstruction requiring a permanent tracheostomy; children who have excessive secretions may benefit from a tracheal diversion.

Routine tracheostomy tube changes should occur once a month or any time there is a suggestion of blockage by secretions or the tracheostomy needs to be cleaned. Some tubes can be reused after cleaning, without increased infection and with decreased cost, by following the instructions outlined in the product insert. Except in the event of an emergency, tracheostomy tubes should be changed with two caregivers present. Tracheostomy ties should be changed weekly, or sooner if soiled. Additional tracheostomy tubes in sizes that the child is currently using, as well as one size larger (in the event the airway has stretched or grown, resulting in a leak) and one size smaller (in case the tube is difficult to replace), should be with the child and readily available. If a different-size tube is required, the child's physician should be notified immediately so that a decision can be made whether an airway evaluation or examination needs to be done. In addition, the child's physician should be notified anytime any of the following occur:

- Blood is suctioned from the tube, possibly suggesting tube erosion through the airway into a vessel.
- Tissue at the ostomy site is puffy, cracked, red, weeping, or oozing.
- Excessive gagging or coughing is observed.
- Difficulty in passing a suction catheter is observed.
- There is a change in secretion color, amount, and consistency.

Mechanical Ventilators

Ventilators used outside of the hospital are significantly less sophisticated than machines used in hospitalized patients. Home ventilators usually are used in the volume mode with pressure limits set. Tidal volumes are usually set to deliver 8 to 10 mL/kg. The ventilator rate is set depending on the amount of spontaneous ventilation the child is capable of providing. The arterial carbon dioxide tension ($PaCO_2$) may vary depending on the patient's underlying disease and whether the patient is being weaned from mechanical ventilation. Children with underlying lung disease, such as severe bronchopulmonary dysplasia, may tolerate a higher arterial carbon dioxide tension, but it generally should not exceed a level of 70 torr. Appropriate ventilation strategies are determined to avoid the development of pulmonary hypertension and to optimize calories to be used for growth rather than breathing.

Positive-end expiratory pressure (PEEP) of less than 10 cm H_2O can be used in the outpatient setting by adding an air compressor. Because many ventilators cannot be transported with PEEP, the child must be able to tolerate a period of time without PEEP for this therapy to be practical. Newer generation mechanical ventilators can provide PEEP without additional equipment.

▶ Oxygen

Oxygen can be used up to a concentration of 30% by using an E cylinder in line with the inspiratory circuit on the ventilator for transporting the child or with an oxygen generator for home use. Higher levels of inspired oxygen require the use of liquid oxygen. A child who requires higher amounts of oxygen to maintain an oxygen saturation of greater than or equal to 92% may not be ready for discharge, unless the child's disease is expected to be terminal.

▶ Batteries

All ventilators used in the outpatient setting have internal batteries with a charge life of about 1 hour. In addition, they can be supported with an external battery for longer trips away from an electrical outlet. If run off a marine battery, a home ventilator can work for 6 to 8 hours, while a car battery can last up to 36 hours. For patients who live in areas with frequent power outages, an auxiliary generator may be indicated. Prior to discharge, the electrical capacity of the home needs to be checked to ensure that the home circuitry can support the needed equipment.

Transporting a child on a ventilator usually results in a 4- to 8-hour absence from home. Before discharge, the child's ventilator should be set on the transport settings for 4 to 6 hours to assess how well this mode is tolerated. This allows for necessary adjustments to make trips out of the home as safe as possible.

▶ Nocturnal Ventilation

There are certain cases for which nocturnal ventilation is the best strategy to use. These include the patient who is being weaned off the ventilator but still needs some support at night, the patient with a neuromuscular disease in the early stages, and the patient with central hypoventilation. Most of these patients, especially younger children, still will require a tracheostomy for nocturnal positive-pressure ventilation. However, with older children, there are other noninvasive ventilation techniques that can be used.

▶ Bi-level Positive Airway Pressure

Bi-level positive airway pressure (BiPAP) nasal mask ventilation is a noninvasive mode of controlled positive-pressure ventilation that has been shown to be effective in children. This therapy requires the use of a mask that covers the nose and is secured with a harness that fits behind the head. For patients who are mouth breathers, a chin strap also may be needed to establish a seal around the mask. A good seal is essential as the BiPAP device is triggered by the patient's spontaneous inspiratory effort. Inspiratory and expiratory pressure levels are set, each depending on the individual patient's need. Common settings for inspiratory pressure are 12 to 20 cm H_2O and expiratory pressures are between 2 to 5 cm H_2O. Inspiratory time and rate are also patient specific and are determined in the same fashion as in positive-pressure ventilation to maintain adequate ventilation and oxygenation. Supplemental oxygen can be bled in and many machines have the capability of humidifying the inspired air, which increases patient tolerance of this therapy. In addition, new BiPAP devices have a ramp mode that can be set for up to 30 minutes, allowing the patient to fall asleep while the device achieves the maximum pressure set for the patient. This technique requires a highly motivated patient-therapist team to achieve success because the mask can be awkward to use and the perceived appearance may result in a child's refusal to use the device.

▶ Cuirass

Other techniques that may allow for noninvasive ventilation include cuirass ventilation and diaphragm pacing. Cuirass ventilation requires an external "suit" in which the child is placed and a negative-pressure vacuum is attached. By setting the negative pressure, cycling time, and rate, negative-pressure ventilation is achieved. Supplemental oxygen can be provided via nasal cannula. Disadvantages include requiring the patient to remain relatively still while sleeping, redoing the fit of the suit with growth, and the noise of the negative-pressure pump.

▶ Diaphragm Pacing

Diaphragm pacing can be used for nocturnal ventilation and for central hypoventilation in the older child. The pacer must be set at bedtime and is usually well tolerated. Diaphragm pacing also can be used during the day in the older child who is quadriplegic and requires full-time ventilation. Pacing can decrease the amount of equipment needed for transporting the patient and potentially improve life quality. The greatest disadvantage to this therapy is that, over time, the phrenic nerve, which is paced, can become scarred, leading to increased resistance to the pacer current. This may result in replacement of the pacer wires closer to the diaphragm. This scarring of the phrenic nerve is accelerated by the frequency of impulses, so full-time pacing is not recommended because pacer lifetime is shortened greatly.

Other Medical Considerations

In addition to specialized care, it is important that children who are dependent on a ventilator receive routine medical care such as immunizations. In addition, hearing, speech, and feeding need to be monitored closely and appropriate care recommended.

▶ Routine Medical Care

Routine medical care should be the responsibility of the child's primary care pediatrician. Subspecialists should directly manage the aspects of the child's care that fall into their area, but also must actively coordinate the care with the primary care physician. Immunizations should be started in the hospital as soon as the child is medically stable, and any catch-up immunizations should be given as soon as possible. The family should know who to contact for what types of problems.

▶ Hearing and Speech

Hearing and speech are essential to the development of all children and should not be overlooked in the child with complex technological needs. Hearing assessments should be performed sequentially throughout the child's hospitalization, as well as after discharge, with acoustic aids provided as indicated. Children with tracheostomies can vocalize even while on mechanical ventilatory support. Minimal leaks can allow for coordination of speech with the cycling of the ventilator. Once the child no longer requires PEEP, a one-way speaking valve can be attached to the tracheostomy of even a very small child, as long as a leak is also present. This type of device requires some adjustment because it causes increased resistance to airflow. In addition, it may be affected by increased secretions because its use prohibits the user from spontaneously clearing the airway. It is important that a skilled pediatric speech pathologist works closely with the child and family to achieve success with this type of device, which can improve clarity of speech and language acquisition.

These therapies, as well as other educational therapies, can begin in the home, but once family has become comfortable with transporting the child, therapy and education in group settings is recommended. Once the child reaches 3 years of age, integration into the school system should begin. If the child is the first with a ventilator in the school system, advocating on behalf of the child becomes a responsibility of the family and all others involved in the child's care, including the child's physicians.

▶ Feeding

Predicting which infants and children who require chronic ventilation will need accessory feeding devices is difficult and often requires a "wait-and-see" attitude on the primary caregiver's part. Almost all infants and children who have had endotracheal tubes in place for extended periods of time and have had tracheostomy tubes placed develop some degree of oral aversion, which can be overcome with time and diligence by exposing the patient to different types of foods with different consistencies and textures. Feeding difficulties are related to an uncoordinated suck and swallow reflex and underlying neurologic dysfunction, which can lead to aspiration. A modified barium swallow with videofluoroscopy in the presence of an experienced speech pathologist can be extremely helpful in determining the reason for the child's feeding problems and can aid in choosing the time and type of feedings the child may tolerate. Transitioning to oral feeds can take an extraordinary amount of time if the child has developed a significant oral aversion, a hyper-gag reflex, or both. In addition, reflux can be a significant problem and evaluation should occur prior to making any decision about a gastrostomy. The type of workup is often at the discretion of the surgeon and can include any or all of the following:

- Clinical signs and symptoms of reflux including but not limited to vomiting, gagging, and coughing
- Barium swallow
- pH probe
- Milk scan

If reflux is significant, a gastric fundoplication can be done, usually at the same time as the gastrostomy. Depending on the size and indications, the feeding tube can be placed surgically or percutaneously. To limit the number of anesthetic episodes for the child, it is helpful to combine as many procedures as can be performed safely and logistically. It is not unusual for a child to have a tracheostomy, gastrostomy with or without a fundoplication, and a central venous catheter placed for long-term management. The needs and timing for these procedures should be determined for each child.

The child's caretakers need to be trained in the care of the child's ostomy site and techniques for feeding. Recently, gastric buttons introduced for use in small children decrease the temptation of the child to pull on the tubing irritating the ostomy site, which could possibly dislodge the tube. Buttons simplify dressing the child because they sit flush to the skin. The greatest disadvantage to gastric buttons is that they are quite expensive and are often not covered by insurance.

Oral stimulation/desensitization therapy should begin as soon as it can be tolerated by the child to aid the child and family in transitioning to oral feeds. Although begun in the hospital, this process must continue at home if oral feeds are to be successful. Techniques that are helpful in making this transition include the following:

- Holding the child during feeding and providing oral stimulation to make it more pleasant for both the child and caregiver
- Using nocturnal feeds to provide calories and allowing the child to eat ad libitum during the waking hours
- Feeding the child with other family members to expose the child to the social aspects of eating

For those children who require parenteral nutrition for some or all of their calories, cycling on and off the infusion can allow for easier ambulatory activities without the infusion pump and can encourage some oral feeds.

Caloric Requirements

Caloric requirements for children dependent on a ventilator are somewhat different from other children. Studies have found that for those children weighing less than 6 kg, calories required for growth are dependent on continued need for mechanical ventilatory support, while for those children weighing more than 6 kg, caloric requirements are dependent on neurologic function and activity level (Table 28-1).

TABLE 28-1. Caloric Requirements for Children Who Are Chronically Ventilated

Ventilated	2-6 kg	All	125-150 cal/kg/d
Non-ventilated	2-6 kg	All	115-130 cal/kg/d
Ventilated/Non-ventilated	>6 kg	Active*	100-125 cal/kg/d
Ventilated/Non-ventilated	>6 kg	Inactive†	60-100 cal/kg/d

*Neuromotor activity allowing for spontaneous movement that overcomes gravity.

†Neuromotor activity incapable of spontaneous movement that overcomes gravity and/or severe anoxic brain injury.

Close monitoring of all growth parameters (ie, weight, height, growth velocity, and head circumference) is essential, especially when the child is discharged from the hospital. Monitoring can be done in many ways, including having the home nurse routinely measure and plot the results or by having the child come to the office.

Home Nursing and Durable Medical Equipment

Home nursing for children dependent on a ventilator requires trained pediatric nurses who are familiar with tracheostomies and ventilators. It is best to bring the nursing director and at least one of the assigned nurses to visit with the child and family prior to discharge so that consistency in care and expectations can be discussed. A representative of the medical equipment supplier must visit prior to discharge and have experience with the specific ventilator prescribed for the child. Prior to discharge, the respiratory therapist should visit the home to determine if utilities are adequate, if the room designated for the child has adequate space for supplies, and if there is adequate access to the home. The utility and phone companies need to be notified that there will be a child who is medically fragile in the home and priority for service restoration needs to be designated. The home respiratory therapist usually follows the family home to make sure everything is set up correctly and to answer any final questions.

Weaning From Ventilatory Support

Weaning from the ventilator usually does not occur until the child has been home and stable for several months. With this in mind, only children expected to be on the ventilator for more than 3 months should be considered for home ventilation, after efforts to wean off the ventilator prior to discharge have been maximized. Before any weaning occurs, the patient should show continued consistent growth and increased tolerance of daily activities. Weaning oxygen can occur at home using intermittent pulse oximetry. It usually is safest to bring the child into the hospital to begin weaning from the ventilator during an overnight stay so that oxygenation and ventilation parameters can be monitored closely. With this type of weaning schedule, few complications arise and weaning can be accomplished safely.

Summary

When considering the possibility of caring for a child dependent on a ventilator at home, keep the following thoughts in mind:
- The care of the child who is dependent on a ventilator can be challenging yet quite rewarding. It is important to develop a multidisciplinary team to focus on discharge planning for the child even while in the acute critical care area.
- Re-enfranchising the family members in the care of and responsibility for the child and empowering them with the skills to advocate for the child can make home ventilator care a successful venture.
- Relying on the primary care pediatrician for continuity care and on the subspecialists for care within their areas of expertise allows for a more normalized approach to childhood health and disease states.

- Focusing on growth and development while using the ventilator places the concerns in the appropriate order and allows for more rapid ventilator weaning. Seeing these children years later off the ventilator and doing everyday things makes all the time and effort behind this type of care worthwhile.

Bibliography

American Academy of Pediatrics, Ad Hoc Task Force on Definition of the Medical Home. The medical home. *Pediatrics*. 1992;90:774

American Thoracic Society. Care of the child with a chronic tracheostomy. *Am J Respir Crit Care Med*. 2000;161:297-308

Fortenberry JD, Del Toro J, Jefferson LS, Evey L, Haase D. Management of pediatric acute hypoxemic respiratory insufficient with bilevel positive pressure (BiPAP) nasal mask ventilation. *Chest*. 1995;108:1059-1064

Goldberg AI, Faure EA, Vaughn CJ, Snarski R, Seleny FL. Home care for life-supported persons: an approach to program development. *J Pediatr*. 1984;104:785-795

Kinnear W, Hockley S, Harvey J, Shneerson J. The effects of one year of nocturnal cuirass-assisted ventilation in chest wall disease. *Eur Respir J*. 1988;1:204-208

Lawless ST, Cook S, Luft J, Jasani M, Kettrick R. The use of laryngotracheal separation procedure in pediatric patients. *Laryngoscope*. 1995;105:198-202

McMahon J, Storgion SA. *Estimating Caloric Requirements of Technologically Dependent Children* [poster]. 17th Clinical Congress of the American Society of Enteral and Parenteral Nutrition; 1993

Messineo A, Giusti F, Narne S, Mognato G, Antoniello L, Guglielmi M. The safety of home tracheostomy care for children. *J Pediatr Surg*. 1995;30:1246-1248

O'Donohue WJ Jr, Giovannoni RM, Goldberg AI, et al. Long-term mechanical ventilation. Guidelines for management in the home and at alternate community sites. Report of the Ad Hoc Committee, Respiratory Care Section, American College of Chest Physicians. *Chest*. 1986;90:(1suppl):1S-37S

Passy V, Baydur A, Prentice W, Darnell-Neal R. Passy-Muir tracheostomy speaking valve on ventilator-dependent patients. *Laryngoscope*. 1993;103:653-658

Schlessel JS, Harper RG, Rappa H, Kenigsberg K, Khanna S. Tracheostomy: acute and long-term mortality and morbidity in very low birth weight premature infants. *J Pediatr Surg*. 1993;28:873-876

Storgion SA. Care of the technology-dependent child. *Pediatr Ann*. 1996;25:677-684

Tolep K, Getch CL, Criner GJ. Swallowing dysfunction in patients receiving prolonged mechanical ventilation. *Chest*. 1996;109:167-172

US Congress, Office of Technology Assessment. *Technology Dependent Children: Hospital v Home Care—A Technical Memorandum*. Washington, DC: US Government Printing Office; 1987. Publication OTA-TM-H-38

Chapter 29

Bronchopulmonary Dysplasia

Howard Panitch, MD

Introduction

The care of infants with bronchopulmonary dysplasia (BPD) in the home requires an understanding of the pathophysiology and course of the disease. The care of these infants can be challenging without an appreciation of the clinical issues that can affect their health.

Clinical Manifestations

Bronchopulmonary dysplasia refers to unresolved lung disease following acute lung injury in the neonatal period. It was originally described in a group of premature infants who required mechanical ventilatory support and high concentrations of supplemental oxygen for treatment of hyaline membrane disease. Subsequently, clinical features of BPD also have been described in newborn infants who required artificial ventilation and supplemental oxygen for a variety of neonatal lung disorders, including meconium aspiration syndrome, sepsis or pneumonia, pulmonary hypoplasia, congenital diaphragmatic hernia, persistent pulmonary hypertension, congenital heart disease, severe apnea, and tracheoesophageal fistula.

The heterogeneity in gestational age and etiology of initial acute lung injury of patients with BPD results in a large variation in clinical presentation, from infants with only intermittent signs of wheezing during acute viral illnesses to children with chronic respiratory insufficiency who require prolonged courses of mechanical ventilatory support. Despite the initial severity of the disease, the clinical course of the infant with BPD should be one of gradual improvement in respiratory status, along with catch-up in somatic growth and acquisition of developmental milestones. When such improvements do not occur, one or more clinical problems or complications that typically occur in patients with BPD may exist and should be investigated. These include hypoxemia, apnea, uncontrolled asthma, central airway obstruction, acute viral lower respiratory tract illnesses, systemic and pulmonary hypertension, cor pulmonale, growth failure, metabolic derangements, visual and hearing deficits, and neurodevelopmental delay.

Hypoxemia

Hypoxemia (oxygen saturations [SpO_2] less than 95%) in BPD most commonly results from abnormal ventilation-perfusion relationships. A reduction in the number of pulmonary capillaries, along with a decrease in alveolar number and simplification of the alveolar spaces, also results in less cross-sectional area available for gas exchange. Additionally, in some patients, intrapulmonary right-to-left shunts develop in areas of chronic inflammation or through bronchial artery collaterals and are a cause of persistent hypoxemia.

Hypoxemia contributes to tachypnea and is associated with poor growth. Acute episodes of hypoxemia cause both bronchospasm and pulmonary artery vasoconstriction. Chronic hypoxemia can cause or contribute to pulmonary hypertension and lead to cor pulmonale. Infants with BPD who demonstrate normal oxyhemoglobin saturations while at rest and awake may have episodic hypoxemia with saturations less than 90% during sleep, during or following feedings, or with activity. Episodic sleep hypoxemia occurs especially during rapid eye movement stages of sleep. Sleep hypoxemia has been associated with an increased frequency of episodes of central apneas and periodic breathing, as well as more disturbed sleep architecture in infants and young children with BPD. Such abnormalities can be corrected or made less frequent with restoration of normal oxyhemoglobin saturation. Autonomic function, as measured by heart rate variability, also is negatively impacted by hypoxemia.

Infants with BPD demonstrate an abnormal response to hypoxic challenge. Although it has been reported that infants with BPD were at increased risk to die from sudden infant death syndrome (SIDS), this association has not been upheld in more recent studies when episodic hypoxemia has been corrected. Those infants with severe BPD who have experienced prolonged or repeated episodes of hypoxemia, however, may acquire abnormal peripheral chemoreceptor responses to hypoxemia and may not mount an appropriate response to an hypoxic challenge. There appears to be a direct relationship between severity of BPD and duration of the period before which the peripheral chemoreceptors reset to normal. Those infants with the most severe pulmonary disease may be at increased risk for apparent life-threatening events or SIDS.

▶ Treatment

Hypoxemia can usually be corrected by administration of supplemental oxygen. The feasibility and benefits of home oxygen programs for infants with BPD have been described for more than 2 decades. There are no data that establish the absolute minimum oxyhemoglobin saturation allowable that will prevent cardiovascular complications or growth failure. As a guideline, therefore, normal oxyhemoglobin saturations (95% to 98%) should be the goal of therapy. Saturations that are routinely lower than 95% suggest inadequate therapy or a change in the underlying respiratory status. Similarly, a sudden or gradual increase in the concentration of supplemental oxygen required to maintain a normal oxyhemoglobin saturation reflects an acute infection or inadequate control of other complications such as asthma, gastroesophageal reflux, or fluid retention. Saturations that routinely range between 98% and 100% indicate that the concentration of supplemental oxygen can be reduced. Measurements of oxyhemoglobin saturation of patients dependent on oxygen should be taken at each office visit during quiet wakefulness with and without supplemental oxygen and, if possible, during sleep and feedings.

As a guideline, therefore, normal oxyhemoglobin saturations (95% to 98%) should be the goal of therapy.

There is no consensus among practitioners about the use of home pulse oximetry monitoring, with opponents citing frequent false alarms and delay in weaning supplemental oxygen because of false low oximetry readings as major detractions. Proponents of home oximetry monitoring cite the ability to wean patients while ensuring normal oxyhemoglobin saturation levels, as well as the observation that a decrease in saturation can be an early sign of respiratory deterioration, as benefits of home monitoring. Most infants and children with BPD who have been discharged to the home with supplemental oxygen therapy, however, do not require continuous pulse oximetry monitoring. Instead, spot-checks during sleep, activity, or intercurrent illness can help guide therapy.

Weaning of supplemental oxygen should occur only when the infant demonstrates normal oxyhemoglobin saturations as well as reasonable growth velocity and stamina for play or activity during therapy sessions. Usually, supplemental oxygen is weaned during awake hours with monitoring by pulse oximetry. Decreases in amount of supplemental oxygen should be followed by several days of observation to ensure that the infant's weight gain and activity level are sustained. Slowing of growth velocity, decreased endurance, or irritability are signs that continued weaning of supplemental oxygen should be delayed. When discontinuation of nocturnal oxygen supplementation is considered, a sleep study or overnight pulse oximetry study should be obtained without the use of supplemental oxygen. Episodic or sustained hypoxemia should be resolved before supplemental oxygen therapy is discontinued.

Central and Peripheral Airway Obstruction

All airways from the larynx to alveolar ducts are variably affected in patients with BPD. Wheezing occurs because of large and small airway narrowing. Direct trauma to the airway from endotracheal tubes and suction catheters can result in stenosis or granuloma formation of the subglottis, trachea, or main bronchus. The extremely compliant characteristics of the immature airway wall, together with its exposure to deforming forces of positive-pressure ventilation, place the infant with BPD at risk for acquired tracheobronchomalacia. A number of histopathologic changes described in patients with BPD, including smooth muscle hypertrophy, increased wall thickness, mucous gland hypertrophy, and reduction in the number of alveolar septal attachments to the small airway wall, may accentuate airway narrowing following smooth muscle stimulation and shortening.

▶ Clinical Manifestations

Dynamic extrathoracic lesions cause inspiratory stridor, while fixed lesions produce biphasic noise. Lesions involving the vocal cords may result in a hoarse cry, although the voice still may be normal. Subglottic lesions will result in diminished voice amplitude if the lesion causes narrowing severe enough to impede airflow. The clinical manifestations of extrathoracic lesions will be exacerbated by upper respiratory illnesses, and some acquired lesions may not become clinically evident until the infant experiences an upper respiratory illness.

Dynamic intrathoracic central airway lesions cause homophonous wheezing that is accentuated with increased breathing effort and may be less severe or inapparent with decreased effort (ie, during sleep). Dynamic central airway collapse also is accentuated by small airway obstruction; the infant must overcome the peripheral airway obstruction with active expiratory effort. The wheezing does not respond to and may be made worse by administration of bronchodilators. Conversely, obstruction can be decreased by administration of bronchoconstrictors. Tracheomalacia and bronchomalacia also are responsible for some cyanotic or BPD spells. Fixed lesions such as granulomas or stenoses cause persistent areas of atelectasis or hyperinflation that occur more frequently in the right lung.

Neonatal injury causes small airway damage, which results in fixed peripheral airway obstruction. This results in hyperinflation and contributes to ventilation-perfusion mismatching and hypoxemia. Patients may demonstrate crackles or heterophonous wheezing and increased work of breathing. Episodic bronchospasm also causes peripheral airway obstruction and occurs in association with acute respiratory infections, gastroesophageal reflux, or fluid imbalance. Airway constriction in infants with BPD has been reported in response to cold air or hypoxia. A substantial number of infants with BPD demonstrate clinical improvement following administration of bronchodilators or diuretics. Both fixed and reversible airway obstruction are present in school-aged children and young adults with a history of BPD. Determining the source of wheezing in the younger child with BPD, however, can be complicated; central and reversible peripheral airway obstruction can coexist, so the response to a bronchodilator aerosol may not be predictable.

▸ Treatment

Infants with BPD who develop chronic or recurrent stridor, weak cry, or biphasic noisy breathing should undergo endoscopic evaluation of the extrathoracic airway. Acquired lesions such as subglottic cysts or webs can be corrected at the time of the evaluation. More extensive lesions such as subglottic stenosis may require a staged repair, depending on the extent and severity of the lesion. Bronchoscopy should be considered in any patient who develops persistent lobar atelectasis or emphysema to rule out intraluminal granuloma or airway stenosis. Patients with significant tracheomalacia may benefit from the use of cholinergic agonists like bethanechol chloride.

Bronchodilators

Because the majority of patients with BPD have a component of reversible airway obstruction, a bronchodilator aerosol should be administered to any patient who has chronic symptoms of tachypnea, coughing, or wheezing. Response can be determined by critically observing for changes in respiratory rate, oxyhemoglobin saturation, degree of air entry, presence of retractions, use of accessory muscles of respiration, and change in the character of wheezing.

Chronic administration of a beta-agonist may be useful to minimize the work of breathing, respiratory rate, and supplemental oxygen requirement. Inhaled medications are preferred because they act more quickly than oral medications and can be used at a lower dose. Frequency of inhalation therapy can be increased to every 3 to 4 hours and the standard dose can be doubled during acute exacerbations if necessary.

Anticholinergic inhaled bronchodilators have been shown to be effective in infants with BPD and can be added to the regimen if routine therapy with inhaled beta-agonists fails to maintain clinical stability. Ipratropium bromide should be administered 20 minutes before albuterol to maximize the effects of the two drugs. It is unusual for a patient to require oral beta-agonist therapy in addition to the inhaled regimen. Occasionally, however, theophylline may be used concomitantly to maintain stability. Theophylline is a weak bronchodilator agent, but it does stimulate central respiratory centers, increase responses to $PaCO_2$ levels, and may strengthen skeletal muscle (diaphragm and intercostal muscle) contraction.

Bronchodilators should be weaned or discontinued after prolonged periods of stability in patients who no longer require diuretics or supplemental oxygen. Oral medications are discontinued first. After several weeks of observation, if there is no increase in cough or work of breathing, the frequency of inhaled medications is decreased. Each change in the medical regimen should be assessed by weeks of observation.

Anti-inflammatories

The role of anti-inflammatory therapy in established BPD is not well studied. For those patients with a prominent history of reversible airway obstruction, however, the risk/benefit analysis favors the use of anti-inflammatory aerosol drugs. Nebulized cromolyn sodium, a nonsteroidal anti-inflammatory agent, is the least potent of the anti-inflammatory drugs, but it has the fewest side effects. If breakthrough wheezing occurs frequently, a trial of nedocromil sodium, another nonsteroidal anti-inflammatory agent, may avoid the need to introduce inhaled corticosteroids. Nedocromil is more efficacious than cromolyn, but comes only in an MDI form.

Inhaled corticosteroids are the most potent inhalational anti-inflammatory agents available, but there are more side effects associated with their use. Oral thrush, hypothalamic-pituitary axis suppression, and alteration of bone metabolism have been described in asthmatic children, but the incidence of most side effects is dose dependent and many can be minimized with the use of a spacer device. An additional theoretical concern about their use in infants and young children with BPD relates to the inhibition of alveolar development. In contrast, if the child requires repeated courses of systemic corticosteroids to control asthma symptoms, the use of inhaled steroids actually may decrease systemic exposure to the drug.

Other Therapies

If appropriate asthma therapy fails to control wheezing symptoms, other causes of airway narrowing should be evaluated and treated. Interstitial or airway wall edema resulting from fluid overload, congestive heart failure, pulmonary hypertension, or abnormal pulmonary capillary permeability will accentuate airway narrowing for any degree of smooth muscle contraction, and can cause chronic or recurrent wheezing that is poorly responsive to the administration of bronchodilators. Evaluation for gastroesophageal reflux should be considered in any patient whose asthma symptoms are poorly controlled despite maximum anti-inflammatory therapy or whose respiratory symptoms are most prominent after meals or during sleep. Gastroesophageal reflux, with or without aspiration, occurs frequently in infants with BPD. Vagally mediated reflex bronchospasm resulting from esophageal irritation or direct airway irritation from aspiration of gastric contents can result in recurrent wheezing. Swallowing dysfunction can lead to aspiration during feedings and to inadvertent relaxation of the lower esophageal sphincter with reflux of gastric contents. Children who have pathologic gastroesophageal reflux and tracheostomies are at increased risk to aspirate because they are unable to protect the airway if gastric contents reflux to the level of the larynx. Usual therapy includes use of a histamine$_2$ receptor blocker and a motility agent to enhance gastric emptying or increase the tone of the lower esophageal sphincter.

Bronchopulmonary Dysplasia Spells

Bronchopulmonary dysplasia spells are episodes of acute respiratory distress, usually accompanied by irritability and agitation, with progression to hypoxemia and often to generalized cyanosis. They may be accompanied by end-expiratory apnea and bradycardia. Underlying etiologies of BPD spells include severe airway collapse secondary to tracheomalacia or bronchomalacia, laryngospasm or bronchospasm following aspiration, pulmonary hypertensive crisis, occult heart disease (ie, unexpected right-to-left shunts), or hydrocephalus.

▸ Clinical Manifestations

Bronchopulmonary dysplasia spells usually occur in infants and younger children. They often are precipitated by painful stimuli but can occur during stooling or in association with being upset. Agitation is accompanied by tachycardia and poor air entry even with positive-pressure support. As the spell progresses, hypoxemia, diaphoresis, bradycardia, and cyanosis ensue.

▸ Treatment

Every effort should be made to identify the underlying cause of the spells and institute appropriate treatment before the infant is discharged from the hospital. If an infant continues to have spells following discharge, a few general measures can be taken to support the infant through the spell. The combination of sedation and positive end-expiratory pressure with bag and mask usually will improve ventilation and reestablish adequate gas exchange. Such interventions require special training of caregivers. Simultaneous administration of bronchodilators by aerosol or subcutaneous route also may improve gas exchange.

Cardiovascular Complications

Pulmonary hypertension occurs in some infants and young children with BPD and results from structural and functional changes in the pulmonary blood vessels. There is a reduction in the number of alveolar capillaries in conjunction with the reduced alveolar number. In addition, arterial remodeling may be present, with medial hypertrophy, intimal proliferation, and excessive smooth muscle extending into peripheral vessels. There is heightened pulmonary vaso-reactivity. Vasoconstriction in response to hypoxia, hypercarbia, and acidosis further reduces arterial cross-sectional area. Together, these changes result in elevated pulmonary artery pressures and increased pulmonary vascular resistance, which in turn can cause right ventricular hypertrophy (cor pulmonale). If right ventricular strain becomes excessive, the infant can develop right-sided congestive heart failure. The structural changes in the pulmonary circulation make infants with BPD sensitive to volume challenges even in the absence of baseline cardiac symptoms. Thus, daily volume loads exceeding 150 to 180 mL/kg/day may precipitate respiratory and cardiac distress. The anatomic changes seen in the pulmonary vessels appear to undergo remodeling to a more normal appearance with age.

Systemic hypertension also occurs in infants with BPD with increased frequency. It usually is found within the first 6 months of life and resolves after several months in those infants who do not require antihypertensive therapy. The etiology is unclear. Approximately half of all patients require treatment for systemic hypertension.

▸ Clinical Manifestations

The clinical signs of pulmonary hypertension include dyspnea, ease of fatigue, diaphoresis, exercise intolerance, poor feeding, and cyanosis. Patients with severe pulmonary hypertension are at risk for recurrent episodes of pulmonary edema and congestive heart failure. Acute viral illnesses can result in a pulmonary hypertensive crisis, a temporarily increased requirement for supplemental oxygen or diuretic therapy, or death.

Signs of volume overload or increased pulmonary interstitial fluid volume include tachypnea and tachycardia. Often, diffuse crackles are present and the amount of supplemental oxygen required to maintain normal oxyhemoglobin saturation is increased. Because intrapulmonary fluid is increased, the lungs become stiffer. Intercostal, suprasternal, and sternal retractions are more pronounced because of the acute decrease in lung compliance, and work of breathing will increase as well. Excess fluid in the interstitial space can accentuate small airway obstruction and wheezing. The walls of small airways become edematous and contribute to airway narrowing. Hepatomegaly reflects the increase in circulating volume.

The sleeping heart rate, a measurement that parents can be taught to make or which they can read from a continuous monitor like a pulse oximeter, is a sensitive indicator of subacute volume overload. Normally, there is a physiologic decrease in heart rate into the 80s to low 100s, depending on the age of the infant, during sound sleep. As circulating volume increases, there is a loss of physiologic sleeping bradycardia. As volume overload increases, persistent tachycardia may ensue. Tachypnea or a persistent increase in respiratory rate above the infant's baseline sleeping respiratory rate will develop as well.

▸ Treatment

Therapies are aimed to decrease pulmonary artery pressures, right ventricular work, and myocardial oxygen consumption. Supplemental oxygen is the mainstay of therapy and is used to minimize pulmonary vascular resistance. If hypercapnia and acidosis persist, tracheostomy placement to facilitate chronic mechanical ventilation should be considered. Fluid restriction and diuretic therapy are used to reduce circulating intravascular volume.

Diuretics

If an infant or young child with BPD demonstrates overt heart failure or severe volume overload, a rapid-acting diuretic such as furosemide should be used for acute intervention. A dose of 0.5 to 1 mg/kg orally or intramuscularly two or three times a day will promote marked diuresis and reestablish homeostasis. When volume overload is present and absorption of a drug from an edematous gastrointestinal tract may be compromised, the parenteral form of furosemide should be used in preference to the oral form. Once the diuresis has begun, the oral form of the drug can be used effectively. A child with signs of moderate or marked distress should be hospitalized so that the rate of diuresis can be monitored carefully.

Furosemide enhances calcium excretion in the kidney and can result in nephrocalcinosis, renal stone formation, and hematuria. Any infant requiring long-term use of furosemide should be screened for rickets with determination of serum calcium, phosphorus, and alkaline phosphatase levels. For long-term diuretic use, calcium-sparing diuretics like chlorothiazide can avoid these complications and are better choices. These diuretics waste potassium and chloride, however, so that spironolactone, a weak diuretic with potassium-sparing characteristics, can be added to help offset electrolyte imbalance. In rare instances, chlorothiazide and spironolactone in combination are inadequate to maintain fluid balance. To avoid the effects of long-term use of furosemide, metolazone can be added to the regimen.

Diuretic use contributes to a hypochloremic, hypokalemic metabolic alkalosis. The resulting elevated bicarbonate levels in turn cause a further elevation of the arterial $PaCO_2$. A blood gas determination that shows a normal or slightly alkalemic pH with an elevated $PaCO_2$ confirms the presence of a primary metabolic alkalosis. Administration of supplemental potassium chloride, 2 to 5 mEq/kg/day, replaces the chloride deficit and promotes renal wasting of bicarbonate. The dose is increased based on serum potassium and chloride determinations. In all instances, volume of fluid intake and daily sodium intake must be monitored closely. All diuretics waste sodium to some degree. If the dietary intake of sodium is adequate (3 to 5 mEq/kg/day), hyponatremia usually is the result of volume overload rather than sodium depletion. Providing more than the daily requirement of sodium will only perpetuate fluid retention and the need for diuretics.

▶ The Weaning of Therapy

The order of withdrawal of therapies such as oxygen and diuretics is more a reflection of style than of science. For families who have trouble maintaining nasal cannula oxygen, adherence to therapy will be enhanced if supplemental oxygen is weaned before diuretic therapy. Children can be allowed to outgrow their doses of medications or the drugs can be actively withdrawn. To track clinical response, only one drug should be discontinued at a time, with close monitoring of heart rate, respiratory rate, weight gain, liver span, and oxyhemoglobin saturation. To wean more slowly, a single dose of the drug can be discontinued with a several week observation period before subsequent doses of the drug are stopped. Potassium chloride supplements can be stopped simultaneously with furosemide or chlorothiazide.

▶ Monitoring

Children with documented right ventricular hypertrophy should undergo repeat EKG evaluations every 3 to 6 months to assess for resolution or progression of ventricular hypertrophy. If hypertrophy fails to resolve or progresses, cardiac catheterization with angiography to rule out other unsuspected cardiopulmonary lesions such as large bronchial-to-pulmonary artery collaterals, and reassessment of oxygen needs, including prolonged monitoring or overnight sleep study, should be undertaken. When diuretic therapy is first instituted, electrolytes should be monitored monthly. When the regimen is established and stable, the frequency of monitoring can be decreased to every 3 to 4 months.

Problems With Growth and Nutrition

Adequate growth is the sine qua non of overall good health for the patient with BPD. Growth failure has been correlated with an increased resting energy expenditure in some infants with BPD. Medications such as caffeine, theophylline, and beta-agonists may contribute to an increased energy expenditure as well. Although energy needs may be greater than normal, intake may be significantly lower than normal. Inability to drink well because of respiratory distress, medically imposed fluid restriction, dysphagia from gastroesophageal reflux with esophagitis, swallowing disorders, or dumping syndromes because of loss of bowel in the neonatal period all can contribute to poor nutrient intake.

▶ Clinical Manifestations

The infant with BPD should gain 15 to 30 g/day to maintain adequate growth. To realize catch-up growth, weight gain of 45 to 60 g/day may be necessary. Anthropometric measurements (eg, weight, length, head circumference) should be taken at each office visit and plotted against standard curves. Inadequate growth is signaled by failure to maintain growth percentiles, but optimal growth should be reflected in a greater than normal growth velocity. Correction for preterm birth usually is made on growth curves for weight until the age of 2 and for length until 3 years, but the history of prematurity can continue to affect the growth percentiles up to 7 years of age.

It is unusual to see clinical signs of vitamin deficiency, whereas mineral abnormalities occur more frequently because of concomitant therapies. Infants who develop hyponatremia and hypochloremia also tend to demonstrate lower growth rates and smaller head circumferences.

▶ Treatment

To achieve catch-up growth, nutritional plans must aim to provide supranormal caloric intake, somewhere in the range of 120 to 150 kcal/kg/day while not overtaxing the infant with an excessive volume challenge. This can be achieved by using concentrated formulas up to 30 cal/oz. Caloric density of formula can be increased by concentrating it up to approximately 26 cal/oz. Thereafter, carbohydrate or fat supplements must be added to the formula to increase caloric density. This method of increasing nutrient intake is not devoid of problems; excessive carbohydrate intake increases the respiratory load by liberating more carbon dioxide during metabolism. Fat additives delay gastric emptying and therefore can exacerbate gastroesophageal reflux; they are particularly irritating if accidentally aspirated. For children older than 1 year, there are nutritionally complete formulas that provide 30 cal/oz.

Occasionally, even with the use of high-calorie formulas, the infant is not able to ingest enough to achieve the daily caloric goal. Additionally, the work associated with ingesting all of the daily calories by mouth may be excessive and contribute to growth failure in younger or sicker infants. In such cases, additional calories can be administered in the form of postprandial gavage or continuous drip nighttime feedings. The nasogastric tube usually is considered a short-term (ie, several weeks) method of delivering supplemental feedings. It causes oropharyngeal discomfort and can inhibit or impair efforts at improving oral motor function. Additionally, the nasogastric tube can become displaced and cause accidental aspiration of feedings into the airway. If supplemental feedings will be required for extended periods, gastrostomy tube placement should be considered. Placement of a gastrostomy tube can worsen preexisting gastroesophageal reflux, however, so many patients also will require simultaneous fundoplication.

If the infant fails to demonstrate catch-up growth or shows a slower growth velocity than expected despite these interventions, a 3-day diet record may discriminate inadequate caloric intake from excessive metabolic demands. Unapparent periods of hypoxemia should be suspected if caloric intake appears adequate for growth. If such episodes cannot be found, measurements of resting energy expenditure may be helpful. In unusual circumstances, elective resumption of mechanical ventilation may be required to decrease the energy cost of breathing to promote catch-up growth. Patients requiring diuretic therapy, fluid and electrolyte balance, blood urea nitrogen, creatinine, calcium, and phosphorus should be monitored along with a urinalysis, especially if free water intake is diminished because of the use of highly concentrated formula.

Neuro-developmental Issues

The course of infants with BPD may be complicated by intraventricular hemorrhage, seizures, retinopathy of prematurity, and hearing deficit. The same problems that cause premature delivery, like maternal drug use, young maternal age, absence of prenatal care, gestational hypertension, or maternal infection, also impact dramatically and directly on neuro-developmental outcome. The likelihood of an infant sustaining significant intraventricular bleeding, hydrocephalus, or periventricular leukomalacia is inversely proportional to gestational age. Postnatal risk factors for poor neuro-developmental outcome include poor socioeconomic status, unemployment, and low level of maternal education.

Retinopathy of prematurity (ROP) results from hyperoxic damage to retinal vessels. Following injury, excessive neovascularization occurs in the retina and vitreous cavity. The healing phase of ROP is marked by regression of these blood vessels with maturation of the retina.

▶ Clinical Manifestations

Motor and cognitive functions of infants with BPD are lower than those of premature controls up to 2 years of age. Over the next year, however, dramatic improvement in infants with BPD and abnormal motor or cognitive skills can be seen when compared with preterm controls. By 8 years of age, no statistical differences exist in neurological function between premature infants with or without BPD, although learning scores are lower in the BPD group and scores of both groups are lower than full-term infants' scores. Learning disorders and problems with attention-deficit/hyperactivity disorder become apparent when children with BPD are challenged to learn in regular classrooms by the first or second grade.

▶ Treatment

Efforts are made to prevent overstimulation of and excessive energy consumption for infants with BPD. The infant's personal space should be free from excessive auditory and visual stimulation to avoid sensory overload. Individualized plans must be made to include appropriate interventional therapies such as occupational, physical, and speech therapy. Parents can be taught exercises and interventions to enhance the periodic sessions with professional therapists. Immediately after hospital discharge, many of these therapies can be provided as home based, but ultimately therapies and ongoing evaluations are transferred to center-based programs. Every effort must be made to mainstream school-aged children into regular classrooms, with remedial classes available to aid children with any learning disabilities. Assistive devices are available for children with hearing and speech impairment as well as motor deficits. Any child suspected of having attention-deficit/hyperactivity disorder should be referred to a developmental pediatrician for evaluation and possible pharmacotherapy.

If an ophthalmologist determines that an infant's retina is not yet mature, meticulous attention to the oxyhemoglobin saturation is necessary to maintain it between 90% to 95%. The infants should be monitored frequently by an ophthalmologist to survey for progression of ROP. If progression occurs, vascular ablation therapy in the form of laser therapy or cryotherapy can halt the progression of the disease and prevent blindness. Once the retina is fully vascularized, or if the infant has undergone cryotherapy or laser therapy for ROP, the infant can tolerate modest hyperoxia without additional retinal injury.

Intercurrent Illnesses

Infants with BPD are particularly prone to serious lower respiratory tract illnesses with viral infections. The most common etiologic agent is respiratory syncytial virus (RSV), but adenovirus, influenza virus, and enteroviruses all can cause serious respiratory exacerbations. Lower respiratory illness serious enough to require hospitalization can occur in children with BPD who are older than 1 year of age. They can be reinfected with the same agent in the same season and still develop severe illness. The airway epithelium of patients with BPD is not normal and local defense mechanisms may be compromised. Thus, while most acute lower respiratory tract infections result from viruses, bacterial infections can occur as well. Children with tracheostomies can develop bacterial tracheobronchitis in association with viral lower respiratory infections.

▶ Clinical Manifestations

Respiratory viral illnesses often cause bronchospasm and exacerbate asthma symptoms. Hypoxemia is common, even in patients who have successfully weaned from supplemental oxygen. In patients who rely on supplemental oxygen via nasal cannula, mucosal inflammation and secretions secondary to an upper respiratory tract infection can obstruct oxygen flow and contribute to hypoxemia and tachypnea. Pulmonary hypertension may be worsened during infectious exacerbations, and signs of volume overload or congestive heart failure may be more prominent.

▶ Treatment

During acute illnesses, all therapies may have to be increased; the child may require a higher concentration of supplemental oxygen, more frequent bronchodilator aerosols, and additional doses of diuretics. If the child demonstrates a clinical response to an aerosolized bronchodilator, a 5- to 7-day course of prednisone, 1 to 2 mg/kg/day divided twice a day, can improve respiratory status and prevent the need for rehospitalization.

Viruses remain the most common cause of infectious exacerbations. In the presence of crackles heard in the chest and fever greater than 102°F, however, bacterial lower respiratory infection should be considered. This is especially true in the infant with moderate to severe BPD who requires supplemental oxygen, chronic bronchodilators, and diuretics. Bacterial tracheobronchitis can be inferred in children with tracheostomies when tracheal secretions increase in amount and become purulent, and a Gram stain demonstrates large numbers of white blood cells along with a predominant organism. Children with BPD and chronic tracheostomies usually harbor gram-negative bacteria like *Pseudomonas* and may require specific antipseudomonal therapy.

Well-Child Care

Infants with BPD should receive the regular schedule of childhood immunizations. In addition, infants older than 6 months corrected age should receive immunization against influenza virus. In recent years, passive immunotherapy against RSV has become available. A hyperimmune intravenous (IV) pooled human polyclonal gamma globulin, respiratory syncytial virus-intravenous immunoglobulin (RSV-IVIG), and an engineered intramuscular monoclonal antibody, palivizumab, have been shown to reduce the need for hospitalization as well as the length of hospitalization significantly in infants with BPD who become infected with RSV. Monthly intravenous infusions or intramuscular injections are administered throughout the RSV season. The intramuscular preparation is easier to administer than the IV drug and is not associated with a volume challenge that can occur with RSV-IVIG. In addition, palivizumab is not a blood product, so it can be used in children whose parents have religious objection to the use of RSV-IVIG. On the other hand, because it is polyclonal, RSV-IVIG also offers some protection against other respiratory viruses that palivizumab does not.

Psychosocial Issues

Normal parent-infant bonding is impaired in the perinatal period because the infant is sick and requires several invasive therapies that isolate the infant from the parents. Parents also may view the infant as exceptionally fragile and may be afraid to interact with the infant. Infants who are sick are discharged with complicated medical regimens and often with complex technologies. Parents not only must provide normal support and stimulation for their infant, but they also must assume the role of medical caregiver. Nevertheless, providing families with assessment skills while simultaneously supporting the patient with the technologies and medications necessary to maintain medical stability will make the home situation less stressful and avoid the need for frequent unexpected rehospitalizations. In this way, parents ultimately become more comfortable with the care of an infant who is medically fragile and has complex needs, and they can begin to dwell on more routine aspects of their infant's growth and development.

Summary

- Children with BPD may have multiple medical conditions including airway obstruction, pulmonary hypertension, fluid overload, failure to thrive, and learning disabilities or developmental delay.
- Multiple medical therapies and technologies may be required to maintain clinical stability for the infant and young child with BPD. Recruitment of family members to participate in a comprehensive care plan and use of subspecialist medical consultants and therapists can simplify care of these patients.
- Withdrawal of therapies becomes a by-product of clinical improvement instead of a focus of care. Helping families support their infant until the natural processes of growth and healing allow for removal of medical therapies is one of the most rewarding aspects of caring for infants with BPD.

Bibliography

Abman SH, Warady BA, Lum GM, Koops BL. Systemic hypertension in infants with bronchopulmonary dysplasia. *J Pediatr.* 1984;104:928-931

Abman SH, Wolfe RR, Accurso FJ, Koops BL, Bowman CM, Wiggins JW Jr. Pulmonary vascular response to oxygen in infants with severe bronchopulmonary dysplasia. *Pediatrics.* 1985;75:80-84

Allen MC, Donohue PK, Dusman AE. The limit of viability — neonatal outcome of infants born at 22 to 25 weeks' gestation. *N Engl J Med.* 1993;329:1597-1601

Ascher DP, Rosen P, Null DM, de Lemos RA, Wheller JJ. Systemic to pulmonary collaterals mimicking patent ductus arteriosus in neonates with prolonged ventilatory courses. *J Pediatr.* 1985;107:282-284

Bhutani VK, Rubenstein D, Shaffer TH. Pressure-induced deformation in immature airways. *Pediatr Res.* 1981;15:829-832

Coalson JJ, Winter V, de Lemos RA. Decreased alveolarization in baboon survivors with bronchopulmonary dysplasia. *Am J Respir Crit Care Med.* 1995;152:640-646

Filtchev SI, Curzi-Dascalova L, Spassov L, Kauffmann F, Trang HT, Gaultier C. Heart rate variability during sleep in infants with bronchopulmonary dysplasia. Effects of mild decrease in oxygen saturation. *Chest.* 1994;106:1711-1716

Garg M, Kurzner SI, Bautista D, Keens TG. Hypoxic arousal responses in infants with bronchopulmonary dysplasia. *Pediatrics.* 1988;82:59-63

Garg M, Kurzner SI, Bautista DB, Keens TG. Clinically unsuspected hypoxia during sleep and feeding in infants with bronchopulmonary dysplasia. *Pediatrics.* 1988;81:635-642

Gray PH, Rogers Y. Are infants with bronchopulmonary dysplasia at risk for sudden infant death syndrome? *Pediatrics.* 1994;93:774-777

Groothuis JR, Gutierrez KM, Lauer BA. Respiratory syncytial virus infection in children with bronchopulmonary dysplasia. *Pediatrics.* 1988;82:199-203

Groothuis JR, Salbenblatt CK, Lauer BA. Severe respiratory syncytial virus infection in older children. *Am J Dis Child.* 1990;144:346-348

Harris MA, Sullivan CE. Sleep pattern and supplementary oxygen requirements in infants with chronic neonatal lung disease. *Lancet.* 1995;345:831-832

The IMpact-RSV Study Group. Palivizumab, a humanized respiratory syncytial virus monoclonal antibody, reduces hospitalization from respiratory syncytial virus infection in high-risk infants. *Pediatrics.* 1998;102:531-537

Katz-Salamon M, Jonsson B, Lagercrantz H. Blunted peripheral chemoreceptor response to hyperoxia in a group of infants with bronchopulmonary dysplasia. *Pediatr Pulmonol.* 1995;20:101-106

Kurzner SI, Garg M, Bautista DB, Sargent CW, Bowman CM, Keens TG. Growth failure in bronchopulmonary dysplasia: elevated metabolic rates and pulmonary mechanics. *J Pediatr.* 1988;112:73-80

Margraf LR, Tomashefski JF Jr, Bruce MC, Dahms BB. Morphometric analysis of the lung in bronchopulmonary dysplasia. *Am Rev Respir Dis.* 1991;143:391-400

Miller KE, Edwards DK, Hilton S, Collins D, Lynch F, Williams R. Acquired lobar emphysema in premature infants with bronchopulmonary dysplasia: an iatrogenic disease? *Radiology.* 1981; 138:589-592

Miller RW, Woo P, Kellman RK, Slagle TS. Tracheobronchial abnormalities in infants with bronchopulmonary dysplasia. *J Pediatr.* 1987;111:779-782

Northway WH Jr, Rosan RC, Porter DY. Pulmonary disease following respirator therapy of hyaline-membrane disease. Bronchopulmonary dysplasia. *N Engl J Med.* 1967;276:357-368

Northway WH Jr, Moss RB, Carlisle KB, et al. Late pulmonary sequelae of bronchopulmonary dysplasia. *N Engl J Med.* 1990;323:1793-1799

Panitch HB, Isaacson G. Transtracheal oxygen use in a young girl with bronchopulmonary dysplasia. *Pediatr Pulmonol.* 1994;18:255-257

Panitch HB, Keklikian EN, Motley RA, Wolfson MR, Schidlow DV. Effect of altering smooth muscle tone on maximal expiratory flows in patients with tracheomalacia. *Pediatr Pulmonol.* 1990;9:170-176

Pinney MA, Cotton EK. Home management of bronchopulmonary dysplasia. *Pediatrics.* 1976;58:856-859

The PREVENT Study Group. Reduction of respiratory syncytial virus hospitalization among pre-mature infants and infants with bronchopulmonary dysplasia using respiratory syncytial virus immune globulin prophylaxis. *Pediatrics.* 1997;99:93-99

Robertson CM, Etches PC, Goldson E, Kyle JM. Eight-year school performance, neurodevelop-mental, and growth outcomes of neonates with bronchopulmonary dysplasia: a comparative study. *Pediatrics.* 1992;89:365-372

Sekar KC, Duke JC. Sleep apnea and hypoxemia in recently weaned premature infants with and without bronchopulmonary dysplasia. *Pediatr Pulmonol.* 1991;10:112-116

Sindel BD, Maisels MJ, Ballantine TV. Gastroesophageal reflux to the proximal esophagus in infants with bronchopulmonary dysplasia. *Am J Dis Child.* 1989;143:1103-1106

Tomashefski JF Jr, Oppermann HC, Vawter GF, Reid LM. Bronchopulmonary dysplasia: a morphometric study with emphasis on the pulmonary vasculature. *Pediatr Pathol.* 1984;2:469-487

Wilkie RA, Bryan MH. Effect of bronchodilators on airway resistance in ventilator-dependent neonates with chronic lung disease. *J Pediatr.* 1987;111:278-282

Zinman R, Franco I, Pizzuti-Daechsel R. Home oxygen delivery system for infants. *Pediatr Pulmonol.* 1985;1:325-327

Chapter 30

Guidelines for Home Management and Phototherapy for Neonatal Hyperbilirubinemia

Vinod Bhutani, MD; Ann Schwoebel, MSN, CRNP; Lois H. Johnson, MD

Introduction

Neonatal hyperbilirubinemia, characterized by a total serum bilirubin (TSB) value greater than 12.9 mg/dL, is one of the most common neonatal diagnoses. Usually benign and considered physiological, it has a myriad of pathological etiologies and potential dele-terious sequelae. Nearly 50% of term and near-term neo-nates deemed healthy and discharged from well-baby nurseries may develop neo-natal hyperbilirubinemia during the first week after birth. In about 5% of neonates, the TSB level will be above 17 mg/dL, in approximately 1% the level is above 20 mg/dL, and less than 1% may develop a TSB value greater than 25 mg/dL.

To facilitate the identification, evaluation, and interventions for the complications asso-ciated with hyperbilirubinemia, the American Academy of Pediatrics has recommended consensus-based guidelines for the management of hyperbilirubinemia. Interventions with phototherapy have effectively and drastically reduced the need for exchange transfusions. The relative ease and safety of phototherapy have allowed for the extension of home-based management of hyperbilirubinemia to home phototherapy. This chapter provides an outline of the risks of hyperbilirubinemia, guidelines for patient selection, management options, and strategies for safe and effective use of home-based care.

Neonatal Hyperbilirubinemia

Biological, epidemiological, and clinical factors account for the propensity for visible jaundice in the newborn. Biological reasons include increased bilirubin production, decreased clear-

343

ance, or a combination of both. Epidemiological factors include near-term gestation, male gender, east-Asian ethnic origin, previous sibling with jaundice, seasonal variation, and prevalence in the breastfeeding population. Clinical factors that predispose the occurrence of hyperbilirubinemia are prenatal factors (oxytocin induction), mode of delivery (vacuum and forceps delivery), bruising and birth trauma, maternal medications with breastfeeding, sepsis, dehydration, and hypoalbuminemia. Unconjugated bilirubin (a breakdown product of heme) levels rise soon after birth and generally peak between ages 3 to 7 days. A percentile-based description of TSB values in healthy term and near-term neonates is shown in Figure 30-1.

Clinical Assessment of Jaundice

Variability of jaundice and potential error limit the value of visual assessment of jaundice on the face, chest, trunk, or limbs. Of greater concern is the fact that jaundice that has extended over the entire body is more difficult to recognize than when the cephalocaudal progression is not complete. When newborns are examined for jaundice, the lighting of the room, skin pigmentation of the neonate, confounding effects of polycythemia (ruddiness) and skin characteristics, and the experience of the observer (especially in a home care setting) need to be taken into account. The correlation between the visual assessment of jaundice and the serum bilirubin level remains poor even with experienced observers.

Risk of Complications Associated With Hyperbilirubinemia

Bilirubin-induced toxicity has been a subject of research, inquiry, speculation, and controversy. A gentler and kinder approach had been recommended until recently, in view of the relative lack of clinical research-based evidence of neurotoxicity. However, evidence from an epidemiological reemergence of kernicterus has challenged views about the purely benign nature of neonatal jaundice. The potential reversible nature of acute bilirubin encephalopathy would suggest chronic athetoid cerebral palsy (kernicterus) is not the only sequelae in survivors. A spectrum of bilirubin-induced neurologic dysfunction (BIND) is evident in the acute state, as tabulated

FIGURE 30-1. Bilirubin Care Map (Term and Near-Term Neonates): Universal Total Serum Bilirubin (TSB)/Transcutaneous Bilirubin (TcB) Screen and Follow-up*

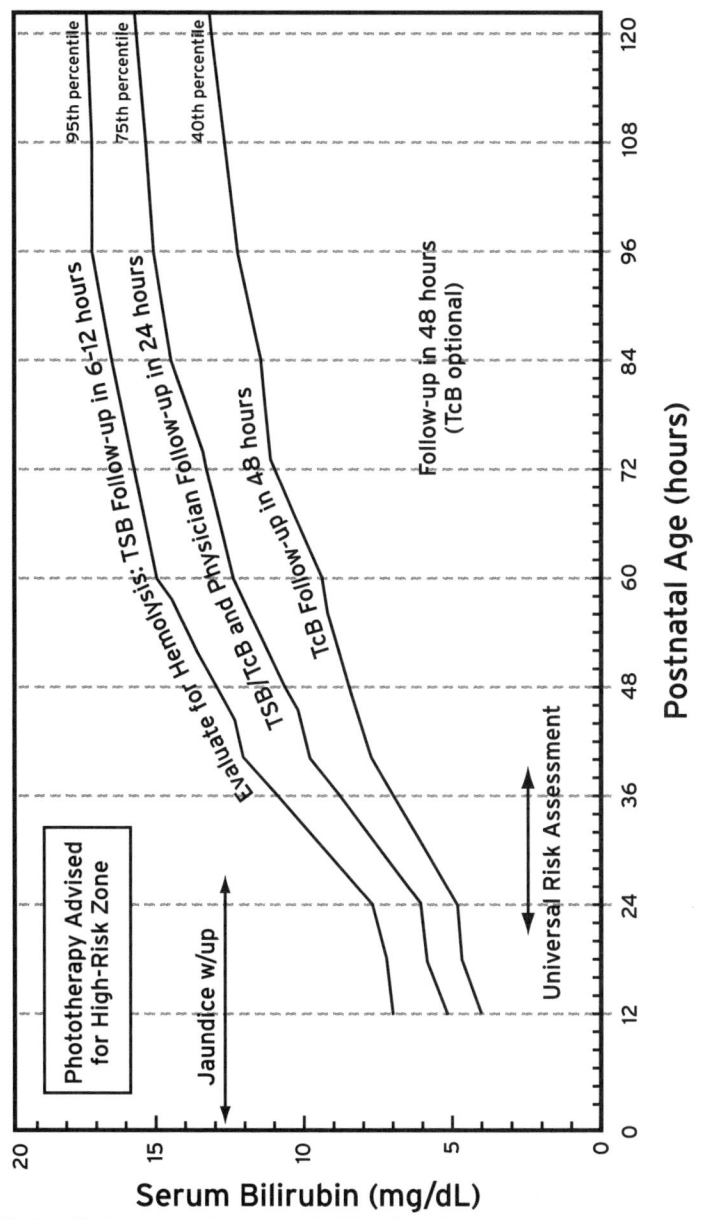

*Based on Bhutani VK, Johnson L, Sivieri EM. Predictive ability of a predischarge hour-specific serum bilirubin for subsequent significant hyperbilirubinemia in healthy term and near-term newborns. *Pediatrics.* 1999;103:6-14. Infants younger than phototherapy age 60 hours were not included in this nomogram.

in Table 30-1. A constellation of suspicious neurologic manifestations historically has been reported in children who have been exposed to excessive hyperbilirubinemia (Table 30-2). Sensorineural hearing loss also is a hallmark of kernicterus, whereas milder sequelae in the form of auditory neuropathy also have been reported. At this stage, there is a paucity of data that would define the risk of BIND following an acute rise in TSB values above the 98th percentile as well as BIND due to persistent and prolonged hyperbilirubinemia in the high-risk zone.

TABLE 30-1. Clinical Features of Bilirubin-Induced Neurologic Dysfunction

Dysfunction Level	Clinical Features		
	Behavior	Muscle Tone	Cry Pattern
Mild	Sleepy, decreased feeding	Variable hypotonia	High pitched
Moderate	Lethargy, irritable Poor feeding	Nuchal or truncal arching	Piercing
Severe	Semi-coma, seizures	Opisthotonus posturing	Inconsolable

TABLE 30-2. Suspicious Neurological Features on Follow-up

- Awkwardness
- Gait abnormalities
- Upward gaze abnormalities
- Failure at fine stereognosis
- Nystagmus
- Exaggerated abdominal and cremasteric reflexes
- Vasomotor abnormalities
- Equivocal Babinski reflexes
- Questionable hypotonia

Risk Assessment for Occurrence of Hyperbilirubinemia

Identification of hyperbilirubinemia in newborns may be done by designating neonates into high-risk, intermediate-risk, or low-risk zones defined by percentile ranks of hour-specific TSB values. When done prior to discharge, a predictive risk assessment is feasible as listed in Table 30-3. For newborns with persistent TSB values in the high-risk zone, special attention must be made to assess neurological status (Table 30-1) and consider an auditory-evoked brain stem response. Other tests have been developed to assess the risk for BIND prior to the onset or neurologic injury. Of these, bilirubin/albumin (B:A) ratio is readily available and has the potential to provide reassurance or identify neonates in the high-risk zone. Presently, the ability to measure free (unbound) bilirubin, which may be helpful in defining the risk of BIND, is not commercially available. Thus, B:A ratio provides an interim and helpful mode to assess newborns with bilirubin values in the high-risk zone (Table 30-4).

TABLE 30-3. Risk of Excessive Hyperbilirubinemia Using Serum Bilirubin

Predischarge Total Serum Bilirubin (measured at age <72 hours)	Probability of Excessive Hyperbilirubinemia
Values <40th percentile track	<1:46 (most likely 0)
Values 40th to 75th percentile track	1:46
Values 75th to 95th percentile track	1:8
Values >95th percentile track	2:5

TABLE 30-4. Risk of Bilirubin-Induced Neurologic Dysfunction Using B:A Ratio*

Low Risk	Indeterminate Risk	High Risk
B:A<5.3	B:A=5.3 to 6.0	B:A>6.0

*Dependent on the hypothesis that bilirubin-induced neurologic dysfunction can be reversible, a more precise risk assessment may be feasible by measuring free bilirubin.

Basis for Interventions

Therapeutic maneuvers to reduce the serum bilirubin and the bilirubin load may be achieved by reducing its production, enhancing its clearance, or providing a neuro-protective mechanism against toxicity. The modes of clinical and experimental interventions are listed in Table 30-5.

TABLE 30-5. Intervention Strategies for Hyperbilirubinemia

	Mode	Method/Drugs
Types of interventions		
Decrease production	Heme-oxygenase inhibitors (experimental).	Tin protoporphyrin, tin mesoporphyrin.
Increase clearance		
Enteral clearance	Decrease entero-hepatic recirculation.	Enhance feeding, use of feed supplements (use of expressed breast milk or formula).
		Encourage stooling (avoid laxatives or cathartics).
Hepatic clearance	Induce glucuronyl transferase enzymes.	Phenobarbital (not usually recommended).
Transcutaneous clearance	Photoisomerization.	Phototherapy (see text).
Vascular clearance	Exchange transfusion.	Arterial/venous exchange or venous exchange transfusion.
Improve neuro-protection	Improve albumin-bilirubin binding.	Albumin infusion.
		Avoid agents that inhibit bilirubin binding: nonesterified fatty acids, ketones, etc.

Rationale for Phototherapy

The goal of phototherapy is to reduce the amount of bilirubin in the neonate with jaundice. In contrast to the effect of sunlight in reducing jaundice (heliotherapy), photo-destruction of bilirubin can be predictable and controlled and is not seasonal dependent. Phototherapy is accomplished by absorption of light by the bilirubin molecule, photo-conversion of bilirubin, and excretion of photoproducts.

▶ Chemical Process

The absorption by bilirubin of a photon from a light source is the initial step that commences the process of photo-destruction. A photon with a wavelength of 450 nm (blue photon) has the highest probability of being absorbed by the bilirubin molecule in vitro. However, in a newborn, the albumin binding characteristics of bilirubin and the effect of long-chain fatty acid co-binding to albumin can change the absorption spectrum of the bilirubin. In addition, the ability of the photons to penetrate the skin and the spectral output of the light source complicates the ideal wavelength at which the best response is to be expected.

▶ Site of Action

Unconjugated bilirubin bound to albumin and deposited in the subcutaneous tissue is the prime target for phototherapy.

▶ Role of Photon Energy

The photon's energy produces an excited state of bilirubin that leads to heat production and a photochemical reaction that actually changes the bilirubin molecule. It is the latter component of the photon's effect that provides a mechanism to reduce the bilirubin load of the neonate. The formation of photoproducts reaches a steady state within 4 hours of the beginning of phototherapy.

▶ Irradiance of Phototherapy

The rate of bilirubin decline is proportional to the dose of phototherapy. The dosage is measured by the intensity of the light at the level of the skin surface and is defined as the irradiance. Handheld compact devices used to measure irradiance accurately that operate on rechargeable batteries are easy to operate. Studies have defined an irradiance of 40 mW/cm^2/nm in the 425 to 475 nm range as being of high intensity.

▶ Spectral Output of Phototherapy

The spectral output of light sources that compare with the absorption spectrum of bilirubin have been studied to define the best light source for phototherapy. The light source itself, dosage of light, characteristics of the neonatal skin, and chemical properties of bilirubin influence the clinical usefulness of the light source. The available light sources can be defined as fluorescent lamps of blue or white emissions, fiber-optic sources (as in the bilirubin blanket lights), and light emitting diode light sources (these are experimental).

▶ Surface Area

Phototherapy should be administered to the largest exposed surface area of the newborn. Because the scalp and torso (front and back) comprise most of the skin surface, these areas should have direct exposure to light.

▶ Duration

The clinical effect of phototherapy should be evident within 4 to 6 hours of its initiation, as the rise of bilirubin is substantially reduced or corrected. Phototherapy should be continued until a substantial reduction in the bilirubin load has occurred and after the newborn has shown evidence of appropriate and physiologic clearance of bilirubin. Upon discontinuation of phototherapy, a rebound level measure of bilirubin should be obtained within 12 to 24 hours to ascertain the continuing decline in bilirubin levels. Phototherapy should be discontinued when the bilirubin level is lower than the 40th percentile track (generally a TSB value less than 12 mg/dL).

▶ Clinical Use of Phototherapy

The newborn is exposed nude (but diapered) to the light. The light source is maintained as close as recommended by the manufacturer to achieve maximum irradiance. The number of light sources will vary according to the neonate's size so that the surface area of exposure is maximized. Based on the ambient lighting at home and the effect of the light on the newborn's skin color, closer observation of the newborn's vital signs is necessary. In view of the side effects of hyperthermia and increased insensible water loss, close observation of the body temperature, fluid intake, and urinary output are recommended. Continuous lights are more effective than intermittent phototherapy; it is recommended that the duration off phototherapy should be minimized. The decline in bilirubin values is dependent on the dosage and duration of phototherapy. The intensity of phototherapy determines the rapidity of the bilirubin decline.

Rationale for Home Phototherapy

The decision to implement home phototherapy needs to be made in an objective manner with appropriate deliberation, parental informed consent, assessment of potential risks, assessment of an anticipated response, and comprehensive and competent supervision. Some of the factors that need to be considered are listed in Table 30-6.

TABLE 30-6. Factors That Influence Home-based Versus Hospital-based Intervention

Factors	Home-based Phototherapy	Hospital-based Phototherapy
Personalize care	Medical equipment and technology at home.	Medical and technological environment.
Prevention of separation	No parental separation.	Parental involvement needs to be facilitated.
Promote breastfeeding	Active maternal role with appropriate lactational support.	Care has to be taken not to inadvertently discourage maternal role.
Intensity of irradiance	Low dose.	High and/or intense dose.
Duration of therapy	Usually 3 to 5 days.	Usually 1 to 3 days.
Parental responsibility	Intense and with parental education. Limited external support.	Supported by a nursery environment and staff.
Cost	Estimated as low cost.	Estimated to be at higher cost.
Accountability	Home care service provider/physician.	Hospital/physician.
Quality assurance	Satisfied parents and no clinical sequelae.	Satisfied parents and no clinical sequelae.

Indications for Home Management for Jaundice

Newborns who are or have been discharged from the well-baby nursery and remain asymptomatic, as well as retain their ability to feed, qualify for home-based management of jaundice provided that

- Follow-up mechanisms are in place for both the neonate and the mother
- Comprehensive discharge education has been provided to parents
- Adequate monitoring of the newborn's intake and output are established
- Home nursing is available

Indications for Home Phototherapy

Excessive hyperbilirubinemia, persistent TSB values above the 95th percentile track (similar to values greater than 17 mg/dL), or an acute rise in levels above the 98th percentile track (similar to values greater than 20 mg/dL) are the recommended guidelines to consider and initiate phototherapy.

Home-based phototherapy may be considered in neonates who are 4 days of age or older and meet the following criteria:
- Individual family motivation established by informed consent
- No apparent signs of hemolytic jaundice
- Asymptomatic for neurologic manifestations
- Absence of clinical sepsis
- Term neonate (more than 37 weeks of gestational age)
- In newborns who already have been treated in the hospital by intensive phototherapy and need continuing phototherapy for less severe bilirubin values

Phototherapy for newborns with serum bilirubin values above the 95th percentile track and prior to 96 hours of age generally is best done in a hospital-based setting, but select cases may be treated in the home. In these newborns the cause of hyperbilirubinemia most likely is a combination of increased bilirubin production (often because of unrecognized hemolysis) and delayed clearance.

Clinical Monitoring Techniques at Home

The home care professional should closely monitor the neonate's clinical status during phototherapy to ensure appropriate hydration, nutrition, and clinical improvement.
- **Nutritional well-being**
  - ~ Intake: record of feeding frequency, volume (or duration if breastfeeding), audible gulping during feeds to indicate sucking and swallowing
  - ~ Urinary: frequency of wet diapers, estimate of "soaking," evidence of "urate" crystals post-voiding
  - ~ Stooling: frequency, relationship to feeds, color and consistency, persistence of meconium
  - ~ Sleeping pattern: duration of sleep during the feed intervals
  - ~ Ability to console following a feed or persistent crying
- **Neurological manifestations:** Serial record and evaluation (see Table 30-1) of the following signs for the duration of phototherapy:
  - ~ Alteration in behavior
  - ~ Alteration in muscular tone
  - ~ Alteration in cry pattern

- **Jaundice assessment:** Phototherapy affects the clinical and visual assessment of jaundice. Thus, hyperbilirubinemia needs to be assessed by serial measurements of TSB or by transcutaneous bilirubin monitoring in the unexposed area of the skin. The first measurement, after initiation of phototherapy, should be done within 6 hours and then subsequently at 8- to 12-hour intervals if the level is unchanged or rising slowly. Once declining, the bilirubin level may be measured at 24-hour intervals.
- **Weight:** In view of the concurrent impact of inadequate oral intake and increased insensible water loss due to phototherapy, it is recommended that the body weight be measured daily to assess the magnitude of weight loss, if any.

Breastfeeding and Home Management of Hyperbilirubinemia

Successful breastfeeding without excessive hyperbilirubinemia may be accomplished by proactive lactation counseling prior to discharge from the hospital. Early support to facilitate latching, education of the mother to detect and recognizing effective latching, consistent sucking, and audible swallowing are fundamental. Promotion of the letdown of milk and the early use of an electrical breast pump facilitate adequate volume of milk production for the third to fifth day when the bilirubin levels are likely to peak.

Breastfeeding should be encouraged during the management of hyperbilirubinemia at home. Care needs to be taken with the maternal use of opioid analgesics (such as codeine) which may depress an infant's sucking and stooling patterns. Mothers should avoid drugs that trigger glucose-6-phosphate dehydrogenase (G6PD)-related hemolysis in families at risk while test results are pending.

During the administration of phototherapy, infants should receive frequent feedings supplemented with expressed breast milk or formula while closely monitoring the urinary output. Rarely, if there is inadequate expressed breast milk, formula supplementation needs to be considered. Intravenous fluids may be necessary only for significant signs of dehydration. The goals of home management of hyperbilirubinemia are to provide enteral nutrition, encourage stooling, and prevent starvation and dehydration.

Nursing Care Plan for Home Care

The nursing care plan should include the following:
- Policy and procedures for instructions in the use of equipment and its safety
- Policy and procedures for indications, contraindications, and patient/family selection
- Guidelines for assessment of the well-being of the newborn, especially in the context of neurological, nutritional, and hydration evaluation
- Policy and procedures for cessation of home phototherapy and emergency admission for hospital-based care
- Policy and procedures for family support respite care and ongoing parental education

Indications for Referral to Hospital Care

- **Total serum bilirubin levels**
  - ~ Rapidly rising value of bilirubin (greater than 0.25 mg/dL/hour) related to unrecognized hemolysis or delayed clearance
  - ~ Bilirubin value greater than 22 mg/dL or those infants being considered for an exchange transfusion
  - ~ Evidence of hypoalbuminemia (value less than 3.4 g/dL)
  - ~ Any bilirubin value with associated neurological signs
- **Feeding difficulties:** If an infant has poor oral intake with signs of dehydration
- **Signs of dehydration:** Based on clinical signs of dehydration, less than 3 wet diapers in a 24-hour cycle, or a weight loss of greater than 15% of birthweight in 3 days
- **Signs of neurological manifestations**

Quality Assurance of Home Phototherapy Programs

Appropriate use of home phototherapy may be assessed by the following indictors:

- Parental satisfaction and well-being survey
- Duration (in days) of home phototherapy
- Incidence of readmission to hospital
- Incidence of an abnormal neurological examination upon readmission to the hospital
- Incidence of hypernatremic dehydration
- Incidence of a need for an exchange transfusion
- Cost assessment of home-based versus hospital-based care for excessive hyperbilirubinemia

Summary

Managing hyperbilirubinemia in the home can be challenging. When assisting in this effort, remember the following:

- Neonatal jaundice predominantly is a benign event. In a small percentage of healthy newborns, excessive hyperbilirubinemia can cause serious and deleterious acute or long-term neurologic sequelae. The risk of such occurrence can be predicted with reasonable foresight.
- Based on a predischarge bilirubin value, lactational competence of a breastfeeding infant, screening for a major cause of neonatal hemolysis, and the tracking of bilirubin values on the bilirubin nomogram, a safe home care plan can be accomplished.
- In those preselected group of infants with excessive hyperbilirubinemia who are not hypoalbuminemic and who do not have rapidly rising bilirubin values, home phototherapy can be implemented safely using a comprehensive program with pediatrician supervision.
- All pediatricians and health care professionals caring for jaundiced infants should reassure the families about the usual benign outcome of hyperbilirubinemia while remaining cognizant of the small potential of neurotoxicity.

Bibliography

American Academy of Pediatrics, Provisional Committee for Quality Improvement and Subcommittee on Hyperbilirubinemia. Practice parameter: management of hyperbilirubinemia in the healthy term newborn. *Pediatrics.* 1994;94:558-565

Bhutani VK, Johnson L, Sivieri EM. Predictive ability of a predischarge hour-specific bilirubin for subsequent significant hyperbilirubinemia in healthy term and near-term newborns. *Pediatrics.* 1999;103:6-14

Brown AK, Johnson L. Loss of concern about jaundice and the reemergence of kernicterus in full-term infants in the era of managed care. In: Fanaroff AA, Klaus MH, eds. *The Year Book of Neonatal and Perinatal Medicine.* Philadelphia, PA: Mosby Yearbook; 1996:17-28

Gourley GR. Bilirubin metabolism and kernicterus. *Adv Pediatr.* 1997;44:173-229

Johnson L, Bhutani VK. Guidelines for the management of the jaundiced term and near-term infant. *Clin Perinatol.* 1998;25:555-574

Johnson L, Brown AK, Bhutani VK. BIND — a clinical score for bilirubin induced neurologic dysfunction in newborns [abstract]. *Pediatrics.* 1999;104(suppl):746

Newman TB, Maisels MJ. Evaluation and treatment of jaundice in the term newborn: a kinder, gentler approach. *Pediatrics.* 1992;89:809-818

Chapter 31

Apnea and Home Cardiorespiratory Monitoring

Alan Spitzer, MD

Introduction

At the present time, many neonates and young infants are monitored in the home. It is estimated that as many as 15% to 20% of the 400,000 premature neonates born annually are treated with home cardiorespiratory monitoring, primarily for clinical apnea and bradycardia but also for the possible prevention of sudden infant death syndrome (SIDS). A significant additional number of infants between the ages of 1 month and 1 year also are monitored because of a history of an apparent life-threatening event (ALTE).

An ALTE is an unexplained episode in which the observer believes that the life of the child may be at risk. Cyanosis, pallor, cessation of breathing, and loss of consciousness often are seen in ALTEs and are terrifying to the parent or caretaker. Because of the fear of sudden death of the child, many of these children are placed on home cardiorespiratory monitors. Lastly, a small, but significant, number of children are monitored for a variety of chronic conditions, such as bronchopulmonary dysplasia (BPD), chronic ventilator dependency, seizure disorders, neuromuscular diseases, maternal drug use during gestation, and cardiac rhythm disturbances.

Although many infants are treated with home cardiorespiratory monitoring, this therapy has not been embraced universally and remains controversial. Advocates of home monitoring believe that it can alert caretakers to episodes of apnea and/or bradycardia before they cause harm, thereby allaying the anxiety of caring for an infant known to be at risk. Opponents of monitoring cite the lack of evidence that these devices substantially alter the outcome for the patients. To date, for example, there has been no prospective study that conclusively proves that monitoring does prevent SIDS. Furthermore, many health care professionals believe that there may be a significant emotional burden associated with monitoring (or not monitoring) an infant. Finally, in this era of decreasing health care reimbursement, the cost of care becomes an important issue in attempting to analyze the risks versus the benefits of home monitoring.

Home monitoring, however, does appear to be effective for some patients when used in a rational and selective manner for certain medical conditions. It is the purpose of this chapter to review the indications and approaches to home monitoring that may be beneficial to some infants.

Patients Who May Benefit From Home Monitoring

There are many infants with an array of clinical conditions who may be considered candidates for treatment with home cardiorespiratory monitoring (Table 31-1). The majority of clinical circumstances in which home monitoring is used occurs during the first year of life. The following discussion will concentrate primarily on the patient populations described in Table 31-1.

▸ Apnea of Prematurity and Infancy

All infants (as well as most children and adults) have occasional apnea as defined by pauses in their breathing. The precise point at which apnea can no longer be considered normal and becomes pathological is unclear. On a statistical basis, it appears that pathological apnea occurs when breathing is interrupted for 20 seconds or longer or for less than 20 seconds when accompanied by a significant decrease in heart rate (bradycardia) or fall in oxygen saturation. Bradycardia for the young infant consists of a decrease of at least one third below the resting heart rate. Because oxygen saturation rarely falls below 85%, even during quiet sleep, a level below that can be considered abnormal. Infants with chronic lung disease of prematurity (ie, BPD) may need the level to decrease to 80% oxygen saturation for it to be considered significant because these infants commonly have reduced resting saturations, even with supplemental oxygen. Furthermore, the fall in saturation must last at least 5 seconds to eliminate the possibility of motion artifact. These definitions, while not universally agreed on, represent significant apnea, bradycardia, and oxygen saturation changes that rarely are seen in normal, healthy premature or term infants.

TABLE 31-1. Clinical Circumstances in Which Home Monitoring Should Be Considered

Premature or term infants with pathological apnea and bradycardia

Acute life-threatening events

Gastroesophageal reflux disease with apnea and bradycardia

Siblings and twins of sudden infant death syndrome victims

Children born to mothers who are substance abusers

Patients with chronic lung disease (bronchopulmonary dysplasia)

Patients with tracheostomies

Seizure disorders with apnea

Cardiac arrhythmias (eg, supraventricular tachycardia)

Apnea is commonly classified as central, obstructive, or mixed. In central apnea, all respiratory effort ceases (Figure 31-1). During obstructive apnea, the infant continues to exhibit respiratory effort, but gas flow to the lungs is prevented by altered anatomical structure or tone within the airway (Figure 31-2). Mixed apnea contains elements of central and obstructive apnea, either within the same apneic pause or at different times during a period of respiratory recording. All forms of apnea are difficult to detect visually, although obstructive apnea may be more obvious to the trained observer because infants may struggle to overcome airway obstruction. For precise diagnostic purposes, multichannel recordings of breathing (most commonly nasal airflow or end tidal carbon dioxide, thoracic impedance, averaged heart rate, and oxygen saturation) are necessary. From published studies, it has been shown that even trained nursing staff will miss more than 50% of episodes of apnea of prematurity (AOP) when compared to multichannel recording.

An alternative form of apnea, periodic breathing, refers to pauses in respiration of less than 10 seconds, separated by periods of breathing of less than 20 seconds, occurring at least three times in succession (Figure 31-3). Periodic breathing occurs as the principal form of apnea in approximately 20% of premature infants. It is not known if this type of apnea has the same significance as other forms of apnea. In healthy premature and term infants, periodic breathing rarely occupies more than 5% of the total sleep time of the infant. Periodic breathing also should be considered significant if it per-

FIGURE 31-1. This home event recording shows central apnea and bradycardia. The top channel reveals slowing of the electrocardiogram beats, the central channel shoes a mean heart rate slowing to approximately 60 beats per minute, and the bottom segment demonstrates no respiratory effort for 18 seconds. Following the apnea, there is an irregular respiratory pattern, which is the result of parental stimulation of the infant to end the apnea episode. The heart rate increases following stimulation.

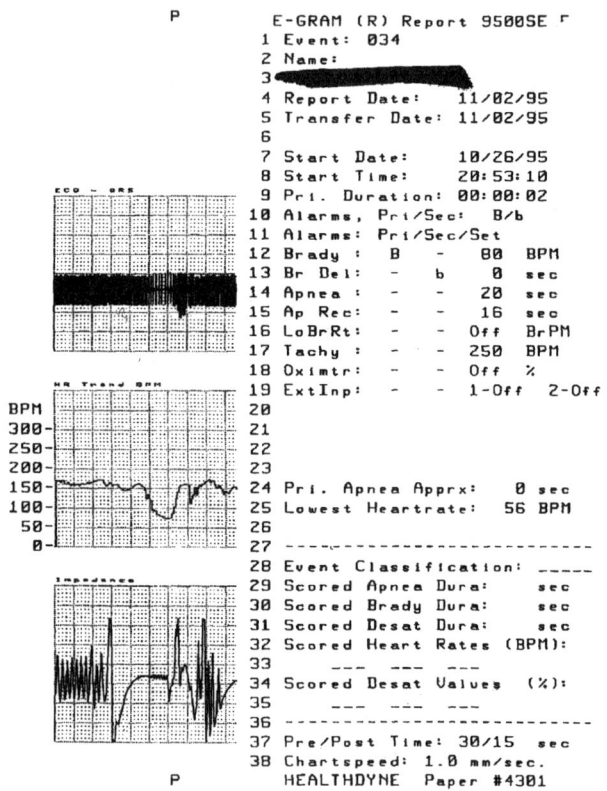

sists longer than 15 minutes continuously or is accompanied by changes in oxygen saturation. Clinical detection of periodic breathing without the recording of several hours of breathing is virtually impossible. Controversy about periodic breathing exists because it is found during sleep in healthy individuals. In normal individuals, however, periodic breathing rarely lasts

FIGURE 31-2. This home event recording shows probable obstructive apnea and bradycardia. The top channel reveals slowing of the electrocardiogram beats, the central channel shows a mean heart rate decrease to approximately 70 beats per minute, and the bottom segment demonstrates continued respiratory effort or bodily movement. Following the apnea, there is an irregular respiratory pattern that is the result of parental stimulation of the infant to end the apnea episode. The heart rate increases following stimulation.

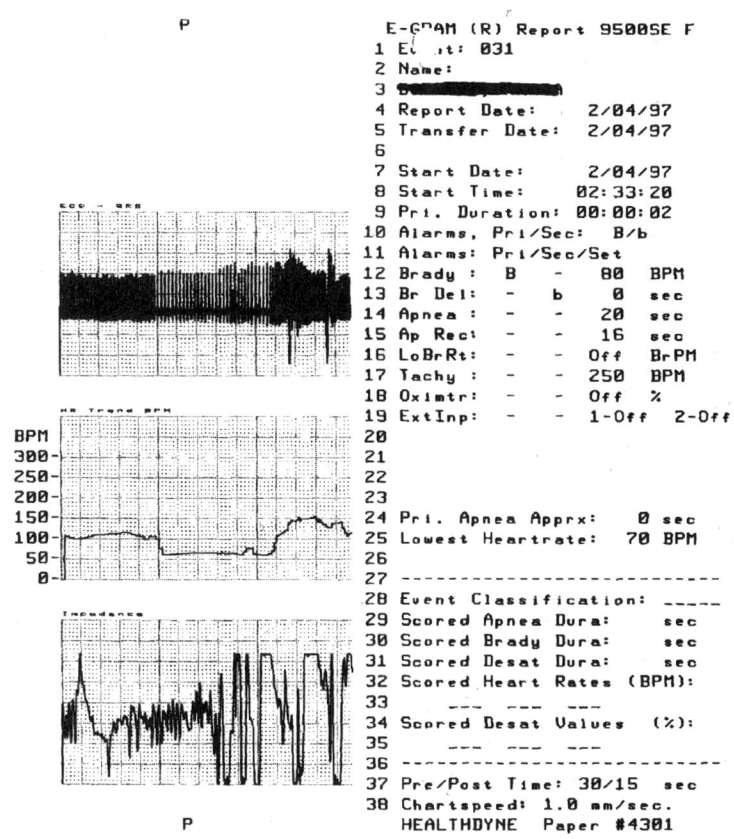

longer than 5 minutes and is not accompanied by changes in oxygen saturation. There currently are no prospective studies that definitively relate periodic breathing to SIDS or adverse outcome of any type.

Apnea can be detected in approximately 70% of infants at 34 to 35 weeks' postconceptional age. While it progressively decreases in frequency over sub-

FIGURE 31-3. A multichannel recording of nasal airflow, thoracic impedance, oxygen saturation, and average heart rate in a premature infant with periodic breathing. There are repetitive cycles of apnea noted in the nasal airflow and impedance channels that last about 10 to 12 seconds, followed by respirations of approximately 10 seconds. The oxygen saturation repetitively drops to 86% to 88%. The heart rate remains essentially unchanged throughout at 150 to 160 beats per minute. This episode continued for an additional 20 minutes. Each box is 5 seconds.

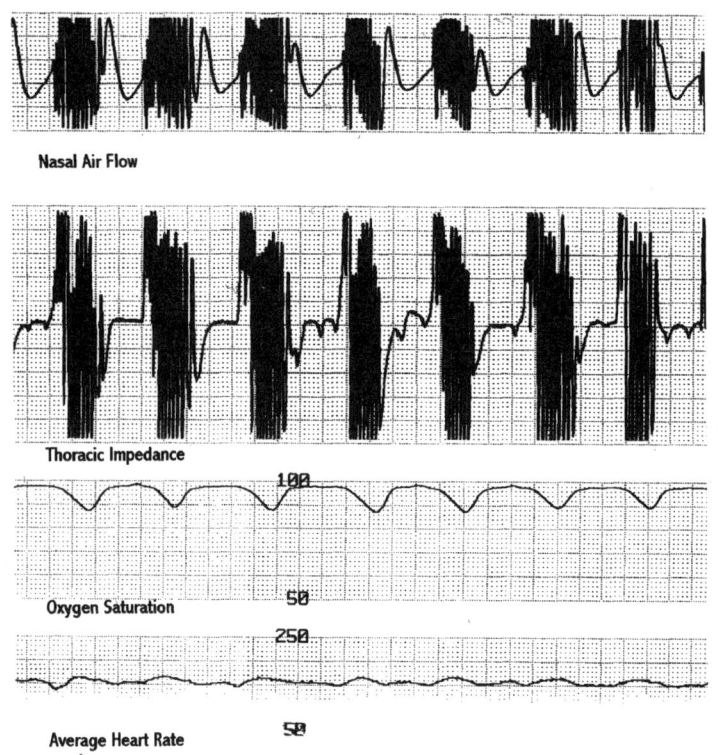

Nasal Air Flow

Thoracic Impedance

Oxygen Saturation

Average Heart Rate

sequent weeks of life, approximately 30% to 40% of infants born prematurely still will demonstrate AOP at the expected due date of the child or 40 weeks' postconception. Significant apnea and/or hypoxemic events have been well documented in premature infants beyond their due date. The mean time to resolution of apnea in premature infants is approximately 50 weeks' postconception. Other recent studies indicate that between 6% and 22% of very low birth weight infants have apnea at term, and 91% of premature infants have apnea of less than 12 seconds duration at the time of hospital discharge. In these infants, 31% also had bradycardia and 6.5% required prolonged hospitalization because of the severity of their apnea and bradycardia. It therefore is evident, contrary to popular belief, that AOP does not resolve at term in many low birth weight infants and may be present for some time after hospital discharge.

In term infants, apnea is seen less frequently. About 2% to 3% of term infants will have demonstrable apnea when studied in the immediate postpartum period. The long-term significance of this apnea is unknown. There are no data that show that term infants with apnea immediately postpartum are at greater risk of an ALTE or SIDS than other term infants. Only 10% of infants who present with an ALTE during the first months of life have an antecedent history of apnea, indicating the highly unpredictable nature of these events during the first months of life. It is precisely for this reason, however, that pediatricians often are concerned about ALTE episodes, because they do not know if they are unique phenomena or have the possibility of recurring until certain circumstances are present.

▶ Apnea, Sudden Infant Death Syndrome, and Home Monitoring

Many physicians have felt great frustration with deaths from SIDS in their patient population, as well as the apparent inability of home monitoring to prevent these deaths in some cases. Such frustration has led to the commonly expressed notion that monitoring has no value whatsoever in the prevention of SIDS. It appears, however, that home monitoring may prevent some deaths from SIDS when used judiciously.

For term infants, it has been acknowledged for some time that the peak age of mortality from SIDS is between 2 and 4 months of life, or a mean of approximately 52 weeks' postconception. The peak age of mortality for the premature infant is approximately 4 to 6 months of life, but at a similar mean of 52 weeks' postconception. The premature infant therefore may have a longer risk period for SIDS following hospital discharge. There is little data that compare risk in preterm infants born at different postconceptional ages with respect to SIDS. The similarity in postconceptional age of mortality for both term and preterm infants, however, suggests the possibility that some neuro-developmental phenomenon may be one of the etiologies of this as-yet-unexplained problem. Although premature infants comprise approximately 10% of the birth population, they account for slightly more than 20% of SIDS deaths. Because immaturity of respiratory control is seen so commonly in the infant born prematurely, it has been suggested that there is a relationship between AOP and the risk of SIDS.

Most unfortunately, there is no simple, accurate method of predicting which infant is likely to die of SIDS at the present time. Many programs have been developed, however, to provide home cardiorespiratory monitoring for infants in an effort to reduce the incidence of SIDS. To date, no prospective, randomized control study has proven that home cardiorespiratory monitoring will prevent SIDS. Anecdotal data from some programs, however, suggest that the incidence of SIDS can be reduced in a population of monitored infants, but it has not been shown that it is home monitoring itself that effects this reduction in the SIDS incidence. It therefore would appear that the judicious use of home monitoring in this era of cost consciousness is a reasonable approach, even if only some deaths can be prevented. For the majority of infants with sporadic episodes of self-revived apnea or periodic breathing, home monitoring may be an effective method for limiting costly prolonged hospitalization.

Siblings and Twins of Sudden Infant Death Syndrome Victims

Although the available data are conflicting, it appears that twins and siblings of former victims of SIDS do have an increased risk themselves for SIDS when compared to the general population. There are a number of reports of twins dying from SIDS within 24 hours of one another. Current evidence suggests a fourfold to tenfold increased risk of SIDS in siblings of victims. Studies of breathing control in this population group also indicate a higher prevalence of apnea than that seen in a control population. Other etiologies of sudden death in families must be eliminated, however, before presuming SIDS as a recurring cause of death in a family. Some of these entities are listed in Table 31-2.

For a variety of reasons (many psychological), some physicians believe that home monitoring is helpful in this unique population of patients. The 1986 National Institutes of Health Consensus Conference on Infantile Apnea and Home Monitoring, however, recommended that siblings of SIDS victims be monitored only when there were at least two prior deaths in a family from

TABLE 31-2. Familial Causes of Sudden Death

Inborn errors of metabolism
- Hypoglycemia
- Carnitine palmityltransferase deficiency
- Aminoacidopathies
- Urea cycle defects
- Organic acid defects

Cardiac problems
- Wolff-Parkinson-White syndrome
- Prolonged QT interval syndrome
- Congenital heart block
- Vascular rings

Congenital central hypoventilation syndrome (Ondine's Curse)
- Spinal muscle atrophy syndromes
- Werdnig-Hoffman disease
- Recurring familial homicide

SIDS. Such conflicting recommendations have proven difficult for physicians charged with the care of such infants to manage. Furthermore, parents who have lost one child to SIDS often need some additional support on the birth of a subsequent child. In such cases, home monitoring may provide an important degree of reassurance. Unless the parents somehow can be convinced about the well-being of their child, they often will pursue a physician who does prescribe a monitor.

Fetal Drug Exposure and Infant Risk of Apnea and Sudden Infant Death Syndrome

The concern about fetal drug exposure and SIDS has existed in the literature for some time. In 1978, Rajegowda reviewed data from New York City between the years 1972 and 1974 and reported that narcotic exposure in utero increased the risk of SIDS 8.7 times compared to that of Manhattan as a whole. Shortly thereafter, Finnegan reported an increased incidence of SIDS in the population of babies born to drug-dependent mothers in Philadelphia. Following these initial observations, Olsen and Lee examined a group of nine infants who were exposed to methadone before birth and reported that they displayed a number of physiological abnormalities that might explain a predisposition to SIDS. These findings included decreased carbon dioxide sensitivity at birth that lasted for some time after birth.

Investigators have found that infants of mothers who are substance abusers have an impaired repertoire of protective responses to hypoxia and hypercapnia during sleep that may play a role in their increased risk for SIDS.

In a meta-analysis of 10 published studies, SIDS occurred in 84 of 12,163 infants with intrauterine cocaine exposure; the variance-weighted estimate for incidence was 5.2 per 1,000 with a 95% CI of 4 and 7 per 1,000. The combined odds ratio for SIDS in cocaine-exposed versus all comparison group infants was 3.9 (95% CI 3 to 5), a significantly increased risk. They concluded that after controlling for the confounding variable of concurrent use of other drugs, the risk for SIDS could not be attributed to intrauterine cocaine exposure alone. The increase in risk for SIDS was found not to be specific to cocaine but to intrauterine exposure to illicit drugs in general. It appears, therefore, that infants of mothers who are substance abusers do have a greater risk of SIDS than that seen in the population as a whole.

Perhaps the single inhalational agent, however, that has been most closely linked with SIDS is cigarette smoke. These studies have suggested that the elimination of cigarette smoking in the home environment (as well as eliminating prenatal exposure) will reduce the rate of SIDS. Parental smoking should be strongly discouraged in all circumstances.

▶ Home Cardiorespiratory Monitoring in Infants Whose Mothers Are Substance Abusers

The use of home cardiorespiratory monitors is very controversial for the treatment of infants whose mothers are substance abusers. Many infants born to mothers who are substance abusers are not identified at the time of birth and few groups of these infants have been studied to determine the value of home cardiorespiratory monitoring for the treatment of the respiratory pattern abnormalities seen. There is no evidence that home monitoring can prevent SIDS in this population, and compliance is a significant problem for any program that treats a large population of these infants. One should not, however, exclude all infants whose mothers are substance abusers from monitoring simply on the basis of the bias and stigma that often are associated with parental substance abuse. Some infants may benefit from the use of home monitoring, particularly if apnea has been identified or if the infant has had an ALTE. It is not appropriate to monitor all infants exposed to drugs in utero. Parents should be trained in the use of the monitor and in cardiopulmonary resuscitation (CPR) when monitoring is initiated. Parents should be informed, however, that monitoring may not prevent SIDS because the causes of SIDS in this population of patients are not completely understood at the present time.

▶ Infants With Bronchopulmonary Dysplasia and Tracheostomies

With increasing survival of low birth weight infants who are critically ill, the population of babies with chronic lung disease of the newborn, or BPD, has increased in recent years. Sudden death in patients with BPD is a well-recognized clinical entity. Although most BPD patients require little more than home oxygen for a limited period of time, some infants are chronically ventilator dependent and have tracheostomies. In addition, infants with a variety of other chronic and often debilitating diseases may require tracheostomies to receive home mechanical ventilation. Monitoring these patients is complex but is predicated on the concept of potentially reducing the morbidity and mortality associated with chronic tracheostomies. The goal of monitoring in such instances is to alert the caregiver to circumstances in which the airway is potentially compromised, ideally at a time early enough to intervene before any harm occurs. For the infant who is ventilator dependent, not only do cardiopulmonary changes in the infant need to be monitored, but equipment failure and ventilator disconnections as well. A separate system is necessary, therefore, to detect equipment failure, ideally before it affects the patient.

Unfortunately, monitors available for the home environment are limited in their ability to detect airway occlusion. At best, they only provide indirect evidence of problems through a secondary warning system such as brady-cardia, often a later component of an obstructive event (Figure 31-2). While some newer techniques may eliminate the false alarms associated with pulse oximetry and allow these devices to be used for tracheostomy monitoring, they are not yet widely available. End-tidal carbon dioxide monitoring, which has significant theoretical advantages in assessing airway occlusion, is difficult to use on a continuous basis because of the accumulation of secretions. In all instances, false alarms are common and add to the stress experienced by the family of the infant. For some infants with extremely critical airways, 24-hour nursing surveillance may provide optimal monitoring.

▶ Additional Candidates for Monitoring

Home monitoring may play a role in the treatment of patients with clinical disorders such as supraventricular tachycardia or seizure disorders. In all such cases, the value of home monitoring should be assessed carefully on an individual basis. Monitoring may be helpful in certain circumstances, especially when apnea, bradycardia, or tachycardia are manifestations of the disease. As with previously described clinical conditions, the use of home monitoring must be initiated with specific goals that can be explained readily to the family. The prescribing of a monitor because it seems like "a good idea" is not appropriate.

The Development of Home Monitoring Technology

Electronic surveillance for cardiopulmonary events, particularly in patients in intensive care units, has been available for several decades. The standard impedance-type home monitor was first introduced in the late 1970s by the Healthdyne Corporation, and soon was followed by a number of similar devices from other companies. Impedance pneumography detects a respiratory signal by using a continuous electrical pulse transmitted between two chest electrodes placed on opposite sides of the thorax. These chest leads are held either in a velcro belt secured around the chest or through electrocardiogram (ECG)-type leads. As the thoracic diameter increases and decreases, the signal varies and the monitor records continuous respiration. Although this method has proven valuable in documenting central apnea, it has serious limitations for the infant with obstructive apnea. This deficiency has been a major cause for concern in the use of home monitoring. Because bodily movement may alter the impedance signal, breaths may be registered incorrectly at times by these monitors, even though the airway is obstructed (Figure 31-2). Because of this limitation, these units also had a second channel that detected heart rate. Although usually a late event, bradycardia often accompanies airway obstruction. Its detection may permit a caretaker to intervene to stop an episode of obstructive apnea.

The standard home monitor detects heart rate by a single-lead ECG through the same electrodes that are used to measure the respiratory signal.

Although ECG signal detection has been used for some time, one of the difficulties with ECG recording with young infants is their mobility during sleep, particularly after the middle of the first year of life. As a result, movement often disrupts the ECG signal. It is the loss of the ECG signal that most commonly produces the false alarms that parents experience with home cardiorespiratory monitoring. Furthermore, unlike the respiratory channel that permits a time delay as long as 30 seconds before alarming, the heart rate channel updates at an average rate of 3 to 4 seconds so that there is no provision for significant delay before alerting the caretaker to an alarm. As a result, brief movement that disrupts heart rate detection for a few seconds may falsely lower the average heart rate and result in a false alarm. Most monitors now are capable of high heart rate detection, but this alarm, particularly when used with preterm infants, may be more worrisome to families than helpful.

▶ Event-Recording Monitors

Rapid advances in computer technology have spurred the evolution of the home monitor. Event-recording monitors use a microchip to record events at home. These events can be downloaded from the patient's monitor to allow the physician to immediately interpret events at home. They also may be stored for later review. With the current computer technology and data transfer capability such as cable modems or T1 lines, information on specific events can be obtained readily in the home and sent to the physician for immediate review and treatment. Any physician who provides care for infants on monitors should have the ability to use the technology that now exists to provide optimal care.

▶ Oxygen Saturation Monitoring

A significant addition to evaluation of the infant on a home monitor is oxygen saturation (SaO_2). The proliferation of saturation monitors in intensive care units and the operating room demonstrate the usefulness of this technology in the care of the infant who is critically ill. Oxygen saturation monitoring, which calculates an SaO_2 value every 3 to 7 seconds (in some cases, with each heartbeat), has major advantages over continuous transcutaneous Po_2 monitoring, which is much slower. The addition of SaO_2 for evaluation of the child with apnea of infancy permits clearer understanding of the physiologic implications of even brief episodes of apnea.

At the present time, most saturation monitors measure a light signal passed through an extremity that determines the wavelength change created by oxygen-containing red blood cells. Most commonly, saturation probes must be placed on fingers, toes, hands, or feet in the young infant, and this often results in movement artifact from signal disruption. This artifact limits the utility of such monitors in the home at the present time. Increasing computer power, however, appears to be on the verge of permitting the use of saturation monitoring for home use. These methods use sophisticated algorithms to eliminate the artifactual movement that has plagued saturation monitoring. The newer generation of monitors may represent an important development for the care of infants with obstructive events and critical airways.

▸ Nasal Airflow Measurement

Nasal airflow measurement, as detected by thermistor or by end-tidal carbon dioxide ($PaCO_2$), has long been a standard modality for inpatient evaluation of the infant with apnea. This technique may be used for evaluation at times during home monitoring as well. Thermistor measurement detects temperature change as air flows past the probe. When the infant inhales, room air temperature is detected; when the infant exhales, body temperature is detected. This temperature variation reflects air movement in and out of the lungs. End-tidal $PaCO_2$ measurements have been used for similar purposes, although the ability to detect $PaCO_2$ in the very young infant, because of the small tidal volume, is difficult and this has limited its usefulness as a home technology. Additional problems with airflow detectors result from the maintenance of their position relative to the infant's airway and their failure from secretions within the detecting device. The constant vigilance necessary for such treatment prohibits use for prolonged periods at the present time.

▸ New Technologies

Some new investigational systems may serve as adjuncts to impedance pneumography in the future. These include inductance plethysmography (piezo belts) and pressure capsules. Plethysmography involves the use of elastic bands placed around the chest and abdomen of an infant. These methods transduce respiratory signals from chest wall and abdominal movement. To date, however, they have not received the widespread acceptance of impedance pneumography. Given the rapid pace of technological change in this field, however, there is little doubt that new procedures for monitoring respiratory pattern abnormalities at home will be available in the future.

Indications for Home Monitoring

The decision to initiate home cardiorespiratory monitoring in an individual infant often is a difficult one for physicians and parents. The decision should be based on the clinical presentation of the child and the subsequent evaluation. A child who presents with one or more life-threatening episodes of apnea or cyanosis is a potential candidate for home monitoring, even if the results of further testing are entirely normal. Appropriate testing should be used, however, to confirm a presumptive diagnosis. As always, treatment should be directed toward eliminating the underlying cause of the events if the etiology can be determined.

For the physician who treats such infants, much of the difficulty arises because certain behavioral episodes or ALTEs in infants appear to defy satisfactory explanation. All pediatricians encounter inexplicable behavioral events in infants during the first year of life. In most instances, the infant appears completely well, the event is benign, and parental reassurance is all that is necessary. Distinguishing such events from more significant ALTEs at times poses serious diagnostic problems, however. It also is not uncommon for a child to have a single severe ALTE and never exhibit any further similar episodes. As a result, many physicians have the understandable difficulty of attempting to discern significance from the benign event. Parental concerns may, at times, be dismissed with little additional evaluation. Unfortunately, on further investigation some infants have demonstrable cardiorespiratory events that are readily detected and often easily treated with home monitoring, appropriate medication, or both.

▶ Evaluation of ALTE

In general, parents appear to be reasonably accurate observers of initial events in infants. Reports of unusual behavior (especially if it involves apnea or color change) should not be dismissed without due consideration and appropriate investigation of the episode. The physician should be aware that most infants with ALTEs may appear completely normal on physical examination, particularly when awake. Because life-threatening events most commonly occur during sleep or around the time of feeding, the physician may first observe the infant at a time during which further episodes are unlikely. The standard physical examination, therefore, may provide only a partial evaluation in such a clinical setting. Given the ready accessibility of programs and equipment for performing home event evaluations in young infants, the physician should refer such patients to appropriate centers if the physician does not feel comfortable evaluating the infant. Basic studies for evaluation of infants with ALTE are indicated in Table 31-3. Not all studies are performed on every infant. Certain characteristics of the history should suggest the appropriate evaluation. For example, the infant with episodes following feeding may be having gastroesophageal reflux-associated apnea. Episodes that are followed by periods of sleepiness may reflect a seizure disorder.

Based on this evaluation, the physician can determine whether home monitoring may be indicated. In many instances, however, an infant can have significant apnea or ALTE with entirely normal studies. Other infants may have episodes of apnea that may be related to metabolic disturbances which are transitory in nature. The necessity for cardiorespiratory monitoring

TABLE 31-3. General Screening Evaluation for Infants With Apparent Life-Threatening Episodes

All infants
- In-hospital observation with cardiorespiratory monitoring
- Careful physical and neurologic examination
- Complete blood count
- Blood glucose
- Chest roentgenogram
- Electrocardiogram
- Electroencephalogram
- Evaluation of cardiorespiratory function by multichannel recording

Selected infants in appropriate clinical circumstances
- Septic workup (blood, urine, cerebrospinal fluid)
- Electrolytes, calcium, phosphate, and magnesium
- Barium swallow
- Lateral neck roentgenogram and otolaryngology evaluation
- Radionuclide milk scan of swallowing
- Esophageal pH study with multichannel recording
- Ultrasound or computerized tomography scan or magnetic resonance imaging of the brain
- Arterial blood gases, especially after the apparent life-threatening event
- Echocardiogram

of these infants is unclear. In such cases, it may be helpful to provide a short course of home monitoring (approximately 2 to 4 weeks) to determine if further episodes can be detected at home. Event-recording monitoring is extremely valuable in this regard. If no further episodes occur, monitoring usually can be discontinued. The physician should be aware that, in general, episodes of apnea tend to cluster, with further events typically appearing within the first couple of weeks after the initial presentation. Furthermore, this brief trial of monitoring can aid in reassuring families and demonstrates the physician's commitment to the child's well-being. Some indications for home cardiorespiratory monitoring currently used are listed in Table 31-4. There is significant disagreement among physicians about the value of home monitoring in some of the listed clinical circumstances. These recommendations are offered as a guide for the practitioner, but should be assessed on an individual basis.

▶ Apnea and Neuro-developmental Outcome

Home monitoring should not be considered solely as a preventive measure for SIDS. Infant apnea, particularly as it may affect the preterm baby, can have significant long-term consequences on neuro-development. Infants with frequent apnea and repetitive bradycardia and oxygen desaturation may be affected adversely in their subsequent childhood development. It is not known at the present time if the reduction of apnea with monitoring and pharmacological agents such as methylxanthines can improve neuro-

TABLE 31-4. Suggested Indications for Home Cardiorespiratory Monitoring

- History of severe life-threatening events or apneic episodes
- Multichannel recording documentation of apnea
- Documentation of increased periodic breathing (>5% of total sleep time)
- Sibling of a sudden infant death syndrome (SIDS) victim
- Twin of a SIDS victim
- Severe feeding difficulties with apnea and bradycardia
- Gastroesophageal reflux-associated apnea
- An infant dependent on technology
- An infant with certain pulmonary, cardiac, or neurologic problems
- Infants of mothers who are substance abusers

developmental outcome in the premature infant. Because of the complex nature of the medical problems experienced by the preterm infant, it is difficult to estimate the contribution of apnea to any developmental disability. Frequent apnea, especially when accompanied by bradycardia and oxygen desaturation, may adversely affect neuro-developmental outcome and should be reduced or eliminated, if possible. Additional work is required to establish this relationship and to determine if monitoring and reduction of apnea can improve neurological outcome.

It is therefore advisable to perform the type of evaluation suggested for ALTE to determine if apnea or increased periodic breathing may be present in an individual infant, especially if associated with frequent decreases in oxygen saturation. If so, appropriate steps should be initiated to monitor these infants at home and treat them with an appropriate medication to decrease the frequency of desaturation. Oxygen supplementation may be required for some infants if desaturation is detected frequently.

▶ The Role of Home Monitoring of Premature Infants

The role of home monitoring of prematurely born infants is unclear from available data. It is recommended that monitoring for premature infants be initiated if respiratory pattern abnormalities are detected during evaluation with multichannel or event recording in the week prior to discharge. Many physicians, however, prefer to have infants remain clinically apnea-free for 8 days, and discharge without monitors. Despite advances in inpatient monitoring during the past decade, it is apparent that the circumstances of hospital monitoring enhance the likelihood of failing to detect episodes of prolonged apnea, even when the apnea occurs relatively frequently. Periodic breathing often is overlooked because the apnea is so brief. Nursing staff may be occupied with other infants who are more critically ill, the multiplicity of alarms in a single patient room may obscure self-revived apnea alarms, the infant may be treated with methylxanthines, and the frequency of false alarms in the intensive care setting may make it impossible for the staff to detect all but the most dramatic episodes of apnea and bradycardia. As a result, reliance on clinical observation alone potentially is hazardous for the infant. If a practitioner does not wish to use home monitoring, multichannel recording should be performed to document that the infant has no apnea or bradycardia prior to discharge.

Furthermore, it also is questionable to keep otherwise well premature infants in the hospital for occasional self-revived episodes of apnea that could be followed successfully at home with monitoring. The risks of nosocomial infection and the cost of such care make this practice suboptimal.

Protocol for Home Monitoring

The plan for home cardiorespiratory monitoring should be discussed clearly with the family at the time of its initiation. It is inappropriate to write a prescription for a monitor without providing the caregivers some idea of the goals and difficulties involved in this therapy. The key to successful care of the monitored infant is the availability of physician, nursing, and technical support throughout treatment.

Once it has been determined that home monitoring is indicated, the protocol shown in Figure 31-4 or Figure 31-5 is initiated (Figure 31-4 is for preterm infants; Figure 31-5 is for ALTE infants). The approaches outlined should serve only as a guideline for care. Physicians should feel free to modify these protocols to meet the needs of the infant and family and the resources available. If monitoring is used, however, parents should be given a copy of the protocol so that there is a clear understanding of the goals of home monitoring and the timetable for its discontinuation.

▶ Initial Monitor Settings

The initial settings for the monitor alarms usually are the following: a 15- to 20-second time delay for the respiratory signal (to minimize false alarms, which occur often with a 10-second delay), a low heart rate alarm of 70 to 80 beats per minute (bpm) for a neonate in the first month of life, and a high heart rate alarm of more than 220 bpm. The low heart rate alarm needs to be readjusted downward by about 10 bpm every 2 months. If oxygen saturation monitoring is used, a saturation of less than 85% is recommended as the alarm level, although numerous false alarms still will be experienced at an SaO_2 of 85%. As a result, saturation monitoring rarely is used on a routine basis.

FIGURE 31-4. An approach to home monitoring for premature infants.

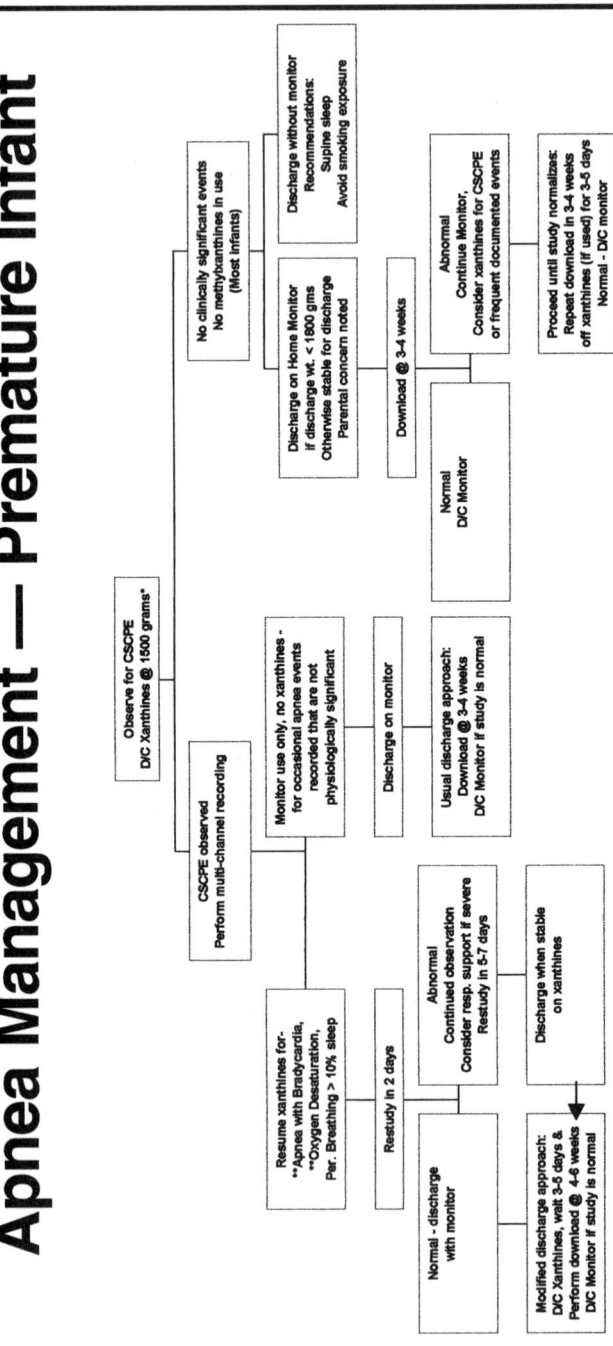

Apnea Management — Premature Infant

Observe for CSCPE
D/C Xanthines @ 1500 grams*

No clinically significant events
No methylxanthines in use
(Most Infants)

Discharge without monitor
Recommendations:
Supine sleep
Avoid smoking exposure

Discharge on Home Monitor
if discharge wt. < 1800 gms
Otherwise stable for discharge
Parental concern noted

Download @ 3-4 weeks

Abnormal
Continue Monitor,
Consider xanthines for CSCPE
or frequent documented events

Proceed until study normalizes:
Repeat download in 3-4 weeks
off xanthines (if used) for 3-5 days
Normal - D/C monitor

Normal
D/C Monitor

CSCPE observed
Perform multi-channel recording

Monitor use only, no xanthines -
for occasional apnea events
recorded that are not
physiologically significant

Discharge on monitor

Usual discharge approach:
Download @ 3-4 weeks
D/C Monitor if study is normal

Resume xanthines for-
**Apnea with Bradycardia,
**Oxygen Desaturation,
Per. Breathing > 10% sleep

Restudy in 2 days

Normal - discharge
with monitor

Abnormal
Continued observation
Consider resp. support if severe
Restudy in 5-7 days

Discharge when stable
on xanthines

Modified discharge approach:
D/C Xanthines, wait 3-5 days &
Perform download @ 4-6 weeks
D/C Monitor if study is normal

*All parents are instructed in monitor use and CPR when child reaches 1500 grams

**To resume xanthines, apnea and bradycardia must occur at least 3 times in 6 hours of recording,
or oxygen desaturation must drop below 85% for at least 5 seconds on three occasions

CSCPE = Clinically Significant Cardiopulmonary Event

FIGURE 31-5. An approach to home monitoring for infants with an apparent life-threatening event.

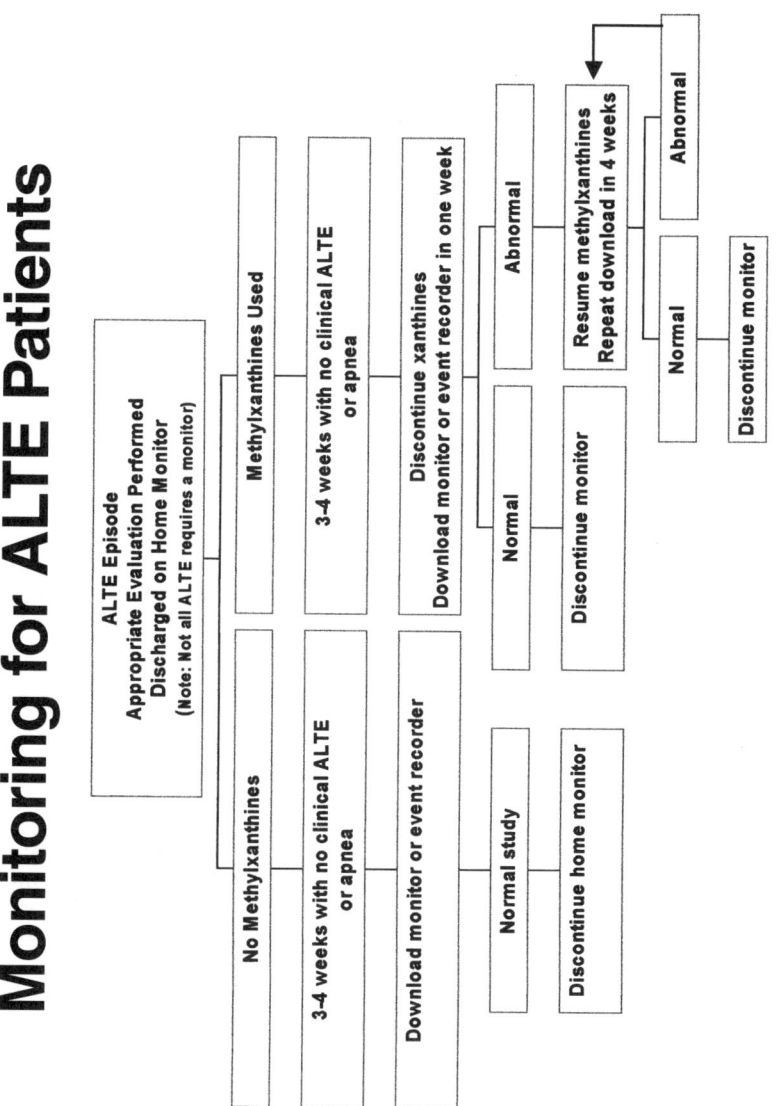

▶ Parental Education

Parents are trained to look at the infant first at the time of an alarm and then intervene after an additional 5 to 10 seconds. It often is difficult to follow these instructions, but the information that they gain through observing the infant at the time of an alarm actually can shorten the course of monitoring. These families rapidly learn to distinguish false alarms from true episodes, making the physician's decision much easier.

The initial intervention should be gentle shaking or tactile stimulation with interruption for further observation. Only if the episode continues beyond 20 seconds after the alarm sounds should parents vigorously shake the infant, being careful to support the head. If this maneuver fails to initiate respiration and color change progresses, CPR should be initiated. Parents should receive CPR training before they are permitted to leave the hospital with their monitored infant. Finally, parents should document all episodes in a diary for comparison with monitor downloading events during evaluation.

▶ Use of Medications

An important initial question in monitoring any infant is whether medication should be used. Methylxanthine therapy is used for preterm and term infants, as well as for the older infant who presents with an ALTE, if they demonstrate frequent respiratory abnormalities, especially when associated with oxygen desaturation. Theophylline may be used; the infant receives an initial oral loading dose followed by intermittent dosing every 8 hours. The provider should obtain a blood level approximately 48 hours after the initiation of dosing to ensure a steady level of 6 to 12 µg/mL. Caffeine therapy may be substituted using caffeine base or caffeine citrate. The loading dose is followed by a single daily dose and a blood level is obtained after 48 hours of treatment. For caffeine, blood levels are kept in the range of 12 to 20 µg/mL. In most infants, methylxanthine doses rarely have to be readjusted once appropriate blood levels are obtained, even though the infant may grow rapidly during the period of home monitoring. Apnea in these infants often disappears during the weeks following discharge, so the infant can be permitted to outgrow the dose of the drug. If parents report an increased frequency of alarms, however, the monitor should be downloaded to see what events are occurring and the drug dose should be adjusted accordingly to reestablish an appropriate blood level. An increase in episodes of apnea that cannot be explained by falling methylxanthine levels may require readmission to the hospital and further evaluation. If methylxanthine therapy is are used in addition to home monitoring, the medication is always stopped prior to discontinuation of the monitor.

▶ Length of Monitoring

At approximately 4 weeks from the time of the initial evaluation, if the infant has had no clinical episodes of apnea, the event monitor is downloaded to determine compliance and to be sure that no events have been overlooked by the family (Figure 31-6). If the event recording is normal, the monitor is discontinued. (Infants in some programs are monitored an average of approximately 6 weeks.)

FIGURE 31-6. Download of monitor compliance use. Each mark represents 20 minutes of use of the monitor. The child is appropriately off the monitor for periods in the daytime hours, but is continuously monitored during the night and nap periods.

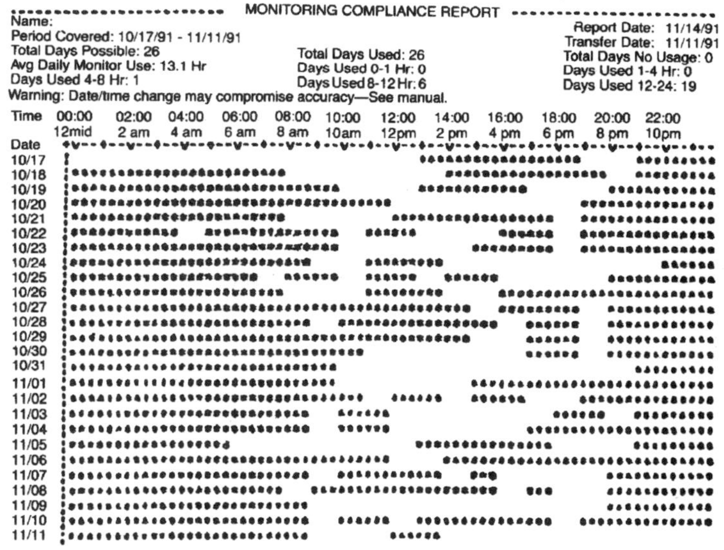

▶ Monitoring of Obstructive Apnea

The infant with obstructive apnea poses unique problems in home monitoring. Because there is no commercially available monitor that accurately detects obstructive apnea at the present time, bradycardia must be relied on as the primary signal for an obstructive event. Because bradycardia may be a relatively late occurrence during the episode in many of these infants, impedance monitoring is less than ideal. Saturation monitoring can be helpful in some of these infants as an adjunct for short periods, but the number of false alarms can be substantial.

Obstructive apnea may be partial or complete, depending on the degree of airway closure that occurs. Obstructive apnea is often associated with gastroesophageal reflux or craniofacial malformation. A number of preterm infants also demonstrate obstructive apnea that is not related to the size of the head and neck flexion. In these infants, it appears that supraglottic closure may occur (from the relatively large tongue size and small oropharyngeal airway volume), with subsequent inability to move air. In cases of obstructive apnea, before the monitor is discontinued, infants may require readmission to the hospital for multichannel recording with nasal airflow and oxygen saturation. Some documented monitoring systems and home monitors, however, now have the capability of measuring nasal airflow and oxygen saturation at home, thereby reducing the need for readmission.

▶ Monitoring of Gastroesophageal Reflux

Gastroesophageal reflux-associated apnea may require additional medication. It should be noted that the diagnosis of reflux-associated apnea must be made with a multichannel recording of esophageal pH, respiration, and heart rate. Radiographic swallowing studies have a notoriously high incidence of both false positives and false negatives.

Positioning of the infant with reflux may help. Infants should be kept upright for a period of time after feeding, if possible. If the infant typically naps on completion of feeding, elevating the head of the bed by 15 to 20 degrees and laying the infant down prone in an anti-reflux sling to eliminate the possibility of rolling down the bed may be of value. For the infant with gastroesophageal reflux that is unresponsive to medication, in whom episodes of apnea or life-threatening events recur, Nissen fundoplication should be considered.

Problems With Home Cardiorespiratory Monitoring

Home cardiorespiratory monitoring in infancy is simple for many families, yet extremely difficult for others. The most common problems encountered during home monitoring are listed in Table 31-5. Perhaps the greatest problems arise when the physician is unclear about the objectives of home monitoring to the family.

▸ Parental Anxiety

Any program that cares for infants on home monitors should have an extensive support system for the family, so that the problems listed in Table 31-5 not only are dealt with effectively, but prevented. Once families are familiar with the technique of home monitoring, compliance with the program improves, false alarms decrease, and length of monitoring is not extended unnecessarily. The family should have a clear understanding of the goals of home cardiorespiratory monitoring. Furthermore, families should understand how the monitor works and precisely what is being evaluated during the infant's care. Parents must be able to troubleshoot a monitor and accurately describe the difficulties that they encounter. Inadequate education in this respect often creates undue anxiety with respect to false monitor alarms. Through a standardized, simple approach, all families, regardless of education or socioeconomic status, can manage home monitoring effectively.

TABLE 31-5. Common Problems Encountered During Home Monitoring

- Inability to distinguish real alarms from false alarms
- Monitor malfunction
- Increasing frequency of false alarms as the infant matures and becomes more mobile
- Increased frequency of alarms during intercurrent illness
- Inability to find alternate caretakers (baby-sitters) for infants on home monitors
- Skin irritation from electrodes
- Sibling jealousy of the monitored infant
- Overdependence on home cardiorespiratory monitoring
- Inability of the family to discontinue home monitoring
- Lack of compliance with home monitoring instructions

▶ Parental Support

The parents should be able to contact a physician or nursing staff involved
with the care of the infant on the monitor at any time. It is not appropriate
to prescribe a home monitor and then leave the family unsupported with
no idea of the objectives or complications of monitoring. It is recommended
that an experienced nurse or physician contact the family on a regular basis
to ascertain what problems there are with home monitoring, answer any
questions that the family may have in relation to home monitoring, and
decide on the timing of appropriate follow-up studies. The home medical
supply company from whom the family rents the device should visit the
home periodically to inspect the equipment, review its use, and be sure that
the family has not prematurely discontinued therapy. Home visiting nurses
are reassuring to many families and help to reduce the anxiety that may be
present. A clinic for evaluation of infants with significant problems related
to home monitoring is extremely valuable, because parents can sit and speak
with a physician about the difficulties they are experiencing and the long-
term prognosis for the infant. Although the commitment to such a program
represents a substantial investment, it does appear to be essential to achieve
best results.

At the time of initiation of home monitoring, parents must be made
aware of the fact that there will be some limitations on their activity while
their infant is monitored. If a parent is alone in the home with the infant,
he or she cannot shower, run the vacuum cleaner, or perform other chores
out of audible range of the monitor. There are several portable devices
(eg, intercoms or walkie-talkies) that allow parents to be alerted to monitor
alarms even while doing some of these tasks. The parents, however, always
should be within 10 to 15 seconds of the infant's bedside in case of an
alarm. Parents must be made aware of the fact that infants reportedly have
died during home cardiorespiratory monitoring when alarms could not be
heard or responded to promptly.

▶ Noncompliance

In many instances of deaths in apnea programs, parents have been non-
compliant, even when physicians were made aware of the fact and the issue
was specifically addressed with the family prior to the infant's death. It should
be noted that among the infants in the Thomas Jefferson University Hospital

program who have died of SIDS, seven of the nine patients were former preterm infants with central apnea and excessive periodic breathing that occurred in more than 20% of their total sleep time. In all cases, parents discontinued medication and home monitoring despite warnings of the potential risk to the infant. It appears that parents of premature infants may represent a special risk category for noncompliance. Because many of these infants were critically ill after birth, the families may perceive that the infant has improved so much by the time of discharge that monitoring may seem more of a hindrance than an essential part of ongoing care.

▶ Discontinuing Home Monitoring

Although the protocol for monitor discontinuation was outlined earlier in this chapter, the actual process occasionally may take longer than intended. Although most infants have their monitors discontinued within 1 month, others take longer. Siblings of SIDS victims often are monitored until 1 month past the age of the prior SIDS event because of the parental anxiety that is encountered. The mean monitor length in siblings of SIDS therefore is about 6 months. Children with BPD or neurological disorders also may have a longer monitor course.

For many families, the monitor becomes such a source of comfort and dependence that the thought of discontinuation produces anxiety. Some of these families persist in using the monitor even after a medical decision has been made to discontinue using the device. Although most parents are amenable to a programmed, gradual withdrawal of the monitor, other families continue reporting episodes of apnea, cyanotic spells, or ALTEs that cannot be detected on event monitor downloading. Inpatient evaluation of these infants typically is completely normal, yet the family claims that they continue to experience events. Direct parent counseling and discussion of concerns may be needed in such cases.

An adjunct to therapy that may be useful in these circumstances is asking the parents to record episodes that they observe. Parents are instructed to set up the camera on a tripod near the infant's bedside or at the site of the infant's typical activity and to begin taping as soon as they observe an event. The tape then is reviewed with the family. On review, parents often quickly cease to observe episodes and request discontinuation of the monitor or they record episodes that are inconsequential. At that point, bringing the family in for further discussion is helpful in allaying their anxiety and aiding in the discontinuation of home monitoring.

Children should not be monitored for apnea beyond 18 months of age. If monitoring is used for the treatment of children who are dependent on a ventilator or neurologically impaired, monitoring may be required for longer periods of time because eliminating it potentially places the child in greater jeopardy.

Goals of Home Monitoring

The following are the goals of home monitoring:

1. To minimize hospitalization and cost of care for infants with apnea and/or ALTE
2. To provide reasonable parental reassurance and security on hospital discharge, especially with very low birth weight infants who are discharged at lower weights and postconceptional ages
3. To enable optimal neuro-developmental outcome unaffected by apnea and oxygen desaturation
4. To act as a diagnostic tool for home events

Summary

The following are important points to remember concerning home monitoring:

- With any use of monitoring, careful follow-up is indicated. If the physician caring for an infant has limited experience with home monitoring or cannot interpret monitor recordings, assistance from a center or program that has such expertise is indicated.
- The mean duration of home monitoring for most infants usually should be less than 6 to 10 weeks.
- Extended monitoring should be reserved for those infants who continue to demonstrate significant cardiorespiratory abnormalities. Only in the rarest of circumstances should any child be monitored beyond 1 year of age.
- Most often, infants who require monitoring in such circumstances have another technological dependency, such as BPDs that require home mechanical ventilation.

- It cannot be emphasized enough that increasing evidence from many countries indicates that there are two key factors for SIDS prevention in term infants: placing infants supine for sleep and avoiding infant exposure to cigarette smoke during and after pregnancy. Unless there are clear contraindications, infants should be placed to sleep in this manner, with smoking avoided during pregnancy and in the infant's environment after birth. These interventions appear to be most significant in their ability to reduce SIDS. Monitoring, however, may be valuable in some clinical situations for the treatment of apnea and to assist families in coping with their infant.

Bibliography

Barrington KJ, Finer N, Li D. Predischarge respiratory recordings in very low birth weight newborn infants. *J Pediatr.* 1996;129:934-940

Beal SM. Siblings of sudden infant death syndrome victims. *Clin Perinatol* 1992;19:839-848

Brooks JG. Apparent life-threatening events and apnea of infancy. *Clin Perinatol.* 1992;19:809-838

Bulterys MG, Greenland S, Kraus JF. Chronic fetal hypoxia and sudden infant death syndrome: interaction between maternal smoking and low hematocrit during pregnancy. *Pediatrics.* 1990;86:535-540

Chasnoff IJ, Burns KA, Burns WJ. Cocaine use in pregnancy: perinatal morbidity and mortality. *Neurotoxicol Teratol.* 1987;9:291-293

Chasnoff IJ, Hunt CE, Kletter R, Kaplan D. Prenatal cocaine exposure is associated with respiratory pattern abnormalities. *Am J Dis Child.* 1989;143:583-587

Cheung PY, Barrington KJ, Finer NN, Robertson CM. Early childhood neurodevelopment in very low birth weight infants with predischarge apnea. *Pediatr Pulmonol.* 1999;27:14-20

Darnall RA, Kattwinkel J, Nattie C, Robinson M. Margin of safety for discharge after apnea in preterm infants. *Pediatrics.* 1997;100:795-801

Eichenwald EC, Aina A, Stark AR. Apnea frequently persists beyond term gestation in infants delivered at 24 to 28 weeks. *Pediatrics.* 1997;100:354-359

Fares I, McCulloch KM, Raju TN. Intrauterine cocaine exposure and the risk for sudden infant death syndrome: a meta-analysis. *J Perinatol.* 1997;17:179-182

Finnegan LP. In utero opiate dependence and sudden infant death syndrome. *Clin Perinatol.* 1979;6:163-180

Henderson-Smart DJ, Ponsonby AL, Murphy E. Reducing the risk of sudden infant death syndrome: a review of the scientific literature. *J Paediatr Child Health.* 1998;34:213-219

Kandall SR, Gaines J. Maternal substance use and subsequent sudden infant death syndrome (SIDS) in offspring. *Neurotoxicol Teratol.* 1991;13:235-240

Klonoff-Cohen HS, Edelstein SL, Lefkowitz ES, et al. The effect of passive smoking and tobacco exposure through breast milk on sudden infant death syndrome. *JAMA.* 1995;273:795-798

Lipsky CL, Gibson E, Cullen JA, Rankin K, Spitzer AR. The timing of SIDS deaths in premature infants in an urban population. *Clin Pediatr (Phila).* 1995;34:410-414

Lipsky CL, Gibson E, Cullen JJ, Cullen JA, Spitzer AR. When does apnea of prematurity resolve? *Pediatr Res.* 1993;33:267A

National Institutes of Health consensus development conference on infantile apnea and home monitoring, Sept 29 to Oct 1, 1986. *Pediatrics.* 1987;79:292-299

Olsen GD, Lees MH. Ventilatory response to carbon dioxide of infants following chronic prenatal methadone exposure. *J Pediatr.* 1980;96:983-989

Oyen N, Skjaerven R, Irgens LM. Population-based recurrence risk of sudden infant death syndrome compared with other infant and fetal deaths. *Am J Epidemiol.* 1996;144:300-305

Poets CF, Meny RG, Chobanian MR, Bonofiglo RE. Gasping and other cardiorespiratory patterns during sudden infant deaths. *Pediatr Res.* 1999;45:350-354

Poets CF, Schlaud M, Kleemann WJ, Rudolph A, Diekmann U, Sens B. Sudden infant death and maternal cigarette smoking: results from the Lower Saxony Perinatal Working Group. *Eur J Pediatr.* 1995;154:326-329

Poets CF, Stebbens VA, Alexander JR, Arrowsmith WA, Salfield SA, Southall DP. Arterial oxygen saturation in preterm infants at discharge from the hospital and six weeks later. *J Pediatr.* 1992;120:447-454

Poets CF, Stebbens VA, Richard D, Southall DP. Prolonged episodes of hypoxemia in preterm infants undetectable by cardiorespiratory monitors. *Pediatrics.* 1995;95:860-863

Rajegowda BK, Kandall SR, Falciglia H. Sudden unexpected death in infants of narcotic-dependent mothers. *Early Hum Dev.* 1978;2:219-225

Samuels MP, Poets CF, Southall DP. Abnormal hypoxemia after life-threatening events in infants born before term. *J Pediatr.* 1994;125:441-446

Shannon DC. Prospective identification of the risk of SIDS. *Clin Perinatol.* 1992;19:861-869

Silvestri JM, Long JM, Weese-Mayer DE, Barkov GA. Effect of prenatal cocaine on respiration, heart rate, and sudden infant death syndrome. *Pediatr Pulmonol.* 1991;11:328-334

Singer LT, Salvator A, Guo S, Collin M, Lilien L, Baley J. Maternal psychological distress and parenting stress after birth of a very low-birth-weight infant. *JAMA.* 1999;281:799-805

Southall DP, Levitt GA, Richards JM, et al. Undetected episodes of prolonged apnea and severe bradycardia in preterm infants. *Pediatrics.* 1983;72:541-551

Spitzer AR, Fox WW. Infant apnea. *Pediatr Clin North Am.* 1986;33:561-581

Spitzer AR, Gibson E. Home monitoring. *Clin Perinatol.* 1992;19:907-926

Spitzer AR, Newbold M, Alicea-Alvarez N, Gibson E, Fox WW. Pseudoreflux syndrome—increased periodic breathing during the neonatal period presenting as feeding-related difficulties. *Clin Pediatr (Phila).* 1991;30:531-532, 535-537

Stefano JL, Anday EK, Davis JM, Fox WW, Spitzer AR. Pneumograms in premature infants: a study of longitudinal data. *Am J Perinatol.* 1991;8:170-173

Ward SL, Bautista D, Chan L, et al. Sudden infant death syndrome in infants of substance-abusing mothers. *J Pediatr.* 1990;117:876-881

Ward SL, Bautista DB, Woo MS, et al. Responses to hypoxia and hypercapnia in infants of substance-abusing mothers. *J Pediatr.* 1992;121:704-709

Ward SL, Schuetz S, Kirshna V, et al. Abnormal sleeping ventilatory pattern in infants of substance-abusing mothers. *Am J Dis Child.* 1986;140:1015-1020

Chapter 32

Home Care of the Child With Asthma

Pamela Wood, MD

Introduction

Asthma, which affects approximately 7% of school-aged children in the United States, is an important cause of chronic morbidity and mortality. Minority children and children living in inner cities are at particular risk for more severe asthma symptoms and higher rates of hospitalization than other children. Asthma symptoms can be controlled when physicians and families work as partners to develop an effective plan for home management. In addition to office-based visits, some children and their families may benefit from home care services provided by a skilled health care professional.

Clinical Practice Guidelines

The National Asthma Education and Prevention Program has developed and disseminated evidence-based practical guidelines for the care of children and adults with asthma (*Expert Panel Report 2: Guidelines for the Diagnosis and Management of Asthma*, 1997). Copies of these documents are available through the National Heart, Lung, and Blood Information Center (see Resource). Certain elements of asthma management are effective in improving health outcomes, including using inhaled anti-inflammatory medicines, using correct inhaler technique, making changes in the home environment, and using a written asthma action plan. Use of inhaled corticosteroids and cromolyn is associated with reduced asthma symptoms, improved peak flow, reduced need for beta$_2$-agonists, and decreased risk of hospitalization. Many parents and children have inadequate skills in using metered-dose inhalers. All patients using metered-dose inhalers should use a spacer, particularly if inhaled steroids have been prescribed. Use of a spacer improves effectiveness of technique. In adults with asthma, better technique is associated with improved health outcomes.

Controlling Asthma at Home

Allergens and irritants in the home environment may adversely affect asthma control. Making changes in the home environment, such as reducing dust mite exposure, may result in improved asthma outcomes. The 1997 guidelines recommend that all patients with asthma have a written asthma action plan. Symptom-based and peak flow-based asthma action plans can improve asthma control.

Unfortunately, there are few data on the effectiveness of home health care for children with asthma. The published evidence is difficult to evaluate because the programs are varied and few programs have been evaluated using controlled trials. Because home care programs are not meant to stand alone, but rather to supplement other health care services, it is difficult to assess the effect of home health programs apart from other interventions that children receive. In one Halifax, Nova Scotia, program, children with asthma who received home visits by a registered nurse had improved health outcomes compared to control group children. However, in addition to the home visits, intervention group children also received care by an asthma specialist and intensive education. Other programs have been less successful. Most data on the effectiveness of commercial home care programs for asthma come from uncontrolled studies and must be interpreted with caution.

Asthma home care programs should include components of asthma education and self-management training. According to the 1997 guidelines, the key messages of asthma education and self-management cover basic facts about asthma, roles of medications, skills training (proper use of equipment and self-monitoring), environmental control measures, and rescue actions (how to use the asthma action plan). Many of these educational activities can be accomplished best in the home environment. Home visits offer an opportunity to make sure that families demonstrate the necessary knowledge, attitudes, and behaviors to manage their child's illness in the real world. Home visits by a health care professional give families an opportunity to practice skills under supervision and to explore the practical issues of integrating asthma management into daily life. A home visit also offers an opportunity for a detailed and accurate assessment of the home environment. The home care worker can identify environmental irritants and allergens and can give the family practical information about how to minimize the effects of environmental asthma triggers.

Home visits address many practical issues that affect behavior change. The home care worker can identify the child's main caretaker(s) and other influential individuals and issues that undermine asthma care (eg, lack of food, shelter, transportation; substance abuse; mental health issues; family discord). The home care worker can contact school or child care personnel to coordinate asthma care that occurs within and outside the home. Finally, the home care worker can help families make small changes that will improve their child's health.

Choosing an Asthma Home Care Program

When choosing an asthma home care program, the physician must consider personnel, program effectiveness, and program content. Home care personnel can be registered nurses, respiratory therapists, or, in some cases, trained lay workers. Because asthma care is complicated and requires extensive practical experience, program personnel must be well trained and experienced in pediatric asthma. Specific individuals should be designated as program staff, and their skills and performance should be monitored by a supervisor who is knowledgeable in asthma management. Asthma home care programs should provide some data on program effectiveness. However, national data may not apply to a local population and data from uncontrolled trials should be interpreted with caution.

Before choosing an asthma home care program, the physician should review program content to make sure that it includes needed elements (eg, home environmental assessment, skills training) and that the materials are appropriate for specific patients. Materials should be age appropriate, written at an appropriate reading level, and sensitive to local issues of language and culture. Written materials should include information about local resources. Finally, the program content should be consistent with the physician's treatment plan and medical practice.

Certain children with asthma and their families may benefit from a home care program. Patients who use health care services frequently (ie, frequent hospitalizations and emergency care visits) and who overuse bronchodilators usually have poorly controlled asthma and may benefit from home visits. Asthma care is more difficult for infants and young children. Their families may need additional home-based interventions. Families who are at risk because of socioeconomic conditions or psychological difficulties also may benefit from home visits. If the physician suspects that there are major environmental asthma triggers, a home-based assessment and intervention may be helpful.

The physician should provide the home care program personnel with results of allergy testing, if available, and a written asthma action plan. The plan can be based on asthma symptoms or on peak flow readings, depending on the age and abilities of the child. Most children older than 6 years of age can use a peak flow meter and peak flow predicted values should be part of the asthma action plan.

Several templates and more information about how to design an asthma action plan are available through the National Asthma Education and Prevention Program. Every child with persistent asthma (daytime symptoms more than twice a week or nighttime symptoms more than twice a month) needs preventive medicine such as an anti-inflammatory. This medicine should be given every day, regardless of symptoms, and should be part of the daily maintenance program used when the patient is well, which is called the "Green Zone Plan." An example of an asthma action plan is shown in Figure 32-1.

There are many barriers to successful implementation of an asthma home care program. Funding rules vary by location and insurance type. In some cases, the physician must write a letter of medical necessity or contact a managed care case manager to obtain authorization for home visits. The physician, family, and home care visitors must work in cooperation. After a home care program has been implemented, the physician should receive reports that include an assessment of skills (eg, use of nebulizers, inhalers, and peak flow meters), an assessment of the home environment, information about actual medications taken and problems with compliance, and information about major social or psychological issues.

Peak Flow Meters

Peak flow meters are inexpensive, portable devices used to measure peak expiratory flow rate (PEFR), the greatest flow velocity that can be obtained during forced expiration starting from fully inflated lungs. Monitoring of PEFR can be used to assess degree of airway obstruction, monitor response

FIGURE 32-1. Asthma Action Plan

Every day, even if you are doing well ("green zone")

Take prevention medicines! _____
(eg, take cromolyn 2 puffs with spacer three times a day)

(Take _____ medicine 20 minutes before physical education/sports.)

For mild to moderate symptoms or peak flow 50% to 80% of predicted ("yellow zone")

Keep taking prevention medicines! _____

Take _____ (inhaled short-acting beta$_2$-agonist).
(eg, albuterol 2 to 4 puffs or albuterol 0.05 to 0.1 mg/kg [max = 2.5 mg] nebulized)

If better, use _____ (short-acting beta$_2$-agonist) every 3 to 6 hours for 12 to 24 hours.

Monitor symptoms and peak flow.

Call doctor if symptoms persist for longer than 12 to 24 hours.

For severe symptoms or peak flow less than 50% predicted ("red zone")

Take _____ (inhaled short-acting beta$_2$-agonist).
(eg, albuterol 4 to 6 puffs [up to 3 doses at 20-minute intervals]) or albuterol 0.1 mg/kg nebulized [max = 2.5 mg])

Start _____ (oral steroid "burst" [1 to 2 mg/kg/day for 3 to 7 days]).

Seek medical care immediately!

If symptoms are very severe, call 911.

---

to therapy, and detect asymptomatic deterioration. Although PEFR correlates with other measures of lung function (eg, forced expiratory volume in 1 second), it measures primarily large airway function. Peak flow is effort dependent and usually cannot be performed by children younger than the age of 6. Predicted values are based on height, gender, and race/ethnicity. Most peak flow meters include a chart of predicted values based on height (Table 32-1). Patients should monitor PEFR for 2 to 3 weeks when their asthma is under good control to establish a personal best value. Current guidelines recommend using a peak flow meter for patients with moderate to severe persistent asthma and for patients with severe exacerbations. Peak expiratory flow rate should be measured before medication is given so that the degree of airway obstruction can be assessed. Measurements of PEFR after medication is given can be used to assess response to therapy. Peak flow meters should meet current standards set by the National Asthma Education and Prevention Program and patients should use the same peak flow meter over time. Newer electronic peak flow meters can store peak flow data and download this information to a central monitoring station or directly to

TABLE 32-1. Peak Expiratory Flow Rate

Normal peak expiratory flow rate (PEFR) values are related to the patient's height as follows:

Height (cm)	PEFR (L/min*)
120	215
130	260
140	300
150	350
160	400
170	450
180	500

*Mean; 2 SD = ±100. An easy-to-remember approximation is PEFR (L/min) = (Height [cm] − 80) × 5.

the physician. The physician should develop an asthma action plan based on peak flow values for children old enough to use this device.

Spacers

Spacer devices are used with metered-dose inhalers to direct smaller particles to the airways, improve hand-eye coordination, and minimize side effects by decreasing the amount of medicine that is deposited in the oropharynx. Many different devices are available, including rigid tube chambers (with or without an attached face mask) and collapsible bags. Current guidelines recommend the use of spacers for all patients using metered-dose inhalers, particularly if the patient is taking inhaled steroids. Dry powder inhalers are designed to be used without a spacer.

The choice of a specific spacer should be tailored to the needs of the child. Infants and young children can use a rigid tube spacer with attached face mask because this device does not require the child's cooperation. The caretaker shakes the metered-dose inhaler and attaches it to the spacer device. The caretaker then places the face mask on the child's face. The mask should fit snugly around the child's nose and mouth. The medication canister is discharged into the chamber and the caretaker waits until the child has taken 6 to 8 breaths before removing the mask.

Collapsible bag spacers allow the caretaker to see that the child has taken a slow, deep inhalation and has held the breath. The caretaker or child shakes the metered-dose inhaler and attaches it to the spacer. The child exhales and places the spacer mouthpiece in the mouth with the lips sealed around the mouthpiece. The caretaker or child discharges the inhaler and the child takes a slow, deep inhalation. The child should then hold his or her breath for 5 to 10 seconds. If the child is not able to empty the bag completely with the first effort, he or she may breathe out slowly into the bag and repeat the effort.

To use a rigid tube spacer, the caretaker or child shakes the metered-dose inhaler and attaches it to the spacer. The child exhales and places the spacer mouthpiece in the mouth with the lips sealed around the mouthpiece. The caretaker or child discharges the inhaler and the child takes a slow, deep breath. The child should then hold his or her breath for 5 to 10 seconds. Most rigid tube spacers have a one-way valve to prevent the child from exhaling into the chamber.

Summary

When considering home care of the child with asthma, be sure to heed the following key points:

- Some children with asthma who receive home care have improved health outcomes.
- Asthma symptoms can be controlled when physicians and families work as partners to develop an effective plan for home management.
- According to the 1997 *Guidelines for the Diagnosis and Management of Asthma*, the key messages of asthma education and self-management cover basic facts about asthma, roles of medication, skills training, environmental control measures, and rescue actions.
- Asthma home care programs should be consistent with the physician's treatment plan and medical practice.
- After a home care program is implemented, the physician should receive reports that include an assessment of the home environment, medication information, and information about major social or psychological issues.

Bibliography

Agency for Health Care Policy and Research. Asthma self-management techniques in home healthcare. In: *Case Studies From the Quality Improvement Support System*. Rockville, MD: Agency for Health Care Policy and Research; 1997:25-30. AHCPR publication 97-0022

Butz AM, Malveaux FJ, Eggleston P, et al. Use of community health workers with inner-city children who have asthma. *Clin Pediatr (Phila)*. 1994;33:135-141

Centers for Disease Control and Prevention. Surveillance for Asthma — United States, 1960-1995. *Mor Mortal Wkly Rep CDC Surveill Summ*. 1998;47:1-27

Charlton I, Charlton G, Broomfield J, Mullee MA. Evaluation of peak flow and symptoms only self management plans for control of asthma in general practice. *BMJ*. 1990;301:1355-1359

Donahue JG, Weiss ST, Livingston JM, Goetsch MA, Greineder DK, Platt R. Inhaled steroids and the risk of hospitalization for asthma. *JAMA*. 1997;277:887-891

Evans R III. Asthma among minority children. A growing problem. *Chest*. 1992;101(6suppl): 368s-371s

Hek G. Child health. Treating asthma at home. *Nurs Times*. 1990;86:64-66

Hughes DM, McLeod M, Garner B, Goldbloom RB. Controlled trial of a home and ambulatory program for asthmatic children. *Pediatrics*. 1991;87:54-61

Mitchell EA, Ferguson V, Norwood M. Asthma education by community child health nurses. *Arch Dis Child*. 1986;61:1184-1189

Murray AB, Ferguson AC. Dust-free bedrooms in the treatment of asthmatic children with house dust or house dust mite allergy: a controlled trial. *Pediatrics*. 1983;71:418-422

National Asthma Education and Prevention Program. *Expert Panel Report 2: Guidelines for the Diagnosis and Management of Asthma*. Bethesda, MD: National Heart, Lung, and Blood Institute; 1997. NIH publication 97-4051. Available at: http://www.nhlbi.nih.gov/guidelines/asthma/asthgdln.htm. Accessed August 30, 2001

National Asthma Education and Prevention Program. *Highlights of the Expert Panel Report 2: Guidelines for the Diagnosis and Management of Asthma*. Bethesda, MD: National Heart, Lung, and Blood Institute; 1997. NIH publication 97-4051A

National Asthma Education and Prevention Program. *Practical Guide for the Diagnosis and Management of Asthma*. Bethesda, MD: National Heart, Lung, and Blood Institute; 1997. NIH publication 97-4053. Available at: http://www.nhlbi.nih.gov/health/prof/lung/asthma/practgde.htm. Accessed August 30, 2001

Pedersen S, Frost L, Arnfred T. Errors in inhalation technique and efficiency in inhaler use in asthmatic children. *Allergy*. 1986;41:118-124

Stout JW, White LC, Rogers LT, et al. The Asthma Outreach Project: a promising approach to comprehensive asthma management. *J Asthma*. 1998;35:119-127

Taylor WR, Newacheck PW. Impact of childhood asthma on health. *Pediatrics.* 1992;90:657-662

Weiss KB, Gergen PJ, Crain EF. Inner-city asthma. The epidemiology of an emerging US public health concern. *Chest.* 1992;101(6suppl):362s-367s

Wilson SR, Scamagas P, German DF, et al. A controlled trial of two forms of self-management education for adults with asthma. *Am J Med.* 1993;94:564-576

Resource

National Asthma Education and Prevention Program
National Heart, Lung, and Blood Institute
301/251-1222
www.nhlbi.nih.gov/index.htm

PART FOUR

Other Considerations for Pediatric Home Health Care

Chapter 33

Home Visits by Physicians

Russell Libby, MD; Alexander Okun, MD; Peter Boling, MD

Introduction

Medicine, as it was practiced throughout the 19th century, primarily was provided at the patient's home. During the Civil War, field hospitals were built to allow for surgical procedures to be performed and for supervised convalescence. The technological advances and centralization of specialized care further spotlighted the hospital as the locus of health care. Primary care physicians, however, continued to provide the outreach to patients in the true tradition of home care. Pediatrician and family (general) physicians would respond to the medical concerns of their patients with a house call. The evaluation and treatment of a patient at the patient's home was a routine part of the workday (which frequently included working into the night).

Social, economic, and professional pressures have driven primary care into an office-based setting, and with that the frequency of home visits progressively has dwindled. Between 1960 and 1975, house calls by US physicians declined from 68 million to 17 million visits per year. A telephone survey of US physicians conducted in 1991 showed that the percentage of physicians making house calls was greatest among family physicians at nearly 63%, intermediate among internists at 47%, and least among pediatricians at 15%. In England and parts of Europe, however, the custom of making house calls still is an active part of practice routines.

The evolution of home care service has allowed for a quicker transition of the care of the patient from the hospital to the home, and even has replaced the hospital as the preferred site for many pediatric conditions. The continuing development of technically sophisticated medical care, specialized nursing care, and ancillary services has inspired some physicians to participate in the ongoing process of caring for their patients at home. The preference of the home over distant, and often intimidating, health care facilities has driven a trend that is appropriate and fitting for physicians serving patients in a variety of medical and social circumstances.

The provider directing the home care is the physician, who supervises
certified nurse practitioners, home care nurses, and other trained outreach
workers. This structure facilitates contact with families from diverse socioeconomic, cultural, and geographic backgrounds. The desired intent of
expanding beyond the medical concept of home care is to improve social
outcomes of children in these households.

Types of Patients

▶ Homebound/Chronic Illness

The home care industry has focused its attention more recently on the
lives of children who are chronically ill, dependent on technology, and con-
valescent, creating a greater need for physician care coordination between
hospital and home. Some examples of the types of children and families for
whom visits can be particularly worthwhile are listed in Table 33-1.

TABLE 33-1. Examples of Patients Who Benefit From Home Visits

Patients Who Are Dependent on Technology
- Respiratory support such as ventilators, oxygen supplementation, suctioning
- Nutritional support using total parenteral nutrition or enteral feeding pumps

Patients Who Require Monitoring
- Apnea monitors for infants who are at risk
- Cardiorespiratory monitoring
- Blood, urine, and stool laboratory needs for various postsurgical, metabolic, or
  other ongoing disease processes

Patients Who Are Technically Challenged
- Respiratory therapies
- Catheter care
- Ostomy care

Patients With Specialized Ancillary Needs
- Speech and oral motor therapy
- Occupational and physical therapy
- Terminally ill in hospice care

Socioeconomic and Cultural Outreach

Work in pediatrics involves children and families from diverse socioeconomic strata, living conditions, and cultural backgrounds that sometimes are vastly different from those of the physician. Though diverse backgrounds may be evident in traditional office-based interviews, nowhere are they more obvious than in home visits. During home visits, families can see that the physician truly is interested and invested in helping and often will feel more comfortable revealing their diversity.

The direct observation of the patient and family in the home setting can lend a great insight into the cause, course, and complications of a medical and/or social problem and may lead to developing the most appropriate approach to treatments or other forms of intervention and support. Advocacy for the child and family can be improved greatly when presented in an accurate context. Table 33-2 lists some examples of children and families who may benefit from socioeconomic and cultural outreach by physicians.

Special Qualities of Home Visits

▶ The Patient and Family

Longstanding relationships between physicians, children, and their families often intensify following a period of involvement around a serious illness or hospitalization. On home visits many physicians find that this relationship has an opportunity to grow similarly without the fears and concerns that dominate a family's experience during the acute illness, particularly in the hospital environment.

TABLE 33-2. Families Who May Benefit From Socioeconomic and Cultural Outreach

- Families from diverse cultures that may be unfamiliar to the physician
- New immigrants who withdraw and avoid sociocultural integration
- Families with large numbers of children and/or multiple generations living in one home
- Dwellings with two or more families living in a space built for one
- Families residing in shelters

During a home visit, the physician is able to see the problems associated with particularly difficult, unpleasant, or painful parts of a home care regimen. Loudon described how in the office, "patients are anxious to please and they may claim startling compliance. In the home, misunderstanding and noncompliance are much easier to discern." With a better understanding of the families' challenges, priorities, and beliefs about their children's care, physicians can collaborate with them toward shared priorities for improved health.

A home visit from the physician may have a positive effect on the patient and family. They may feel more receptive to specific advice about routines, treatments, and follow-up when it is offered with compassionate authority and realistic goal setting from their physician in the home.

The home is a place where key decision makers in the family who are unavailable for office visits can be reached. Often they are less informed about many details of the child's illness and treatment options than those who interact directly with the medical system in the office or hospital, yet they play a dominant role in therapeutic decision making for the child. They benefit from clearer information and a chance to have their questions and concerns discussed directly with a physician. The child benefits from having more informed decision makers.

Home visits have the potential to pose special burdens in some situations. A family may feel ashamed for the physician to see the conditions under which they live or may need to maintain some degree of secrecy about their lives. In an era of fewer home visits by physicians and more investigatory visits by public assistance workers, immigration personnel, and child protection caseworkers, visits by physicians may feel more threatening today than they did years ago. The home visit may be viewed by a family as intrusive or misconstrued as solicitous and of a different intention or intimacy. Physicians must be extremely sensitive to these boundaries and clearly define them.

▶ **The Physician**

The physician is rewarded with many insights and opportunities during home visits. Observing how the family copes with, accommodates, and attends to the child's medical needs can help with determining what forms of treatment have the highest likelihood for success. The positive effects of a home visit also will increase receptivity to advice and better medical compliance. Trust and cooperation will be helpful in times of crisis or if hospital-ization is necessary. According to Goldberg, the physician making home visits can better "understand the advantages and disadvantages, strengths and weak-nesses, and values and limitations of home care."

The potential for advancing the relationship through home visits is valuable particularly in the care of children with terminal or life-threatening illnesses where discussions about withdrawing certain medical interventions may be an option. On home visits to terminally ill patients in general prac-tice, Loudon wrote: "All clearly perceive that the doctor who visits offers comfort without the hope of cure. This is seen as proof that the doctor cares. The process is intimate and familiar and the goodwill that is created is immense and extends far beyond the immediate family." The physician can be helpful in situations where caregivers need support in making difficult decisions about their child who is terminally ill.

The potential for advancing the relationship through home visits is valuable particularly in the care of children with terminal or life-threatening illnesses where discussions about withdrawing certain medical interventions may be an option.

Professional satisfaction can be enhanced greatly by a feeling that one is closer and better able to influence certain patients and families. Physicians usually are thanked warmly and appreciated for the commitment they show in making a home visit. Physicians must not expect any special rewards or gratitude from the family above that which would come naturally from this demonstration of caring.

Many physicians have difficulty conceptualizing how to integrate home visits with their office-based practice. The potential inconvenience, technical limitations, and time requirements are significant and may discourage some physicians. However, there has been considerable effort on the part of the American Academy of Home Care Physicians to establish *Current Procedural Terminology (CPT)* codes and reimbursement standards that are being used with Medicare and other third-party payers. Realistically, economic rewards cannot compare with the beneficial qualities of home visits for the patient and physician.

When visiting the homes of children anywhere, but particularly in inner-city areas, a certain degree of risk exists. Many office-based physicians natu-rally are uncomfortable with these risks. The potential hazards of providing care within a community should be assessed and the physician should determine how these visits will affect the decision about whether, where, and how often to make home visits.

Philosophical Implications of Home Care

Home visitation is one of the most fundamental ways of practicing family-centered care. Working collaboratively and effectively with families and children requires a relationship based on mutual trust, respect, caring, sensitivity, and communication. Families and children often share concerns and feelings about their medical care during home visits with their physician that they otherwise might feel intimidated, reluctant, or afraid to express in the office or hospital. Aware of these issues, physicians can better engage in what Klass calls "empathetic listening," providing support, offering suggestions, and helping with problem solving. For families of children with terminal illnesses, there is no better way to create palliative care plans and help the family to have some control over the comfort-oriented care of their children than to work with them in their homes and help ease their anguish.

Interface With Allied Health Professionals for Continuity of Care

Home visits and the direction of home care services rely on cooperation among all allied health professionals and community-support service physicians. Specialized home health nurses, nursing aids, pharmacists, speech and oral motor therapists, occupational therapists, social workers, home tutors, and child care providers, among others, participate in identifying and carrying out the care of the patient. It is important to understand what each member can contribute and to factor the best balance of effort, priority, and realistic outcomes. The family often gives the best perspective on the frequency, quality, and effectiveness of patient care, providing valuable insight to the physician.

Education and Training

The American Medical Association called for "role models and training experiences" to be "developed for new physicians so that they can integrate home health skills and values into their future practices." Goldberg wrote that in addition to allowing trainees to enrich their knowledge base, home visits offer "learning opportunities to establish attitudes, promote values, and determine essential behavior required of physicians in meeting home care roles and responsibilities."

Despite these recommendations, physician education in home care and preparation for home care practice is inadequate and slow to evolve. Although home health care has become 3 percent of national health care spending and represents a $40 billion industry annually, the average physician has little or no formal, required exposure to home care during medical school, and the average resident may spend 24 hours or less during postgraduate training in activities that specifically focus on home health care. It, therefore, is no surprise that most practicing physicians are poorly informed about home care when they enter practice. Unfortunately, too many remain poorly informed throughout their careers. Home care is not a popular topic for continuing medical education and many physicians perceive home care as an important service for patients that is laden with bureaucracy and has little need of direct physician participation. Despite this relatively dismal history, there are some rays of hope. Throughout the decades, there have been published accounts of teaching through home care in many different medical schools and training programs. These activities tend to be small in scope, led by one or two passionate champions, and may be evanescent, but they keep appearing and thereby reflecting the underlying need. More recently, there have been larger, more concerted efforts to integrate home care into the mainstream. One example is the John A. Hartford Foundation grant program developed by 10 medical schools called the "Expansion of Home Care Into Academic Medicine."

Grant funding of home care education projects is a natural extension of the belief that preparing young physicians for medical practice requires that they experience the settings in which they most likely will be practicing later. Because most medical care is provided outside of acute care hospitals, there has been a shift in emphasis during the past 2 decades, moving resident training from acute care environments to various outpatient settings. Residency review committees (RRCs) have prescribed substantial time commitments for ambulatory care and other settings outside of hospitals. This is particularly true for primary care disciplines, including pediatrics. Some RRCs, such as family practice, specifically require experience in home care and nursing home settings. Other RRCs give program directors greater discretion. Seeking the appropriate balance between inpatient work and ambulatory care and choosing the optimal ambulatory care settings have been central challenges for those who regulate residency training and run the training programs.

Office practices and clinics have seen the most concentrated efforts of curriculum transformation. This is appropriate because this is the setting

Program directors need to encourage and support the allocation of time for home care experiences in a residency program.

where the vast majority of medical encounters occur. However, many residencies have developed programs in nontraditional settings (eg, home care, hospice, and nursing home care). In each case, the basic requirements are easily understood. There must be a strong champion within the residency program and a well-developed clinical service through which residents can rotate.

Residents may resist new and nontraditional training experiences imposed on their demanding routines and may question their value and relevance. It is likely the value may not be perceived until after they have entered their practice setting. Program directors need to encourage and support the allocation of time for home care experiences in a residency program. It will take interested physicians to promote and facilitate exposure to home care, provide teaching opportunities, and highlight home care's clinical and nonclinical attributes.

The American Academy of Pediatrics Section on Home Health currently is working on a formal residency curriculum (*see* Appendix). There is no active medical school component, although exposure during clinical rotations may create opportunities for elective clerkships. The majority of effort and implementation of home care curricula has come from the Geriatrics Interest Group in the Society of General Internal Medicine. While the commonalities between geriatrics and pediatrics sometimes are overstated, the home care, hospice, and nursing home experiences have a great deal in common because of their similarities in care systems and delivery options.

Pediatric residency programs have found that the longitudinal continuity experiences in ambulatory care have greater value than block rotations. This is clearly analogous to the home care experience. Many programs necessarily are built around interdisciplinary teams in which other disciplines provide

much of the education. However, a mentoring physician faculty is essential
for the success of a teaching program. It also is important to recognize that
hands-on, task-oriented elements are more effective than mere observation.

Residents may be anxious about providing care in unfamiliar environments. In home care, this is compounded by fear for personal safety. Although
this fear usually is not well grounded, it tends to be a major hurdle, especially
for urban programs. Traveling in pairs or traveling with others may be an
important issue for some learners. In the nursing home there is a similar issue
in relating to an unfamiliar environment. There also is anxiety associated with
chronic and/or terminal illness that must be overcome. The positive and
rewarding aspects of chronic care should be identified and emphasized.

Every home care curriculum must identify learning objectives and content. These may vary with the institution and its geographic and socioeconomic environment and the types and levels of care available. Opportunities
to participate in home care and all of its venues are important if new graduates are expected to use and derive the benefits of home care in their practice.

▶ Nontraditional Teaching Venues

Hospice programs have mandatory medical direction, so there is a natural
opportunity for teaching young physicians. Hospice programs tend to be
small and the patient care is emotional and intense; small numbers of learners
are essential. Hospice rotations can be arranged as day, week, or month
blocks, depending on the hospice and the students. It is unusual to see
longitudinal hospice activities. In part, the typically short duration of care
for the patients precludes that sort of arrangement, though when it does
occur it often is a powerfully moving experience. Hospice staff tend to be
very protective of their patients, which is an issue to take into account when
trying to negotiate a teaching relationship.

Nursing homes for children are relatively uncommon, but chronic care
hospitals and group homes tend to offer many of the same learning opportunities. These are settings where a longitudinal relationship can be constructed more easily as long as it fits within the other elements of the training
experience. Many facilities welcome medical students and residents because
the socialization that occurs benefits the patients.

Another mobile care venue that can be appealing for learners is an ambulance service. Riding along with an ambulance crew can offer considerable

excitement and drama, as well as a look at a cross section of society. The need to have mentorship may be lessened by the inherent drama of the activity, but the learning aspects are enhanced by having a faculty physician who provides teaching and continuity in the emergency department.

Home care programs tend to be of two varieties: those that draw heavily on home health agencies for structure, and those that are anchored by a physician house call practice. Both can provide beneficial educational opportunities if the importance of physician leadership and mentoring is emphasized. When working with a home health agency, often there are business issues that influence the agency and may limit teaching options. Home care physicians cannot wait around for students who arrive late and they must keep up their pace during visits to complete their clinical assignments. There also is a schedule coordination issue that can be challenging. Time must be carved out at the beginning of the academic year before too many other activities are scheduled.

If available, a physician home visit practice probably is the best setting for teaching residents about home care. Home care faculty can teach in the car so that residents can familiarize themselves with the patient's chart, talk with family members, and perform other necessary tasks once in the home. The faculty member then always must complete and document the basic elements of any billed service. Home care actually can be a relatively efficient teaching venue in the sense that there is not much loss of pace when taking learners along. Overcrowding the home with learners and physicians can become an issue in home care, just as it can in hospice. However, home care is a more forgiving venue than hospice in this regard because of the type of patients. Careful patient selection usually will minimize potential problems.

▶ Curriculum Design

There are many factors to consider in the design of a home care curriculum. Unique yet essential elements to consider include how to conduct a home assessment to determine what service options are feasible for a particular patient, an introduction to the regulatory constraints and requirements imposed on home care for compliance and payment, a lesson on an operational awareness for appropriate ordering and successful use of durable medical equipment, and providing practical medication orders for the family and the home health nurse. In addition, the ability to recognize subtle forms of abuse and neglect needs to be developed, as does the options for appropriate intervention. Table 33-3 lists some unique elements that need to be considered in the home care curriculum.

The experience of established home care curricula indicate that clinical-care–based experiences and problem-solving exercises need to be integrated. Some of this may be best initiated in the classroom and can be enhanced by computer simulation case presentations. There also needs to be some type of learning assessment tool. The Medical College of Virginia House Calls program uses a multiple-choice test and a case-based assessment tool that focuses on a variety of common problems treated and managed by home care physicians. This includes the consideration of when and how to make a home visit, when and how to refer to a home health agency, and the recognition of neglect.

Home Visits as a Part of Your Practice

The recommendation has been made for physicians to visit the homes of patients receiving ongoing home care services and of patients in certain cultural, familial, and socioeconomic situations the physician would like to

TABLE 33-3. Unique Elements in the Home Care Curriculum

Home Assessment
- Technical
- Social

Durable Medical Equipment
- Standards
- Practical realities and problems
- Sources
- Cost

Regulatory Issues
- Medicare/Medicaid
- Fraud and abuse

Privacy Issues

Recognition of Abuse and/or Neglect

understand better (Table 33-2). Indeed, any patient and family might appreciate such a visit. Families with newborns are especially receptive to professional visitation. In many countries throughout the world, health visitors, district nurses, or other providers visit frequently during the neonatal period for the purposes of evaluation and teaching.

Berger and Samet, writing about home visits to pediatric patients, proposed areas for "home assessment" that included "environmental factors" and "family dynamics." Environmental factors included certain aspects of the neighborhood and family home, and the family dynamics centered on interactions between the child and parent and understanding the family's values, routines, and recreational opportunities.

A sampling of the multitude of considerations in assessing the qualities of the home location are listed in Table 33-4. Qualities to consider for the family setting are listed in Table 33-5. Issues to consider for continuing oversight of the home setting are listed in Table 33-6.

▶ Home Visit Program Structure

It is useful to define the home visit activity as a distinct component of the practice organization. Time should be set aside for home visits and there should be a system for scheduling them, along with a system for handling the paperwork and telephone calls that are inherent to home care medicine. Physicians who do not set aside time for home visits somehow find themselves so pressed by other demands that the home visits are deferred too often.

As one example of program structure, consider an office-based primary care physician who has a relatively small population of patients who are chronically homebound and who does not offer urgent home visits. This physician might make home visits one afternoon each week or every other week. An office with five physicians might assign one physician to home-based rounds each afternoon, thereby covering the entire workweek. This also would allow the addition of visits for urgent or unplanned illnesses.

▶ Visit Frequency, Scheduling, and Policies

The office should establish basic policies for the home visit program and make them known to all patients. It is advisable to develop a policy that makes it clear that home visits are provided only to patients who are homebound and who would otherwise have great difficulty reaching the office. Homebound status can be conferred by medical or psychiatric conditions

TABLE 33-4. Assessment of the Home

At the dwelling and inside the home, the physician can look for the following:

- Proximity to major roads and the potential for pedestrian motor vehicle accidents
- Protective barriers between play areas and potential hazards from falls, drowning, electrical, or other injury
- Cohabitation with animals in domestic living and play areas for young children
- Ease of access to living space (eg, by stairs, elevator, ramp)
- General condition of the interior of the home (eg, overall cleanliness, visible mold, odor of mildew, obvious leaks, cracked/peeling paint)
- Obvious presence of allergens and airway irritants, when appropriate
- Source and adequacy of heating, lighting, hot water, air conditioning
- Obvious infestations with rodents, ants, roaches
- Arrangement of durable medical equipment, supplies, and medications
- Safety precautions in the kitchen, around windows, from cleaning solutions and other caustics or toxins, on electrical outlets, and on firearms, if any
- Storage space for foods, dietary choices
- Sleeping arrangements, degree of privacy, and extent of crowding in the household
- Education/entertainment in the home (eg, toys, books, computer, stereo, television)
- Allocation of space for child-oriented play and work
- Smoke detectors, emergency evacuation plan

TABLE 33-5. Assessment of the Family

- Identify the caregiver most knowledgeable about the child's condition and whose level of information most needs advancement.
- Identify how decisions are made about changes in therapies or seeking consultation.
- Identify who interacts most with school and home care personnel.
- Understand how different adults are involved in the child's emotional life.
- Get a sense of the child's and family's day-to-day routines.
- Look for obvious strains and tensions (eg, financial, marital safety, child care).
- Seek opportunities for respite, family recreation, relaxation/leisure, and vacation.
- Listen for expression of health beliefs based in cultural, religious, or family traditions.
- Observe sibling interactions, sharing, and fighting.
- According to Berger and Samet, gauge the degree of "warmth in parent-child interactions," the degree of "restrictiveness," and any "observable punishments."

TABLE 33-6. Assessment for Continuing Patient Care

- **Medications:** Check how they are stored, scheduled, and organized.
- **Supplies:** Check where they are stored and how the family maintains a sense of inventory.
- **Oxygen:** Understand what delivery systems are used, how they are maintained and refilled, what sort of backup there is, how portable and cumbersome they are, and the distance from combustible sources.
- **Equipment:** Check what is there, how often it is inspected and maintained by the home care company, how well it appears to be working, and what backup sources of power and equipment are present and their level of function.
- **Home care personnel:** Understand who visits, how often, how long they stay, what they do, how regular and dependable they are, and how useful and necessary their work is felt to be by the child and family.

and is influenced by the available options for transportation. Sometimes, the inability of a caregiver to transport the patient, such as a mother with many other young children at home, may be a factor favoring home visits. In any case, "convenience" home visits should be discouraged unless home visits are the core operation of the primary practice.

Several other related policies are necessary. For example, a policy on distance limits should be defined clearly and stated. The office should let patients know whether after-hours home visits can be expected, and whether unplanned or urgent home visits are possible. If there is a regular home visit schedule, such as Tuesday afternoon community rounds, this should be made known. A home visit fee schedule should be given to patients just as physicians provide fee schedules in the office. The physician should decide whether to carry medicines on home visits. Generally, it is safer not to announce this practice, particularly if working in an urban environment. Fortunately, unless the home visit team provides urgent care, physicians usually do not need to carry many medications for home medical visits. Planned treatments, such as vaccinations, can be included in the travel bag at the beginning of the home visit session. Small quantities of commonly used items can be included in a procedure kit, such as lidocaine used for local anesthesia. A list of medical equipment and supplies that may be carried by the physician on home visits is in Table 33-7.

The frequency of visits to a homebound patient because of illness may range from one or two per year for a very stable patient to more than 30 per year for someone with frequent exacerbations and co-morbidities.

In a chronic, continuity-oriented, primary care practice, the average rate of home visits probably lies between 6 and 10 annual visits per patient. Remember that these patients are by definition among the most seriously ill in the practice. Being homebound by disease implies a serious illness. About a quarter of these encounters are likely to be unplanned visits for urgent problems. These guidelines for visit frequency also assume that the physician is using home health agencies for interval care when patients need and qualify for home health care.

Maintain a separate list of home visit patients and develop a systematic scheduling approach. Patients or their caregivers usually will call when urgent problems occur, but once someone becomes a chronic house call patient, the onus is on the physician to maintain the interval continuity visits. Without a systematic approach, these patients can fall between the cracks in a busy office practice. To maximize efficiency, visit scheduling should be organized geographically whenever possible.

TABLE 33-7. The Portable Pediatric Office

Essential	Helpful	Optional
Blood pressure cuffs	Blood collection kits	Asthma education kit (with peak flow meter)
Examination gloves	Portable scale	Active media
First aid kit	Rapid streptococcal test	Formula/electrolyte solution
Otoscope/ophthalmoscope	Specimen containers	Intravenous catheter/tubing
Reflex hammer	Surgical tools (scalpel, forceps, scissors)	Lactated ringers solution
Snellen chart (pocket)	Urine dipsticks	Portable device to measure bilirubin, blood gases, glucose, and hemoglobin
Cooler (with thermometer if vaccines are carried)	Stickers, novelties, lollipops	Pulse oximeter
Stethoscope		Kits/procedure tray (burns, eye, catheter, suture, warts)
Tape measure		Dictation device
Thermometer		Laptop
Tongue blades		Patient education material
Vaccines		
Chart forms		
Practice information (with phone numbers)		
Prescription pads		

In the Medical College of Virginia House Calls program, the appropriate interval until the next scheduled visit is estimated and entered into a computer. Each week a database is used to generate the week's visit list, which includes the name of the patients, the usual home visit physician for those patients, and the geographic location of the home (ie, north, south, east, or west). The same scheduling can be done with a manual home visit log or a variety of other methods. Because of the unexpected demands faced each week, it is more practical to set an approximate time frame for scheduled follow-up visits, rather than to give patients a specific time and date in advance. Calls are placed the day before or the day of each planned visit to ask if a visit will be acceptable to the household. If it is not convenient to visit a particular home, another patient is added to the schedule. For offices that have smaller home visit practices and less frequent visits, advance scheduling may work well and be preferable. Notes of specific scheduling issues at particular homes are made. The consideration for working families may require a time when both parents can be at home. It may be efficient to schedule when siblings are at home or, alternatively, when they are at school and cannot create distractions during a visit. Physicians need to remember that they are guests in the home and should make every effort to accommodate the needs of the family. If it is necessary to visit a particular home at a particular time for medical or logistic reasons, physicians sometimes must persuade families to accommodate their needs.

The scheduling of urgent or unplanned visits is more challenging. This usually requires that each physician has a pager and that someone in the office is adept at handling telephone calls. The person in the office must evaluate the information being provided by the caller and determine whether it is necessary to page a clinician. These types of calls generally should be handled promptly to plan the rest of the day and to make sure that truly urgent problems are addressed. If a visit is required and more than one clinician is in the field, it then is necessary to decide who should make the visit. The issues to consider are continuity (which is always valuable) plus the practical issue of who can get to the patient in the most timely and efficient manner. To optimize this type of planning in a practice where there is more than one mobile physician on a given day, the dispatch operator must know approximately where each physician is located when a call comes in. In an office practice, the matter of handling unplanned needs for home visits is similarly challenging. Someone must decide how to redirect physicians to handle the request, whether a home health agency can provide the care, or if the patient should be sent to an emergency room.

▸ Staffing

No matter how the practice is structured, there are some basic staffing necessities. Someone must answer the phone and someone must make home visits. It is important to remember that the person answering the phone may not be a clinician and may need help when deciding if a particular problem is urgent. Office policies and guidelines can be established for this purpose.

A small home visit practice that is nested in an office practice will not have separate staff or offices. In this setting, office clerical personnel and nurses who handle phone calls should be trained and familiar with the home visit program's policies.

In larger practices, there may be dedicated staff for the home visit program. Again, someone must answer the phone; phone calls are common when working with this population. The telephone operator may be a clerical employee or a medical assistant. If it is feasible, the latter option has advantages because there will be a fair amount of clinical complexity involved in some calls.

The home visit providers may be physicians, nurse practitioners, or physician assistants. Nurse practitioners are capable of making initial and continuity home visits and may function effectively as case managers. There must be good support and communication between the physicians and the nonphysician clinicians on the team, and physicians must be available to make home visits on a scheduled and an urgent basis.

Another valuable asset is a team social worker. Patients who are homebound and their families often have substantial social support needs that are time-consuming and may not be within the expertise of the medical physicians. Although home health agencies and other community services can help with these needs, regulatory constraints may limit their involvement and leave the medical team with only intermittent social work help in a particular case. Hiring a social worker may not be feasible for an office-based physician who has a small homebound practice. However, if the homebound practice is larger, or if the physician practice is affiliated with a hospital or medical care system, social work help for the home visit program may be a negotiable option.

Some home visit programs employ drivers who travel with the medical providers. This helps with security if the visits are made in high-risk areas, and it also allows medical providers to use their time more efficiently. While riding, providers can dictate or use a cellular phone to perform case management. In the home, the driver, who usually is a medical technician, can assist with the visit by measuring vital signs, helping move the patient, obtaining specimens or doing diagnostic tests as needed, and performing parts of the home assessment.

▶ Ancillary Relationships

In any home medical practice, a substantial number of the patients are likely to use home care service delivered by other types of providers. Home health agencies and home medical equipment companies are the most common physicians of ancillary services. It is useful to develop relationships with local physicians. Identify organizations that deliver timely, high-quality service and use them as preferred physicians. Along with these home health physicians, several other numbers will be needed in a desktop resource file. Child Protective Services is one, along with pharmacies that will deliver medications, group homes and other alternative living options when home care fails, and various other community agencies that provide support services for the frail and chronically ill. Associations that serve patients with muscular dystrophy or cystic fibrosis are examples.

One of the key elements in building relationships with external providers is developing a good communications system. In the physician's office, the chart of each patient should identify the names and phone numbers of other resources involved in the case. The physician's office also should have an organized system for handling telephone calls and paperwork from external physicians in a responsive and timely manner. Clinical care breaks down when communication breaks down. Furthermore, the outside providers cannot bill when the physician's office delays the paperwork. This creates major cash flow problems for the outside organizations. At the outside agency, similar requirements must be in place. The agency chart for each patient should contain key information about the physician who is directing the patient's care, and the outside agency should have a well-developed strategy for communicating with each physician.

Knowledge of the available physicians, other providers, and services is essential to home care medicine. It usually takes some time to accumulate the critical reference list; this resource file should be maintained actively. In the same vein, the medical home care physicians must be knowledgeable about payer coverage rules and responsive to outside providers with respect to processing the paperwork that is involved. This can be fairly extensive and tedious, but it is a basic responsibility that accompanies work in home medical care.

▶ Internal Communications

When running a mobile team, communication among team members is one of the highest priorities. For this purpose it is advisable to have regular team meetings. Pagers and cellular phones are also valuable.

If a mobile team that has several members has more than one clinician involved in the care of a particular patient, it is critically important that the providers tell one another what needs to be done as they hand off tasks. The office is a good location for these handoffs, but e-mail also works well for this purpose. If e-mail is used, all providers must agree to a set of rules and check messages regularly. Even with these precautions, problems will occur. Computer systems fail temporarily or people neglect to log on. Accordingly, if there is an important message, call the office or page teammates to prevent lapses in patient care.

▶ Medical Records

The format of the home care medical record is much like the format of the office medical record. However, the home care chart should include designated space for information about the home environment that may not be discoverable during office visits. At the very least, this section of the record should be expanded. Other key information, such as directions to the home, caregiver information, and key medical and social support phone numbers, needs to be listed. Documentation templates can make charting more complete and readable, especially if the chart is completed between stops.

The original medical record must be protected. It is best that the version of the chart that goes on home visits is backed up by another copy that remains at the office. It also is important to protect all patients' confidentiality when making visits. This important precept is reflected in the Joint Commission on Accreditation of Healthcare Organizations requirement that charts are kept secure and under the physician's control when the charts are outside of the office.

There are many attractive features to having electronic records; if a system allows this luxury, it may be a very useful asset. However, there are a number of logistic complications that are inherent to developing and using an electronic medical record in home care.

▶ Billing and Reimbursement

If the home visit is more than a rare event, the physician must consider the financial impact on the practice. The clinical justification for making home visits is easy to find; the financial analysis can be more difficult. It is necessary to consider the fee schedules provided by the dominant payers in the practice, and it is essential to know how to determine overhead.

The billing codes for home care have been developed recently with Medicare fee schedules in mind. They parallel evaluation and management (E/M) codes for office visits. These codes apply for visits to the patient home and not licensed domiciliary facilities and nursing homes. Table 33-8 lists these levels of service with standard Medicare rates. Medicaid has not yet incorporated home visits into its fee schedule.

A question frequently is raised about the issue of homebound status and billing for home visits. Home health agencies have been facing increasingly stringent interpretation and oversight on the homebound issue and the federal definition for homebound now is being revised to be more specific. Although homebound status is not mentioned in the *CPT* manual for home visits, supplying a fairly strict definition of homebound when billing for home visits is recommended. Homebound status relates to the difficulty a patient faces when leaving the home and is judged in part by how often the patient leaves home for nonmedical reasons. If the patient is rarely out of the home except when receiving medical care, homebound status is easily established. If the patient leaves home for social or nonmedical reasons multiple times in a week, it usually is inappropriate to claim that patient as homebound. The degree of physical, psychological, or financial burden associated with leaving the home are also taken into account. Bear in mind

TABLE 33-8. 2001 Medicare Fee Schedule*

Code[†]	Medical Decision Making	History	Physical Examination	Problem Severity	Approximate Payment[‡]
Home Visit, New Patient					
99341	S	PF	PF	L	$62
99342	L	EPF	EPF	M	$92
99343	M	D	D	M-H	$139
99344	M	C	C	H	$181
99345	H	C	C	H/unstable	$220
Home Visit, Established Patient					
99347	S	PF	PF	S-L	$48
99348	L	EPF	EPF	L	$77
99349	M	D	D	M-H	$121
99350	M-H	C	C	M-H	$176

*S, straightforward; L, low; M, moderate; H, high; PF, problem focused; EPF, expanded problem focused; D, detailed; C, comprehensive.

[†]CPT five digit codes, nomenclature, and other data are copyright 2001 American Medical Association. All Rights Reserved. No fee schedules, basic units, relative values, or related listings are included in *CPT*. The AMA assumes no liability for the data contained herein.

[‡]Payment will be adjusted by the geographic index.

that a patient can be homebound solely on the basis of a psychiatric condition such as a severe phobia.

To determine the level of service to bill within each family of *CPT* codes, consider the intensity of work involved in the three basic elements of each visit: history, physical examination, and medical decision making. New patient codes are used for patients who are new to the practice or patients who have not been seen for a long time (3 or more years between visits is the Medicare guideline). All follow-up visits use established patient codes. These are the same rules that are used for billing office-based encounters. It is vital that documentation matches the level of service that has been billed. Retroactive review of billing compliance by payers is becoming increasingly common.

Note that each payer has its own fee schedule for these *CPT* codes and some payers, such as Medicaid, may vary considerably from state to state. Home visits are a group of codes that have lacked attention for many years.

It may be worth an effort to make sure that someone in the state government has recently reviewed the home visit codes to see whether the state's rate of reimbursement in the Medicaid program is appropriate.

Care plan oversight (CPO) is another billable service. This code was designed for patients with Medicare home health care. Physicians must determine whether their local Medicaid program or private carriers reimburse for CPO. The basic rules state that a physician may bill for certain services within a calendar month if the physician provides 30 minutes or more of overseeing the home care process. This work can involve phone care to other professionals, reviewing records or test results, and completing paperwork. Care plan oversight does not include conversations with caregivers or the work done by the physician's staff. There are other rules that relate to medical directors of home care agencies and hospice organizations, physicians who direct dialysis for their patients, and surgeons. More details on CPO are available in the American Academy of Home Care Physicians booklet, *Making Home Care Work in Your Practice*. The *CPT* codes for CPO are **99375** for home health care patients and **99378** for hospice patients, but many were recently revised by the Centers for Medicare and Medicaid Services (CMS) (formerly the Health Care Financing Administration [HCFA]) to CMS Healthcare Common Procedure Coding System (HCPCS) code G0181 for home care and G0182 for hospice to allow more inclusive language when billing for these services.

Procedures and diagnostic testing performed during the course of a home visit also can be billed. For example, immunizations, antibiotic injections, nebulization treatments, and wound care services are billable procedures. Some physicians carry portable diagnostic testing equipment and these services are billable. Additional rules apply to transportation fees for some of these tests, and, for certain portable laboratory equipment, a Clinical Laboratory Improvement Act (CLIA) license may be needed. These details are most important for a physician that has a large homebound practice and employs a lot of portable equipment.

Risk-bearing contracts are an important consideration for some practices, and they create an ideal opportunity to demonstrate the value of home visits. The cost of a home visit is small compared to the cost of an ambulance ride and emergency room visit or hospital stay. As long as the targeted criteria used to select patients for the home medical program are well chosen and the decision about when to make home visits is made carefully, financial managers can be convinced that the efforts are cost-effective as a result of cost avoidance. One key is identifying a reasonable comparison group. The positive effect from a well-structured home visit program can become apparent with even a few patients.

Depending on payment method, cost reduction is another strong argument for a home visit program. Shortening hospital stays and reducing costs by strong case management and through the availability of reliable, high-quality, in-home follow-up care is a positive feature of such programs. If the hospital or health care system is paid prospectively for inpatient care, as is true with Medicare diagnosis-related groups (DRGs) or global case rates for specialized services, home visits again make good sense.

Remember that the overhead costs should be low in home visit programs, running perhaps 25% to 35% of gross revenue (as opposed to 65% in office practice). These efficiencies are not possible if home visit activity is a small part of an office practice where the office overhead follows the physician. However, if there is a greater commitment to home visits, office costs can be proportionately lowered by reducing the number of rooms and support staff. Under these conditions, using the Medicare fee schedule as a basis for developing the business pro forma, it is feasible to break even or make money in a home visit program. This does not have to be a purely charitable undertaking as long as it is remembered that, like any business, controlling costs and providing efficient service are vital considerations.

▸ Practice Management and Staff Issues

The development and operation of a home visit team becomes increasingly complex as the team increases in size and takes on more involved care delivery. Providing ancillary service also adds a layer of administrative complexity. It usually is best to start small and grow from there.

A few staff issues bear mention. One issue is the obvious need for providers (physicians, nurse practitioners, or physical assistants) who are interested in making home visits a regular part of their clinical roles. Such clinicians are not prevalent in today's professional world and any practice seeking to move actively into home visitation must take provider availability and recruitment into account. Turnover may present the same issue periodically.

To minimize turnover, several strategies may help. One is to provide clinical staff with good office support. Another is to have regular team meetings. This will encourage professional collegiality and will create a forum for team problem solving. It also is important to staff and design the home visit program with the awareness that there will be unexpected peaks and valleys in the level of demand. Thus, the program must be staffed for the average and it must be understood that there will be some times when the demands on the practice are light and the staff can relax. Home visit work is particularly demanding and some opportunities to relax are valuable.

The presence of a strongly committed, charismatic team leader is helpful in building and sustaining a home visit program. Within a large health system, it is important to have the support of the administration.

Patient Examples

Physicians without home visiting experience may wonder what type of patients can be seen in the home and what type of care can be provided. The following patient examples illustrate the practical benefit of physician home visits.

▶ Example 1

A 4-year-old boy with moderate, persistent asthma, in kinship foster care with his great grandmother following sexual abuse by the mother's boyfriend 2 months prior, was visited by the resident who had been providing longitudinal outpatient care prior to the episode of sexual abuse. The resident understood that he had no pets, smokers, carpets, or mold in the home and that he used cromolyn sodium by nebulizer three times daily and albuterol by nebulizer as needed. At the home visit, a kitten bolted out the front door as the resident entered. The great grandmother and mother were smoking. The mother was present even though she was not permitted to see her son without supervision from caseworkers. The apartment was dank, dusty, and carpeted throughout. The mother stated that there was a nebulizer "in storage" that she was unable to access because of the legal proceedings against her and her boyfriend. Another resident along on the visit began wheezing after 15 minutes. Following the home visit, the primary care physician realized the need to reorient asthma education back to the very basics, considered contacting the caseworker to ensure appropriate supervision in the home, and advocated for a move to a better housing environment.

▶ Example 2

A 1-year-old girl with profound developmental delay, seizures, and recent hospitalizations for pneumonia and wheezing was visited by the resident providing longitudinal primary care since the neonatal period. The child lived with her 15-year-old mother, the 32-year-old grandmother, and an uncle with chronic mental illness in an apartment building with many abandoned units. The mother reported recent visits to emergency rooms for wheezing, at each of which a written management plan had been issued, along with prescriptions. None of the three written plans recommended the same inhaled anti-inflammatory medication, and two different preparations of nebulized albuterol were prescribed. The caregivers did not appear to be confused by these discrepancies. The grandmother was worried by a potential conflict with attending the girl's intake appointment the next day at a developmental evaluation center. The resident encouraged the caregivers to discard two of the plans and segregated the medications pertinent to the third, demonstrating how to draw up the appropriate dosages. Attendance at the evaluation was urged.

▶ Example 3

A 10-year-old boy with autoimmune polyglandular syndrome was visited at home by the attending pediatrician caring for him for the past year. He was affected by hypoparathyroidism, hypoadrenalism, hypothyroidism, and mucocutaneous candidiasis, and calcium levels had been abnormal for 6 months in spite of 1,25-dihydroxyvitamin D absorptive capacity. He lived with his mother, 2-year-old sister, and stepfather in a one-bedroom basement suite of a private house with lush vegetable and flower gardens in a middle-class section of the city. The maternal grandmother watched his sister and him while the mother worked in the afternoons and evenings, but she was ill from human immunodeficiency virus. No one regularly supervised the administration of the evening doses of his multiple medications. A pill box had been suggested as a way to organize and remember to adhere to the regimen, but the boy did not like the idea because his grandmother used one for her medications. At the visit, the boy proudly showed the physician the section in his armoire for some of his clothes and videotapes. Following the home visit and expression of concern for his well-being, the boy's calcium levels normalized for a 3-month period. Subsequently, he became easily fatigued, fell acutely ill with vomiting and dehydration, and acquired deeper pigmentation during winter months. When given double doses of hydrocortisone by his mother as prescribed by episodes of fever, he felt well. He had orthostatic vital sign changes at serial office visits. He and his mother were confronted about regular adherence with adrenal replacement. The mother denied the possibility of non-adherence, then became tearful at her isolation and inability to recruit help supervising his medical regimen. They missed subsequent follow-up for several months. The previous expression of genuine concern on the pediatrician's part had been effective at restoring adherence but was not sufficient to protect against the alienating effects of the subsequent confrontation.

▶ Example 4

A 5-month-old surviving twin girl conceived by in vitro fertilization, born at extremely low birth weight, and discharged 1 month earlier on oxygen, diuretics, and cardiorespiratory monitoring was visited at home by the resident caring for her in continuity clinic. The parents, from Ghana, lived in mixed-income housing in an airy apartment overlooking three city bridges and much of the city. Her mother remained indoors all day in her bedroom, by the infant's crib, with the infant tethered to the oxygen supply by tubing roughly 6' in length. A source of liquid oxygen was presented for travel to appointments. Playing on the portable stereo on the bureau was one of a set of tapes with sermons in a native dialect, entitled, "How to Be a Good Wife." Bottles of fish oil, cod liver oil, and gripe water were seen in the medication tray beside the bottles of diuretics, multivitamins, and iron. The mother was pleased and proud at her infant's progress and weight gain. The total daily dose of vitamin A being administered was found to greatly exceed the recommended amount, and stopping the fish oils was discussed. The resident encouraged the mother to take walks outside during pleasant weather, to leave her bedroom from time to time, or at the least to ask for breaks from other women in the apartment. After the visit, a plan was made to speak to the father and discuss this advice with him to permit greater freedom for the mother. Longer extension tubing was ordered for the stationary oxygen source.

▶ Example 5

A 9-month-old girl, born at extremely low birth weight and discharged at 4 months of age on oxygen, diuretics, nebulized bronchodilators, caffeine, and cardiorespiratory monitoring, was visited at home. Her young parents always had come neatly dressed and on time to the office and seemed articulate, polite, concerned, and informed. The mother lived with her sister and maternal grandfather in a two-bedroom apartment in aging projects. The halls of the apartment were not navigable unless one turned sideways to slip past columns of cartons and piles of clothes. Laundry was strewn over the sink, shower rail, tub, and toilet tank. The living room was chilly because of a cracked window and insufficient heat, and was half filled to the ceiling with furniture piled up. A summons for the aunt to appear in criminal court sat atop a tower speaker near the entrance to the living room. The father returned from the kitchen with a vial of palivizumab, which the attending had been ordering from a pharmacy that delivered it to the office. He said that a man from a pharmacy had brought this vial to their home and told them to keep it refrigerated and call their doctor about it. A parallel prescription was discovered that had been initiated on nursery discharge, and one supply of palivizumab was stopped. The attending and resident involved had been unaware of the living conditions the family endured and helped them advocate for better public housing placement.

▶ Example 6

A 14-year-old boy from Gambia who was neurologically devastated from adrenoleukodystrophy has been visited every 1 to 3 months for 4 years by his primary care pediatrician or nurse practitioner. He lived in a bedroom with his mother on the bottom floor of a six-bedroom duplex apartment in modern projects in the city, together with his father, six half siblings, and his father's three other wives. At the afternoon visits, men congregated in the living room to eat, smoke, and talk while women prepared food in the kitchen or tended to children downstairs. Although the boy was wasted, lacked cutaneous sensation, and had frequent seizures, his skin was immaculate, his mouth was clean, and he remained well hydrated. During the visits, the physicians reviewed his care plan, oriented toward comfort, diminution of seizures, and reduction of aspiration risk, with his mother and home health aide. The father declined to discuss his son's medical care, believing his condition had been caused by the brain biopsy performed before his diagnosis was established. The boy lived in this steady state with a do not resuscitate (DNR) order before succumbing to pneumonia.

▶ Example 7

A 13-year-old boy with severe myasthenia gravis, unimproved by immuno-modulatory therapy or thymectomy, had become wheelchair bound and suffered four respiratory crises requiring intubation in the 18 months prior to a home visit. Born in Puerto Rico, he had lived with his parents and older brother since age 2 in a two-bedroom, first-floor apartment in a semi-attached house with a newly installed ramp in front. The father rarely came to appointments or to the hospital but greeted visiting professionals warmly, making them coffee, showing off his chickens in the backyard and the home renovations he had created. The mother did not read or easily follow the doctors' explanations of the medicines' actions, but was believed to supervise the medication regimen with excellent adherence. She brought her son to weekly appointments to an osteopath of cervical manipulation intended to aid the flow of lymph and other fluids in the lungs. At the visit, the father explained to the visitors that he viewed his son's major recent difficulties as caused by mucus accumulation in the throat and lungs. He had prepared a nostrum of aloe, lemon, garlic, and olive oil for his son to drink whenever congested and found it to be as effective as the bronchodilators prescribed. The parents would not agree to discuss the options of a DNR order, although the boy contemplated refusing intubation at the next myasthenic crisis. Renewed attention was paid to the boy's respiratory secretions in the hope that it would facilitate the future exchange of ideas about management issues the family seemed likely to face in the future.

Summary

- The evolution of home care has allowed for a quicker transition of the patient from the hospital to the home, even replacing the hospital as the preferred site for many pediatric conditions.
- Patients who are dependent on technology, require monitoring or specialty care, or who have special ancillary needs benefit from home care.

- Socioeconomic and cultural outreach benefits physicians and patients alike.
- Observing a family at home allows the physician to assess the home and family, then determine treatments that are the most likely to be successful.
- Physicians who plan to integrate home visits into their practice must define those visits as a distinct component of the practice. They must ensure they have systems in place for scheduling visits, handling paperwork and phone calls, staffing, handling ancillary relationships, and handling medical records.
- Home care education is being integrated gradually into the medical school curriculum. One example is the John A. Hartford Foundation grand program developed by 10 medical schools called, "Expansion of Home Care Into Academic Medicine."

Bibliography

American Academy of Pediatrics, Committee on Bioethics. Appropriate boundaries in the pediatrician-family-patient relationship. *Pediatrics*. 1999;104:334-336

American Medical Association, Council on Scientific Affairs. Educating physicians in home health care. *JAMA*. 1991;265:769-771

Berger LR, Samet KP. Home visits: extending the boundaries of comprehensive pediatric care. *Am J Dis Child*. 1981;135:812-814

Boling PA. *The Physician's Role in Home Health Care*. New York, NY: Springer Publishing Co Inc; 1997

Boling PA. The value of targeted case management during transitional care [editorial]. *JAMA*. 1999;281:656-657

Goldberg AI, Gardner G, Gibson LE. Home care: the next frontier of pediatric practice. *J Pediatr*. 1994;125:686-690

Klass CS. *Home Visiting: Promoting Healthy Parent and Child Development*. Baltimore, MD: Paul H. Brooks Publishing Co; 1996

Loudon ISL. Visiting patients in their homes. *JAMA*. 1988;260:501-502

Making Home Care Work in Your Practice. Edgewood, MD: American Academy of Home Care Physicians; 1998

Naylor MD, Brooten D, Campbell R, et al. Comprehensive discharge planning and home follow-up of hospitalized elders: a randomized clinical trial. *JAMA*. 1999;281:613-620

Chapter 34

Ethical Issues in Pediatric Home Care

Ronald M. Perkin, MD; Robert Orr, MD; Dennis Deleon, MD

Introduction

The ethical principles that guide medical decision making in home care are similar to the principles used in other health care settings. Ethical theories and principles provide a foundation for ethical analysis and moral reasoning. Theories that focus on consequences (eg, various utilitarian theories), motives (eg, virtue theories), and duties (eg, deontologic theories) guide the reasoning process. Ethical principles, such as beneficence (doing good), non-maleficence (avoiding or minimizing harm), veracity (telling the truth), justice (ensuring fairness or equality), fidelity (keeping promises), and autonomy (deciding for oneself), are commonly applied to clinical situations.

Principles provide an organizing framework by offering a guide for understanding ethically relevant information in a troubling situation. They also suggest direction, offer proposals to resolve competing claims, and often supply the reasons for justifying moral action. Ethical principles are universal in nature, but they are not absolute; even these principles have exceptions in certain situations. Ethics is not a majority issue.

Principles of Decision Making

All of the above principles are important in discussing a moral framework for decision making involving children, but this chapter will focus on the principles of beneficence and its corollary non-maleficence, respect for people, and justice. Based on the principles of beneficence and non-maleficence, health care professionals seek to promote the well-being of their patients and to reduce or alleviate harm. Choices among alternative treatments should benefit the infant or child and clearly outweigh the associated burdens and harms. Even though children are not autonomous or self-determining, respect for people still is required in decisions about their care because

the lives of children have unique meaning. To treat children with respect is
to acknowledge and value who they are outside of a medical context, rather
than to treat them only according to how professional goals and values are
advanced. Justice demands that individual patients be treated fairly and that
decisions are not made based on subjective criteria such as race, age, sex,
diagnosis, or socioeconomic status.

Autonomy implies the importance of the individual in making his or
her own life decisions. This concept is accepted for adults and children, but
vicarious decisions necessarily must be made for infants and children.

A triangle of understanding needs to be established among the child,
family, and health care team. In children with chronic health care problems,
this triadic relationship often is complex. Instead of one physician, there may
be a health care team whose chief may change on a regular basis; the home
health nurse often provides most of the vital sense of continuity. Instead of
two involved parents, there may be a single teenage mother, or the parents
may already be separated or divorced, each accompanied by a new partner.
The parent(s) often are accompanied by a variety of family members with
differing philosophies. The child is not yet autonomous but completely
dependent on others for care, love, and decisions. In the setting of an acri-
monious family, the ethical health care team must constantly think of what
is best for the child.

Parental decision making on behalf of children can provoke questions
about parental rights versus the rights of children, parental rights versus the
duty of the pediatric professional, and the interests of the decision makers
versus those of the state.

Parental Rights and Responsibilities

As a rule, the law protects the natural rights of parents to raise children
free from unwarranted state interference, presuming that parents will act
in the best interest of their children. Accordingly, parents are allowed considerable latitude for medical decisions on behalf of their children, even if
the choices may not concur with the physician's recommendation. These
rights are conditional on parental fulfillment of the duty to provide necessary care for minor children. Even more important than parental rights are
parental responsibilities. If parents fail to provide their children with at least

a minimum standard of medical care, the state may assert its interest in protecting the welfare of children by involving child protection statutes to override parental wishes.

Courts regularly uphold such interventions when parental refusals, even when genuinely motivated by strong family convictions, may be life threatening. However, when the consequences for the child are grave but not life threatening, states have differed in their willingness to intervene, reflecting the continuing struggle to balance the rights of individual children and family privacy. Many state child-protection statutes include exemptions for parents who seek nontraditional forms of treatment based on religious convictions, although the American Academy of Pediatrics has urged states to repeal such provisions. It must be emphasized that the central principal guiding decisions should be what protects the best interests of the child and not mere parental preference.

Disclosure

Considerable guidelines exist about the disclosure of a chronic illness to a child. In general, disclosure is geared to a child's level of cognitive development and psychosocial maturity. For most illnesses, young children receive simple explanations about the nature of their illness and what their responsibilities are in caring for themselves. The exact diagnosis and prognosis of the disease are less important in early discussions with young children. As children mature, they should be fully informed of the nature and consequences of their illness and encouraged to participate actively in their own medical care. Children with a variety of chronic diseases, including cancer, have exhibited better coping skills and fewer psychosocial problems when appropriately informed about the nature and consequences of their illness.

Self-determination

The commonly accepted concepts of parental consent and parental right to refuse consent raise serious ethical problems when they compete with the responsibilities of health care professionals to their minor patients who have the capacity to consent for their own medical treatment. Historically, the right of self-determination is recognized at the legal age of maturity, defined as 18 years. Many legislatures and courts have expanded minors' rights to consent to medical treatment. In most states a child may acquire status as an emancipated minor entitled to treatment as an adult through marriage, judicial decree, military service, parental consent, failure by the parents to meet legal responsibilities, living apart from and being financially independent of parents, and motherhood. In addition, statutory mature minor rules uphold the validity of consent given by minors if the treatment is appropriate and the minor is considered capable of comprehending the clinical circumstances and therapeutic options. As a child's powers to interpret and integrate life's experiences evolve from a characteristically concrete, shortsighted perspective to an appreciation of abstract, future-oriented concepts, concomitant expansion of decisional rights involving increasingly complex and risky alternatives may follow. Though it is well recognized that age alone is not an adequate gauge of maturity, some developmental psychologists suggest that most children older than age 15 have the ability to make their own medical decisions, and many between 11 and 15 years of age also have this capability. Professionals even have been encouraged to obtain consent for treatments from children as young as 7 years and, in the interest of promoting children's rights, to consider persistent expressions of dissent by young children. Courts have recognized the rights of minors approaching the age of 18 years to participate in decision making, including choices involving life and death consequences.

Distributive Justice

Decisions about what will benefit individual patients should be separated from decisions about how society will allocate its health care resources in general. While health care professionals have a moral mandate to be involved individually and collectively to promote efforts to meet the health needs of groups of patients and of society in general, such decisions are not suited for the bedside but belong within the context of a larger societal debate. Distributive justice is a policy, rather than a clinical concept. However, when marginally beneficial treatments are considered, health care providers have a responsibility to allocate resources in a fair, fiscally responsible manner.

Societal good clearly is achieved by the restoration to health of a child with an illness or disability who then can be expected to reach adult life and become a full member of society. When an infant has severe birth defects, especially with associated mental retardation, the picture is intuitively less clear. In the United States, legislation resulting from the Indiana Baby Doe controversy (see Pless in Bibliography) states that treatment should not be withheld unless the infant is chronically and irreversibly comatose; the provision of such treatment would be futile in that it would merely prolong dying or would not be effective in ameliorating or correcting all of the infant's life-threatening conditions; or treatment would be virtually futile in terms of survival and would be inhumane. The Department of Health and Human Services construed these provisions narrowly to specifically exclude any consideration of the potential "quality of life" of the affected infant. This ruling accepts that societal good is dependent not on whether the infant will become a productive member, but on the preservation of the life and well-being of the disabled patient. The rights of personhood are intrinsic to the individual and not dependent on an extrinsic measurable property such as physical ability, personal productivity, or intelligence.

Ethics and Advocacy

Addressing ethical concerns begins with an understanding of the advocacy role of professionals. Advocacy means assisting patients or, in the case of children, their surrogates, to make informed choices and to act in the child's best interest. Advocacy is not acting instead of someone else, and it should not be confused with "rescuing" someone. At times, professionals become confused about the boundaries of their advocacy role. They may begin to make decisions for the patient instead of with the patient. This paternalistic approach usurps patients', or their surrogates', authority to act for themselves. The appropriate advocacy role involves advising, sharing specific information, and offering recommendations to enable patients to make their own decisions. It embodies an authentic model of shared decision making that presumes equal power and authority.

The goal of advocacy is to enable the patients and families to adjust to the changes in health of their loved one in their own unique way. The health care professional's actions are directed toward maximizing the control exerted by the patient and family while assisting them in this process. In this way, the health care professional advances the sense of personhood, self-worth, and dignity of the child and family, consistent with a family-centered philosophy

of care. Successful advocacy demands that the health care professional engage
in trusting relationships with patients and families and appreciate their
unique values and life goals within the context of their culture, religion,
and belief system.

Moral Sensitivity

Moral sensitivity refers to the individual's ability to recognize that a moral
problem or conflict exists. In the broadest sense, it means being attuned to
the moral dimensions of the situation, or being able to recognize what is
morally significant in the context of a particular situation. Paying attention
to one's emotional barometer and intuitions and using such information to
articulate moral tensions and questions can enhance such attunement.

Clarifying personal and professional values and societal norms is a related
and essential prerequisite for sound ethical deliberations. Value clarification
involves examining one's personal and professional values. It includes examining the origin of certain values and testing their application in various
clinical situations. Health care professionals should engage in an ongoing
process of self-reflection and assessment of their values about issues such
as life, death, disability, and relationships.

Futility

The concept of futility implies that treatment may be discontinued or
withheld if efforts to prolong life will not be effective or (some would say)
merely result in meaningless existence. Decisions involving this concept
are made almost daily in active intensive care settings in the presence of
irreversible brain damage from various causes. Like most ethical concepts,
this is easier in the more extreme situations. There are now generally
accepted objective criteria for a diagnosis of death by neurologic criteria
(brain death). The child who has no cortical function and no conscious
ability to respond to the external environment, but who does not fulfill
the criteria for neurologic death, presents a more complex case because
the only possible purpose of treatment of the child is the prolongation of
physical survival or the hope of an error in the diagnosis. Careful neurologic
examination with reference to the cause and circumstances of the illness
or injury can make misdiagnosis extremely unlikely. Because such children

presumably cannot experience suffering or joy or interact with their environment, they have no interest in continued survival. However, from
the child's perspective, it is not clear whether death would be preferable to
life. In this case, the best interests standard may not be helpful. Many have
expressed the belief that patients who are in a permanent vegetative state,
and therefore lack the ability to think, communicate, give or receive love,
and appreciate pain or pleasure, have no interests to be considered except
the right to be treated with dignity. Therefore, society should have the
authority to preclude the use of technological intervention to sustain life
in such patients, regardless of their age.

When there is doubt about the possibility or duration of survival, or over
the implications of a particular disability's influence on a child's chances for
a meaningful life, unanimity may be lacking and serious divisions may arise
among individual health team members, the family, and others. Divisions
tend to arise most often in three critical situations. First, the medical facts
are unknown or in dispute; a consensus can only be built on what all know
to be the truth. Second, the concept of meaningful life cannot be agreed
on for the individual child. Third, the moral, ethical, and philosophic viewpoints of the team and family are unknown, are at variance, or have not yet
been properly discussed. After the medical facts are known with clarity, a
consensus needs to be established. This takes time and empathy. Discussion
with an ethics committee or an ethics consultant may help clarify the true
facts and points at issue and return the child to the central role, a role sometimes lost sight of in prolonged heated arguments. Parents faced with such
tragic circumstances may be counseled to withhold or withdraw all life-
sustaining medical treatments from their children not based on medical
futility, but on the perception of the interests of the child and the potential
benefits of the treatment. The child is and must remain the apex of the
triangle of understanding.

Role of Home Care

Home care is an exceptionally diverse endeavor covering a wide range of
initiatives, from the care of those dependent on extremely complex technology to the continuing management of a person who needs assistance in the
basic activities of daily life, such as feeding, ambulating, and personal hygiene.

Some children require a significant amount of daily care and much of that care has moved from hospitals into homes. Home care now includes the use of tracheostomy tubes, intravenous transfusions and infusions, peritoneal dialysis, and the long-term use of ventilators. The burden of care has shifted to the family, assisted to various degrees by home care nurses, therapists, and equipment companies. One distinctive ethical issue, broadly construed, of high-technology home care is the tendency to medicalize the home environment, subjecting the traditionally private sphere of home to the intrusions of medical personnel, timetables, and equipment.

Families often prefer home care because they believe it has benefits for the child and family and represents a safer, more normal environment than the hospital. In some cases, the life of the child may be prolonged, whereas for others, home is a more acceptable place to manage the final stages of a terminal illness. Home care provides many personal, social, and financial benefits, but it also presents the family with problems. The personal, social, structural, and financial barriers to successful home care can be overwhelming, and sources of support may be limited.

One distinctive ethical issue home care is the tendency to medicalize the home environment

Families with more resources often experience serious limitations in maintaining careers and preferred personal and family lifestyles. Some homes are not conducive to the successful provision of home care. The worst home is not necessarily better than the best medical institution. Children in these circumstances remain in institutions until alternatives can be found. The success of home care depends on the determination and resourcefulness of the family, and the quality of the support network that can be marshaled to assist them.

Fundamental ethical dilemmas arise when one set of problems (for the patient) is solved at the cost of creating a new set of problems (for the patient and caretakers). The relatively recent popularity of home care for patients who are chronically ill or dependent on technology has moved professionals into unfamiliar settings with great rapidity, often without time for contemplation of the significant changes in attitudes and priorities home care demands.

A main factor, which has encouraged complex care in the home, is the development of sophisticated medical technology. High-tech, safe equipment has permitted the introduction of a variety of treatment and mechanical support in the home.

However, the technology itself is largely responsible for the stress that families experience. The transition from hospital to home can be felt by patients and family members as a shift from technology overload to technological isolation. At home, some patients and their families can feel cut off from or even abandoned by the system of intensive medical supports present in the hospital. This lack of connection can be experienced by families as a profoundly alienating and isolating experience. Thrown back on their own resources and instincts, families must rely on impressions and guesswork rather than data. The ensuing magnification of uncertainty can be a source of great worry and anxiety.

The advantages of high-tech home care include the following:

- The presence of family and familiar surroundings. Institutionalization interferes with the ability to form normal, interpersonal family and community relationships that are important for normal growth and development.
- Fewer infectious complications.
- Generally less expensive.

The following are major disadvantages of high-tech home care:

- Increased burden on the family. Home becomes an intensive care unit with physical, emotional, and often financial burden on the family.
- Loss of privacy.
- Impact on other family members such as siblings.
- Potential out-of-pocket costs for family.
- Absence of immediate professional help.

The goal of a home health care program for infants, children, or adolescents with chronic conditions is the provision of comprehensive, cost-effective health care within a nurturing home environment that maximizes the capabilities of the individual and minimizes the effects of the disabilities.

Careful review of the patient's status and needs should be made by each professional participating in the patient's care. Each discipline should formulate goals and objectives for the patient. Eligibility for home health care should be based on a comprehensive analysis of the capabilities of the home health care program, whether the child's therapeutic needs can be met by home care, the potential benefits and risks, and the available resources. Families should not face excessive pressure to enroll their children in a home care program if such a move would be detrimental to the child or family.

Understanding the personal, professional, economic, medical, psychological, and social forces of which pediatric home care is a part and to which it contributes is essential; there must be congruence among these various realities and the knowledge, expectations, and goals of professionals and families alike to achieve a successful home care program. Coerced or uninformed choices will predict failure or, at the very least, continual conflict and psychological discomfort for all or some of the parties involved in a given home care plan.

Technologic capacity does not ensure or equate with benefit to patients or their families (ie, doing more does not necessarily mean doing better). Health care professionals and families are obligated to make difficult choices in the care of patients dependent on technology. Survivability and available technology should not be the only criteria by which the choice for long-term support is made.

Nature of Home Care

Home care is mostly chronic care. It differs markedly from acute care, which focuses on short-term, cure-oriented treatment. Chronic care is ongoing, uncertain about prognosis, varied (even diffuse) in its modalities, and often directed at palliation and functional support rather than cure and return to normal function.

Because home care tends to be chronic in nature, it is not simply or even predominantly medical. Ethical problems arise, in less dramatic fashion, within the routines of daily life, and these dilemmas often are quite different from those encountered in the acute care setting. The home setting, the role of family as caregivers, the nonmedical dimensions of care, and the limited reimbursement system all create special problems that press ethical reflection beyond the standard acute care discussion.

Unfortunately, home care is relatively poor in status and resources; it often is ancillary and marginal. It functions with very little physician involvement, relies on nursing and social work supervision, and is heavily dependent on ancillary formal caregivers and a large but often "invisible" force of informal caregivers (mainly family members).

One of the principal policy motivations for the development of home care has been the claim, or at least the hope, that by providing a less expensive alternative to institutional care, it would lower overall costs of health care.

Informed Decision Making

Decisions for or against long-term home care usually are made in the acute care setting and almost always in the intensive setting. These decisions must be based on adequate and thorough information provided to patients and families. Once the information is provided and digested, a decision based on the collective best interests of patient and family should be sought. The decision must weigh the benefits and burdens primarily for the patient, but also for the family members. Investigation and assessment of the family's ability to provide the environment as well as the many duties required of patients who are dependent on technology must be conducted by clinicians experienced in chronic home care. One must search for the existence of psychological, social, or cultural barriers to effective care.

A number of issues related to the potential effects of having a child who is severely ill at home need to be explored with the family, including issues of privacy, physical burdens of care, impact on other family members such as siblings, time demands of home care, role of the parents in coordinating care, and the social and financial aspects, including issues of confidentiality.

Placing complex life-support systems in the home may create extraordinary challenges for parents and families. In the face of these challenges, one cannot simply judge parents acceptable if they provide recommended health care or neglectful if they do not. Professionals must be careful in deciding how vigorously to try to convince parents, explicitly or by implication, to assume obligations for such care.

The patient's general condition, including associated functional or cognitive disabilities and other medical problems, and ability to participate in social and academic activities need to be weighed in the light of the natural history of the disease process to decide about benefits of long-term support. This judgment is fundamentally subjective, but it requires consideration by parents and caregivers. In this situation, informed consent must be seen as a dynamic process whereby both caregiver and patient/family benefit from each other's thinking, not as a finite moment in time. The home care process must allow decisions to be reviewed and revised and take into account the family's quality of life. Without a process to change decisions, families may resort to making their own decisions, such as implementing privately sanctioned do not resuscitate orders that are later explained as equipment failures or accidents. The home care movement must advocate a system of continuing assessment of the patient and family. High-tech home care contracts with the family should be renegotiable throughout the course of the patient's care.

Families and the Challenges of Home Care

Families face difficult moral issues in attempting to understand the nature and the extent of their obligations to provide care. The extent of family caring indicates widespread recognition that families have a serious duty to provide care. On the other hand, families often are deeply perturbed by the inescapable need to set limits to this care. As the disabilities and dependencies of their children increase, many families face emotional and moral exhaustion. Trying to balance the demands of care against their own dwindling resources, they are caught between imperative duties and impossible demands.

Individual family members caring for loved ones regularly confront questions on their own identity and social roles. Parents caring for children dependent on technology naturally wish to maintain and foster an exclusively loving, nurturing, and comforting relationship with their child. Their natural role is to protect, to safeguard from harm, and to reassure. But these same parents, in their role as dispensers and maintainers of high-tech medical treatments, sometimes must inflict serious pain and suffering on their own children. In this second role, they must act more like doctors than parents, or more like technicians than nurturing mothers and fathers. Many may wonder whether their child who is dependent on a ventilator might be better off elsewhere, perhaps in a comfortable residential setting, where the child may focus his or her rage against others, and the family members may be better able to retain their identity as caring nurturers.

Faced with such challenges, family caregivers have a real stake in decisions affecting the focus and level of care for their children. Decisions about home care can seriously alter the lives of family caregivers, infringing on their independence, autonomy, and commitments to others. Depending on the extent and impact of family members' caregiving, their autonomous interests can move into the foreground of decision making. This is not to suggest that home care requires a move from a model of patient as primary agent to one of family as primary agent. The ethical problem for home care becomes one of determining how the autonomy and interests of family members should counterbalance those of the child receiving care. When family members heavily share the challenges of care, decision making becomes a horizontal, interactive process involving negotiation, mediation, compromise, and recognition of values. The traditional, patient-centered moral framework must give way to a new ethic for chronic home care based on the notion of reasonable accommodation of competing legitimate interests.

In home care, family caregivers play crucial roles that have no parallel in acute care. These roles and their distinctive ethical challenges deserve fuller description and analysis. The following issues stand in the foreground: the basis of family obligation to provide direct care; the limits of this obligation; the relation between familial obligation and wider societal obligation to provide home care; and the nature of autonomy and beneficence, as well as independence and paternalism, within family caregiving.

Formal Caregivers

Most home care patients receive formal (health care professionals) and informal (family) care and, therefore, the cooperation of family members is crucial to the success of care plans. A model for hospital discharge and home care planning should clarify relationships among physicians and establish mechanisms of accountability for all involved in caring for the child. It must be community based and include physician involvement at the tertiary and local levels. Roles and responsibilities should be established, to the extent possible, for the physician based in the tertiary care center and the community-based physician before hospital discharge. The community-based physician should be identified early in the planning process and should have the opportunity to supply input into the home care plan and to receive training, if needed, at the tertiary care center.

Once the child is home, physicians are part of a team that includes parents, community health care professionals, home medical equipment providers, funders, and others. The physician, in partnership with the parents and other team members, should help define those roles and provide support in the maintenance of those guidelines and any subsequent changes. Caring, compassionate, and knowledgeable pediatricians must address the needs of their patients and all children in the context of the community.

Children with chronic illnesses and disabilities can comprise 20% of a primary care pediatric practice. Providing care to these children can be frustrating and challenging for pediatricians serving this vulnerable and complex population. At the same time, this aspect of practice can be rewarding to all the professionals involved.

The frustrations generally fall into three categories: time, information, and coordination. First, quality primary care services for children with chronic conditions are time-consuming. As the managed care industry thrives, primary care physicians receive the same capitation rate for children with complicated problems as they do for other children. There is little financial incentive under most managed care plans to spend extra time on complex problems and some insurers discourage primary care physicians from attracting children with high-cost health care needs into their practices.

Children with chronic illnesses and disabilities can comprise 20% of a primary care pediatric practice.

Second, many primary care physicians feel inadequately informed about managing chronic illnesses and disabilities. Well-trained informal caregivers may be more knowledgeable about the management of the technology and even more expert in disease assessment for their unique patient than the primary pediatrician who joins the care team relatively late in the endeavor.

Finally, children with chronic illnesses often require extensive care coordination that involves the entire community. Communication between health care professionals can run the gamut from fair to inadequate. Sometimes there is no coordination at all; in other cases children have multiple case managers who fail to communicate with one another.

Within communities, efforts should be made to develop effective and efficient chronic condition management programs. Pediatric practices can strengthen their services to children with special health care needs with a well-planned management approach that is part of the medical home model. This type of program earmarks specific children for extra services in the primary setting and improves the following: access to office services, responsiveness to family needs, care coordination, ongoing education, and office efficiency and reimbursement.

Providing care in a home environment is very different from hospital-based care for a number of reasons. One of the main differences centers around the environment itself. Within the hospital setting there are prescribed standards of practice and a controlled area in which to carry them out. Rules are established to maintain control over the patient's medical care. In the home environment, the standards of care are more ambiguous and the "where, how, and who" aspects of delivering that care are less formal. In the home, the professional caregiver has much less control over the child's nutrition and exposure to communicable diseases, the hygiene of the home, the quality of care, and the equipment available to the child. Even in relation to meeting the developmental needs of the child, caregivers are confined to the limitations of the home environment (eg, physical space and financial resources).

In addition, the home environment is a secondary setting for formal providers and the primary setting for the family. This is a paradigm shift from the hospital where formal caregivers were in control. In the home setting, parents are in the primary position of authority and, in the past, did not consult with others about how they functioned or the decisions they made about their child. In fact, to take the child with a disability home, they were required to become expert in their child's care and in most situations were lauded by the medical profession for their skills. This reversal of authority and narrowing, or even reversal, of the professional-parent expertise gap may cause conflict because it is a role foreign to the professional health care provider and parent. This role change is necessary in the home care environment where the emphasis is on empowering parents to make critical decisions about their child's care, but it may be very uncomfortable for and even threatening to the physicians involved. A more subtle issue relates to the fact that parents are the employers. They have the authority to hire and fire formal caregivers and to establish guidelines as to how they wish services to be provided to their child.

The goal of a therapeutic relationship is to have well-defined boundaries among the health care professionals, child, and family that promote the family's control over the child's health. The ability to maintain a therapeutic relationship in the home often is compromised by the informal environment and the natural tendency of many families to integrate the health care professional (usually the nurse) into their lives. In addition, the health care professional may confuse boundaries because the family participates in the child's care in the same manner that colleagues in the hospital do.

When formal caregivers' boundaries are unclear or diffuse, they may become over-involved in their job. In the home care environment, they may manifest this by negotiating care for the sick child on their time off or modifying policies established by the agency that employs them. Other problems that can occur when professionals' boundaries are unclear include caring for siblings or performing household tasks while parents are away.

The autonomy and authority of formal caregivers can be muted by the home setting, the nature of the care provided, dependency on family caregivers, and tensions created by family supervision of care. Caregivers face sharp conflicts when patients and families, emboldened by these elements, press to control care in an unreasonable fashion. Even in less contentious situations, authority and control remain underlying problems.

The various tensions between caregivers, patients, and families require more than a strict ranking of autonomy and authority. The ethical equation becomes more complex, and it often is helpful to focus on goals of therapy rather than the ethical principles. The recognition of common, corresponding, or at least cohabitable goals often may be more productive than the determination of whose goal finally wins. In daily home care, autonomy is acutely protected by accommodation, the recognition of interdependence, mutuality, and the sharing of challenges.

Home Care Agencies' Responsibilities

Although the services of the home care agency are contractual, monitored by state inspectors, and open to regulatory citation, judicial suit, and the canons of professional practice, family caregivers are comparatively free of outside scrutiny. This creates problems when an agency finds that a family's caregiving is inadequate because it is substandard or delinquent. An agency cannot simply mandate better care from family caregivers, and it may be unable to encourage or indirectly elicit it. While the agency remains responsible for the overall status of its patient, it does not control the care situations as institutional caregivers do. In the cooperative endeavor of home care, the agency's covenant with family caregivers exists mainly in the moral and not the legal order. Responding to family failure in care is strategically difficult and ethically complex. The cooperative nature of home care argues not for standoffs between the competing autonomies of formal and informal caregivers, but for mediating the varied obligations and self-determined interests.

Formal caregivers working for or through a home care agency often struggle with the ethical dilemma of whether to continue to participate in what they assess to be substandard care, so that the patient will have at least some professional oversight, or to withdraw from the situation as a matter of professional conscience, fearing that the patient will be even less well served. Either action may be subject to concerns of moral complicity and/or legal liability. Resolution of such dilemmas sometimes requires compromise from ideals, but should always focus on what is best for the individual patient.

Home care agencies are corporate moral agents of a special sort, and the moral dilemmas they face need full examination. Many of these dilemmas fall under the ethics of strained resources, such as lack of reimbursement for critical services to patients, fiscally driven access and discharge problems, staff shortages and turnover that affect quality of care, and conflicts created by the dual advocate/gatekeeper role. When ethical problems are examined from the perspective of home care professionals, the most common problems cited are difficulties with payer regulations and the competence of coworkers. In general, home care provides rich territory for exploring issues such as distributive justice, covert rationing, the right to health care, and the relative priorities of medical and social forms of assistance. In home care, the reality of these overarching issues is most powerfully felt in the experiences of home care agencies. Home care agencies should consider in-service education and discussion of ethical issues, the development of ethics committees, and consultation or mediation services to deal with ethical conflicts and dilemmas. Given the limited resources of many home care agencies, the development of multiagency or regional ethics committees might be a productive strategy.

There is little doubt that pediatric home health care will continue to grow. High-tech care at home has become increasingly feasible, and more patients and families desire care in the home environment. It is critical that this rapid growth be accompanied by ensurances that pediatric home care is age appropriate and of high quality.

Periodic Review

At intervals during the child's home care program, there should be a coordinated review of the patient's and family's needs, how the family is managing, the progress toward home care goals, and other available relevant information. This is important because the child's and family's medical, social, and financial needs likely will change over time.

Principles of program review should include the analysis and improvement of key clinical, social, and financial outcomes, with evaluation of the ultimate value of the care provided. Follow-up and outcome assessments need to be based on the following:

- Survival
- Need for subsequent hospitalizations and other mobility
- Developmental progress
- Course of the underlying disease
- Actual utilization of resources with comparison to expected utilization
- Financial experience
- Effect on family members, including siblings

Funding

Private long-term insurance provides exceedingly limited coverage, and most patients and their families are not able to meet home care costs. Restricted and fragmented resources create ethical problems. The paternalistic physician pressing for aggressive medical treatment is not a looming threat in home care, where patient autonomy is threatened more by lack of options and limits on service than by coercion to accept treatment. Enhancement of autonomy is more crucial than noninterference with it.

▶ Managed Care

Children with chronic illnesses and disabilities increasingly are joining managed care arrangements. The rapid expansion of managed care has unknown consequences for children with chronic conditions and disabilities.

Although a paucity of research exists on the effects of managed care on children with chronic conditions, it is clear that organized systems of care have potential advantages for children with chronic conditions and their providers. For example, health maintenance organizations (HMOs) and other organized systems offer the potential for improved coordination of care as well as better preventive services and health care maintenance. There also are necessary procedures in most managed care arrangements. Proponents of managed care argue that it can offer improved access to primary care.

There are potential disadvantages for children with chronic conditions enrolled in managed care. For example, access to and choice of specialist services may be reduced in managed care settings. Customary doctor-patient relationships may be disrupted for many families as they enter organized systems of care. Pediatricians increasingly will be asked to serve as gatekeepers for the service system; at the same time they will experience reduced autonomy in choosing courses of treatment for their patients. Moreover, if physicians are given economic incentives to reduce service use, they may no longer be in a position to serve as effective advocates for patients who are chronically ill.

Beyond the direct effects on pediatric patients and providers, enrollment in managed care also may carry significant indirect ramifications for families. For example, the limited deductibles and co-payments common to managed care, especially in HMOs, should mean that many families will see their out-of-pocket expenses for medical care decline, freeing resources for other family needs. Other families may experience increased outlays for medical care and related services, especially if they are obtained from providers outside the plan.

To date, researchers and policy makers have garnered little more than anecdotes and speculation concerning the impact of managed care on children with chronic conditions. There is a critical need for this population to identify its strengths and weaknesses. As managed care is likely to become the predominant mode of medical practice for children with special health care needs, information gained from a thorough assessment of existing models of managed care would be helpful in indicating adjustments and modifications that could result in improved outcomes for this population.

The home health care team should evaluate the projected cost of the child's care and the available methods of financial support and resolve funding problems before hospital discharge of the child. There should be continuing review and dialogue among the home health care team, insurers, and public programs to help ensure the financial coverage of home care. Creative financing approaches include negotiated arrangements among a diversity of health care and social service funding sources.

Increasing interest in home care for children who are dependent on technology arose from a combination of rising hospital costs, reduced payments by private and public payers, improved technology, increased numbers of survivors of serious pediatric illnesses, and adverse effects of prolonged hospital stays on normal child development. Home care for children who are dependent on technology is felt to be more cost-effective than institutional care.

▶ Cost Shifting

Cost shifting to families is a particularly insidious aspect of cost saving for institutions. There has been insufficient attention given to the financial effect that high-tech home care can have on families. The material cost to families in terms of lost income, leisure, career opportunities, and interaction with other family members needs to be calculated over time. A survey of parents of children assisted by a ventilator showed that 71% of parents were unable to pursue career choices, education, or job changes because of care requirements of their child. Home care may not be less expensive than institutional care for some patients if the long-term economic impact of home care on the patient's family is taken into consideration.

Parental Employment Issues

Another recent study demonstrated that having a child assisted by technology may force many parents to quit employment, diminishing family resources at a time when financial needs may actually increase. These findings support the need for strengthening several family resources, including social and other supportive services, and providing financial assistance to replace lost income. The Supplemental Security Income program for children and adolescents provides financial aid to low-income households with children having severe mental, developmental, or physical disabilities. The use of home care social workers experienced in coordination of care as well as counseling may help families to make decisions about care at home and out-of-home work schedules and aid family adaptations. Employment outside the home not only may be important economically, but may have implications for the mental health of parents or guardians.

The data also indicate the importance of improving nursing and child care services for this population, recognizing the complex nature of the health conditions. Lack of respite care, child care, or after-school programs for children assisted by technology seemed to be a major problem for the families in this study. Community-based programs should aim at the inclusion of children with chronic conditions and those assisted by technology. These services may particularly benefit parents who remain employed. In addition, certain labor policies, such as flexible time arrangements or additional sick leave to take care of a sick family member, also may help to alleviate stress in families with children assisted by technology.

If moving children from the hospital to the home depletes the financial and emotional resources of their families, no benefit is gained by society or third-party payers. Ethical analysis demands that there be accurate assessment of the motivations behind a movement that appears grounded in principles of beneficence. Although home care for high-tech patients indeed can be beneficial, there must be a preservation of options to ensure optimal patient and family functioning. Costs, while clearly a vital component of sound health care policy, should never be the exclusive or preeminent factor in decision making.

Conflicts With Resource Use

The reorganization of health care is profoundly influencing the roles, responsibilities, and even the loyalties of physicians. The accelerated disappearance of the solo practitioner has been matched by an increase in the number of physicians who belong to various complex organizational groupings, including independent practice associations (IPAs), physician-hospital organizations (PHOs), and group- and staff-model HMOs. No matter what the physician reimbursement mechanism is in each plan (fee-for-service or global capitation), plan administrators expect individual physicians or groups of physicians to stay within a fixed budget for their panels of patients. To achieve this goal, many try to persuade physicians to make caring for their entire group of patients a higher priority than caring for each individual patient. In doing this, physicians are expected to adopt what has been called a distributive ethic, in which the principle is to provide the greatest good for the greatest number of patients within the allotted budget.

Now more than ever, new fiscal constraints in health care challenge physicians to do more with less. During the 1990s, public attention was focused on the financial conflicts inherent in capitated reimbursement settings, particularly those in which financial incentives were created by managed care organizations to reduce utilization of expensive resources. A conflict of interest in this context exists when a physician has obligations that involve divided loyalties; ie, situations in which the fiduciary duty to patients conflicts with a contractual duty to a third party, such as an HMO, employer, or government agency. Examples include any payment incentive that may interfere with clinical decision making, such as restricting treatment provided to the chronically ill; "gag rules" that restrict patient alternatives; and gatekeeping activities that potentiate denial of payment for services rendered.

Under these circumstances, there is a great temptation to manipulate or bypass the system altogether to obtain the care a patient needs. Falsification of the severity of an illness, shaping the diagnosis to fit the eligibility criteria, and raising the level of severity of symptoms are temptations to which even conscientious physicians are subject. Deception is never justified even to serve the good of the patient. Society must question the validity of any system that forces the physician to deceive to ensure patients have access to needed care.

In fee-for-service medicine, physicians can earn more money by performing more tests and ordering more therapies that may or may not be in the patient's best interest. The obvious direct financial benefit to the physician and the potential overuse of medical resources diminishes confidence and trust in the physician. Additionally, it generates an unjustified greater health care expense. The conflict of interest occurs only when the physician is unduly influenced by financial gain and patient welfare becomes a subordinate consideration. Whether financial incentives in the fee-for-service system provoke physicians to do more rather than less, or managed care arrangements encourage them to do less rather than more, physicians must not allow such considerations to affect their clinical judgment. The principles of beneficence, fairness, and non-maleficence must be applied, while acknowledging that health care resources are limited. Physicians must seek to affirm that the medically appropriate level of care takes precedence over financial compensation imposed by an individual physician or group practice, investments, or financial arrangements. In addition, all physicians who practice emergency medicine are bound by the Emergency Medical Treatment and Active Labor Act, which requires a basic screening examination to be provided to all patients seeking care. Therefore, it is unethical, as well as illegal, to withhold therapy from patients just because they may not be able to pay. Because trust is the central tenant of the physician-patient relationship, physicians must be cognizant of all of the aforementioned influences, and appropriate use should be guided by fairness, truth, and honesty.

▶ Conflicts of Interest

The fundamental ethical values of medicine are based on the belief that physicians are competent, are compassionate toward the sick, and will put the interests of their patients before their own. Conflicts of interest, however, are an inherent hazard of all compensation systems. Every method of paying physicians, including fee-for-service and salary arrangements, involves incentives that influence physicians' clinical judgment and effort in ways that may compromise the care received by an individual patient. Therefore, a central ethical imperative is to integrate into the design of compensation systems safeguards that minimize potential conflicts as much as possible. Conflicts of interest, which inevitably remain despite these safeguards, sometimes can be mitigated by honest disclosure of such conflicts to regulatory bodies and even to patients and families.

▶ Physician Self-referral

Physician self-referral is pervasive in some specialties. Physicians should not refer patients to an outside facility in which they have invested financially or at which they stand to gain direct financial benefit through care not directly provided by themselves. Although many physicians who participate in self-referral would argue that they provide only tests and therapeutic interventions that are medically indicated, there is sufficient data to support that self-referral generates greater utilization of ancillary services and greater costs. An exception is applicable only when the capital funding and necessary services otherwise would not allow an essential resource to be made available to patients.

The intent of the Stark I law, named after its primary author, Rep Pete Stark of California, and enacted by Congress in 1989, was to restrict physician self-referral of Medicare clinical laboratory services. Another piece of legislation, the Stark II statute enacted in 1993, curbed Medicare and Medicaid physician referrals in a broader sense to entities in which the doctors or immediate families had financial interests, such as home health facilities. Though these laws intended to restrict the inappropriate self-referral practices discussed above, their actual implementation, especially in the case of Stark II, has proven so complex that the federal government itself proposed rules intended to put Stark II into effect only in January 1998. Objections to Stark II and the proposed cumbersome enforcement rules have been so widespread that the House Ways and Means Health Subcommittee and Representative Stark himself are considering a repeal or rewrite of the legislation. Despite the practical difficulty of writing legislation that prevents inappropriate self-referral while still allowing communities of patients to benefit from necessary services, it is critical that physicians who provide home health care avoid situations in which their financial gain could be reasonably construed as clouding their professional judgment. The possibility of such a scenario unfortunately is commonplace in today's complex medical environment.

Alternatives to Home Care

The use of intermediate or chronic care facilities may be considered as an alternative to home care. The choice of home care or alternative care must be based on a thorough evaluation of the needs and wishes of the family and the expected course of the illness. Effective care planning requires the development of a continuum of care options and the evaluation of alternate types of care. Components of a care plan include the spectrum of care that may be required over time depending on changing circumstances.

Though it seems intuitive that a child's well-being could be better served in the home, where at least some of the care is provided by family members, rather than in an institution, where care is provided almost entirely by "strangers," individual patient and family circumstances and capabilities vary. Home care may be the best choice for some patients, but institutional care may be the better option for others. Families should be helped with this very difficult initial decision and should not be made to feel guilty about choosing institutional care.

In some situations, a trial of home care may be tried and found to be too burdensome or otherwise unworkable. Transition from home to institution should then be facilitated, again without imposing or implying guilt.

Termination of Professional Relationships

Occasionally, home care agencies or individual formal caregivers may wish to terminate their professional relationship with a particular patient or family because of nonpayment for care, noncompliance by the informal (family) caregiver, or both. Prior to termination, legal and ethical issues must be considered.

First, if termination of home care is contemplated, the issue of potential liability for abandonment must be addressed. To establish abandonment, it must be proven that termination of the professional-patient relationship was unilateral, occurred without reasonable notice, and occurred when further attention was needed by the patient.

As long as the agency gives reasonable notice, services can be terminated without liability for abandonment. Of course, the key issue is, what is reasonable notice? In most cases, reasonable depends on the facts and circumstances of individual cases. To account for unique facts and circumstances of the case, the agency should hold a meeting including all members of the treatment team. At the meeting, the following circumstances should be considered: (1) patient's clinical condition; (2) patient's mental status; (3) the wishes of the family; (4) the patient's wishes; (5) possible alternative sources of care; and (6) the availability of other primary caregivers. Other circumstances that the staff considers relevant also should be considered.

If the team decides to terminate services, it also must determine a reasonable notice period, considering all of the facts and circumstances identified in the team meeting. Notice to the family must be given in writing and a copy placed in the chart. The patient's physician should be notified (if not involved in the team meeting) of the agency's decision. Care for the patient on the day of termination must be planned.

The agency should report immediately any possible abuse and/or neglect of patients by family or professional caregivers. The duty to report is determined by state statute so health care professionals must review the law in their states to make final determination about their obligation to report.

Withdrawal of Therapy

Ethical and, potentially, legal dilemmas develop when withdrawal of therapy from a child is contemplated. Patients and their families should be informed at the onset and reminded occasionally that a decision for long-term care is not irreversible. After a trial of therapy in the hospital or home, if the patient with decisional capacity decides that the challenges of therapy outweigh the benefits, the patient may decide to discontinue the therapy. If the decision appears to be motivated by concern about the burden of the program to the family, additional support or an alternative setting should be sought. A decision to stop therapy that is life-sustaining should not be made impulsively. Caregivers should assure themselves that the decision is coming from the patient or from an appropriate surrogate who is seeking the patient's best interests and that this decision persists over time. The ethical principles of autonomy, beneficence, and non-maleficence should be the basis for withdrawing life support in chronically/terminally ill patients.

Many adolescents with chronic medical conditions want to participate in the treatment decisions, especially decisions about life-sustaining medical interventions. Such chronic medical conditions often worsen over time (eg, certain kinds of cancer, neuromuscular diseases, cystic fibrosis, acquired immunodeficiency syndrome, complicated types of heart disease). Having experienced years of physical and psychological suffering, gone through multiple hospitalizations and numerous treatments, probably experienced depression, and probably observed the dying of several hospitalized friends with similar medical problems, these adolescent patients are frequently mature beyond their chronological years. They have had, at the very least, multiple opportunities to think about the inescapable anguish that characterizes their lives, the features of life that make it worth continuing, the benefits and challenges that accompany medical treatment, and the prospect of death. At least some of these adolescents want to give voice to their values; provide directions for parents, physicians, and nurses regarding end-of-life care; and be assured that their wishes and preferences will be respected and carried out should their medical conditions deteriorate to the point that they will not longer be able to communicate their deeply felt views.

Advance Directives

Advance directives, which were developed for this very purpose in adults, can help meet this goal for pediatric patients with chronic conditions. Enabling adolescent patients with chronic, life-threatening conditions to communicate their wishes about treatment options through oral or written advance directives can provide ethical justification for such decisions, which should then provide a measure of legal protection of physicians. Pediatricians, family physicians, and others caring for such patients would be able to document the specific end-of-life treatment wishes of these patients and their conversations about the use or nonuse of life-sustaining treatment that had taken place with the patients and their parents. Though no jurisdiction gives statutory authority for minors to complete written advance directives, the unique situation of chronic care makes them important ethical tools to be considered by professional caregivers.

Advance directives should be respected by emergency medical technicians (EMTs) in the out-of-hospital setting. Prehospital advance directives are regulated through the state or local emergency medical services (EMS) authority. Optimally, there should be clear policies for out-of-hospital advance directives. Until the legal authority is established for advance directives completed by minors, it may be necessary to have explicit discussions between primary physicians and the local EMS caregivers to avoid unwanted emergency interventions.

The directive usually requests limitation of treatment such as refusal of resuscitation measures, including cardiac compression, endotracheal intubation, advanced airway management, and defibrillation. The use of a standard form, in which the patients, the primary care physician, and a witness sign the document, helps to avoid confusion. In addition, the form should contain a picture or other identifying data so that the EMTs are clear that it is the correct patient involved.

The question usually arises as to why EMS were called for a patient who does not want resuscitative procedures. There are multiple factors involved in calling EMS. The patient who does not wish to have resuscitation procedures performed may desire standard emergency treatments for reversible diseases such as pneumonia, asthma, or congestive heart failure. Even in circumstances where an informed decision has been made to forgo life-prolonging interventions, 911 or the local emergency number may be called by a family member who encounters an unanticipated complication. In these situations, assistance with emergency comfort measures still may be appropriate without the automatic cascade of transport, emergency room, intensive care unit, etc. When there is confusion, disagreement among family, or any question about the legitimacy of an advance directive applying to patient's present condition, the recommendation is that EMTs err on the side of life and institute appropriate treatment, including resuscitation.

Summary

- Home care should be endorsed as one reasonable option in a continuum of alternatives to acute hospitalization. Home care should be seen as a beneficial choice when it is desired by the patient and the family.
- Home care cannot mean abandonment of the family. The care plan must include supportive services, a continuing mechanism to evaluate and monitor the initial goals, opportunities for reassessment of site of treatment, and the ability to change directives when there is alteration in patient status or wishes or when the family no longer can provide the necessary care.

Bibliography

American Academy of Pediatrics, Committee on Bioethics. Guidelines on foregoing life-sustaining medical treatment. *Pediatrics.* 1994;93:532-536

American Academy of Pediatrics, Committee on Bioethics. Informed consent, parental permission, and assent in pediatric practice. *Pediatrics.* 1995;95:314-317

American Academy of Pediatrics, Committee on Bioethics. Religious objections to medical care. *Pediatrics.* 1997;99:279-281

American Academy of Pediatrics, Committee on Child Health Financing. Guiding principles for managed care arrangements for the health care of infants, children, adolescents, and young adults. *Pediatrics.* 1995;95:613-615

American Academy of Pediatrics, Committee on Child Health Financing. Principles of child health care financing. *Pediatrics.* 1998;102:994-995

American Academy of Pediatrics, Committee on Children With Disabilities. Guidelines for home care of infants, children, and adolescents with chronic disease. *Pediatrics*. 1995;96:161-164

American Academy of Pediatrics, Committee on Children With Disabilities. Managed care and children with special health care needs: a subject review. *Pediatrics*. 1998;102:657-660

American Academy of Pediatrics, Committee on Children With Disabilities. Pediatric services for infants and children with special health care needs. *Pediatrics*. 1993;92:163-165

American Academy of Pediatrics, Committee on Children With Disabilities. Why supplemental security income is important for children and adolescents. *Pediatrics*. 1995;95:603-608

American Academy of Pediatrics, Committee on Community Health Services. The pediatrician's role in community pediatrics. *Pediatrics*. 1999;103:1304-1307

American Academy of Pediatrics, Committee on Pediatric AIDS. Disclosure of illness status to children and adolescents with HIV infection. *Pediatrics*. 1999;103:164-166

Arras JS, Dubler NN. Bringing the hospital home. Ethical and social implications of high-tech home care. *Hastings Cent Rep*. 1994;24:S19-S28

Bartholome WG. A new understanding of consent in pediatric practice: consent, parental permission, and child assent. *Pediatr Ann*. 1989;18:262-265

Carraccio CL, Dettmer KS, duPont ML, Sacchetti AD. Family member knowledge of children's medical problems: the need for universal application of an emergency data set. *Pediatrics*. 1998; 102:367-370

Clemens CJ, Davis RL, Novack AH, Connell FA. Pediatric home health care in King County, Washington. *Pediatrics*. 1997;99:581-584

Collopy B, Dubler N, Zuckerman C. The ethics of home care: autonomy and accommodation. *Hastings Cent Rep*. 1990;20(suppl):1-16

Cooper R, Koch KA. Neonatal and pediatric critical care: ethical decision making. *Crit Care Clin*. 1996;12:149-164

Fields AI, Coble DH, Pollack MM, Kaufman J. Outcome of home care for technology-dependent children: success of an independent, community-based case management model. *Pediatr Pulmonol*. 1991;11:310-317

Fields AI, Rosenblatt A, Pollack MM, Kaufman J. Home care cost-effectiveness for respiratory technology dependent children. *Am J Dis Child*. 1991;145:729-733

Fleischman AR, Nolan K, Dubler NN, et al. Caring for gravely ill children. *Pediatrics*. 1994; 94:433-439

Goldberg AI, Gardner HG, Gibson LE. Home care: the next frontier of pediatric practice. *J Pediatr*. 1994;125:686-690

Goldberg AI, Monahan CA. Home health care for children assisted by mechanical ventilation: the physician's perspective. *J Pediatr.* 1989;114:378-383

Grebin B, Kaplan SC. Toward a pediatric subacute care model: clinical and administrative features. *Arch Phys Med Rehabil.* 1995;76(12 suppl):sc16-20

Haddad AM. Ethical problems in home healthcare. *J Nurs Adm.* 1992;22:46-51

Hays RM. Health care ethics and pediatric rehabilitation. *Phys Med Rehabil Clin N Am.* 1991;2:743-763

Hilton T, Orr RD, Perkin RM, Ashwal S. End of life care in Duchenne muscular dystrophy. *Pediatr Neurol.* 1993;9:165-177

Hogue EE. Child neglect in home care: weighing legal and ethical issues. *Pediatr Nurs.* 1993;19:496-498

Jessop DJ, Stein RE. Who benefits from a pediatric home care program? *Pediatrics.* 1991;88:497-505

Kassirer JP. Managing care—should we adopt a new ethic? *N Engl J Med.* 1998;339:397-398

Keens SE, Jansen MT, Lipsker LE, Gilgoff IS, Keens TG. Lifestyle alterations in families with ventilator dependent children at home [abstract]. *Am Rev Respir Dis.* 1989;139:A195

Khaneja S, Milrod B. Educational needs among pediatricians regarding caring for terminally ill children. *Arch Pediatr Adolesc Med.* 1998;152:909-914

King NM, Cross AW. Children as decision-makers: guidelines for pediatricians. *J Pediatr.* 1989;115:10-16

Klug RM. Clarifying roles and expectations in home care. *Pediatr Nurs.* 1993;19:374-376

Kohrman AF. Chimeras and odysseys. Toward understanding the technology-dependent child. *Hastings Cent Rep.* 1994;24:s4-s6

Lantos JD, Kohrman AF. Ethical aspects of pediatric home care. *Pediatrics.* 1992;89:920-924

Leiken S. A proposal concerning decisions to forgo life-sustaining treatment for young people. *J Pediatr.* 1989;115:17-22

Levine C. The loneliness of the long-term care giver. *N Engl J Med.* 1999;340:1587-1590

Levine C, Zuckerman C. The trouble with families: toward an ethic of accommodation. *Ann Intern Med.* 1999;130:148-152

Lundberg JA, Noll ML. The long-term acute care hospital: a new option for ventilator-dependent individuals. *AACN Clin Issues Crit Care Nurs.* 1990;1:280-288

Mallory GB Jr, Stillwell PC. The ventilator-dependent child: issues in diagnosis and management. *Arch Phys Med Rehabil.* 1991;72:43-55

McPherson M, Arango P, Fox H, et al. A new definition of children with special health care needs. *Pediatrics.* 1998;102:137-140

Nelson LJ, Nelson RM. Ethics and the provision of futile, harmful, or burdensome treatment to children. *Crit Care Med.* 1992;20:427-433

Newacheck PW, Stein RE, Walker DK, Gortmaker SL, Kuhlthau K, Perrin JM. Monitoring and evaluating managed care for children with chronic illnesses and disabilities. *Pediatrics.* 1996; 98:952-958

Newacheck PW, Stoddard JJ, Hughes DC, Pearl M. Health insurance and access to primary care for children. *N Engl J Med.* 1998;338:513-519

Newacheck PW, Strickland B, Shonkoff JP, et al. An epidemiologic profile of children with special health care needs. *Pediatrics.* 1998;102:117-123

Parent S, Shevell M. The 'first to perish.' Child euthanasia in the Third Reich. *Arch Pediatr Adolesc Med.* 1998;152:79-86

Pearson SD, Sabin JE, Emanuel EJ. Ethical guidelines for physician compensation based on capitation. *N Engl J Med.* 1998;339:689-693

Perkin RM, Orr R, Ashwal S, Walters J, Tomasi L, Winslow G. Long-term ventilation in children with severe central nervous system impairment. *Semin Neurol.* 1997;17:239-248

Pless JE. The story of Baby Doe. *N Engl J Med.* 1983;309:664

Quint RD, Chesterman E, Crain LS, Winkleby M, Boyce WT. Home care for ventilator-dependent children. Psychosocial impact on the family. *Am J Dis Child.* 1990;144:1238-1241

Rosenbach ML, Irvin C, Coulam RF. Access for low-income children: is health insurance enough? *Pediatrics.* 1999;103:1167-1174

Sahler OJ, Greenlaw J. Pediatrics and the Patient Self-Determination Act. *Pediatrics.* 1992;90:999-1001

Sanders AB. Advance directives. *Emerg Med Clin North Am.* 1999;17:519-526, XIII

Sevick MA, Bradham DD. Economic value of caregiver effort in maintaining long-term ventilator-assisted individuals at home. *Heart Lung.* 1997;26:148-157

Shatin D, Levin R, Ireys HT, Haller V. Health care utilization by children with chronic illnesses: a comparison of Medicaid and employer-insured managed care. *Pediatrics.* 1998;102:E44. Available at: http://www.aap.org/cgi/content/full/102/4/e44. Accessed August 9, 2001

Sprung CL, Eidelman LA, Steinberg A. Is the physician's duty to the individual patient or to society? *Crit Care Med.* 1995;23:618-620

Stein RE, Jessop DJ. Long-term mental health effects of a pediatric home care program. *Pediatrics.* 1991;88:490-496

Storgion SA. Care of the technology-dependent child. *Pediatr Ann.* 1996;25:677-684

Thyen U, Kuhlthau K, Perrin JM. Employment, child care, and mental health of mothers caring for children assisted by technology. *Pediatrics.* 1999;103:1235-1242

Wade SL, Taylor HG, Drotar D, Stancin T, Yeates KO. Family burden and adaptation during the initial year after traumatic brain injury in children. *Pediatrics.* 1998;102:110-116

Walsh-Kelly CM, Lang KR, Chevako J, et al. Advance directives in a pediatric emergency department. *Pediatrics.* 1999;103:826-830

Weir RF, Peters C. Affirming the decisions adolescents make about life and death. *Hastings Cent Rep.* 1997;27:29-40

Chapter 35

Quality Improvement in Pediatric Home Care

William Wenner, MD

Introduction

Home health care has a tradition of quality improvement (QI) that equals and frequently exceeds that of inpatient care. Evaluating and improving the level of care has always been part of home health care. Initially, home care had to prove an ability to provide the same or better care than traditional inpatient care. Home care is now an accepted component of the health care continuum. Currently, QI continues to make sense because a competitive environment requires optimal performance, regulatory agencies such as the Centers for Medicare and Medicaid Services (CMS) (formerly Health Care Financing Administration [HCFA]) and the Joint Commission on Accreditation of Healthcare Organizations (JCAHO) require institutional QI, and, most significantly, it serves as a protective measure for the child.

Formal, institutional QI is a mandated component of home health care. The US Department of Health and Human Services (DHHS) rules for conditions of participation for the Medicare and Medicaid programs (section 484.65) require that a home health agency demonstrate improved performance. The US Department of Health and Human Services has distilled the requirements into four core conditions: patient rights, patient assessment, care planning and coordination of services, and quality assessment and performance measurement. These core conditions derive from the DHHS standard that a home health agency is to "attain and maintain the highest practicable functional capacity for each patient."

None of the major influences for home care QI have a pediatric focus. The CMS and the JCAHO are predominately agencies of adult care, and the unique aspects of pediatric QI often are lacking. These unique aspects need to be championed by pediatric care providers. However, with proper modification, adult home care structures can serve as models for pediatric QI.

Components of a Pediatric Home Care Quality Improvement Program

Home care QI programs must serve separate but overlapping institutional roles. Quality improvement/quality assurance (QA) helps the organization meet external standards and provides the structure by which an organization understands what it does, what it accomplishes, and how to better meet its objectives. For a QI program to serve these roles, the proper structure must be in place.

▶ Resources

The proper resources for QI include time and money. Some quality experts estimate that 0.5% to 1% of an organization's budget should be committed directly to improvement. Some organizations may find it productive to commit higher levels of resources and may achieve a higher level of return.

The resources available to the quality process are not just for committee meetings, storyboards, and regulatory compliance. If there is to be real improvement, the quality process must be directly linked to the institutional resource allocation system. Quality improvement projects should influence resource allocation. Nothing reflects lack of institutional integrity more than repeated quality projects that have no effect on care because of a lack of resources to implement the corrective process.

▶ Staff

Adequate personnel must be committed to QI. It rarely can be done on a part-time basis or as an additional responsibility to an already overworked staff. Precise resource allocation should be flexible. There are no absolute numbers but general experience suggests 1 to 2 full-time equivalents (FTEs) per 100 children per year.

Quality improvement staff must be experienced in pediatric home care. Previous experience in providing pediatric care enhances the ability to direct QI activity in productive methods.

▶ Information Technology

An adequate information system is mandatory. There is a need for a mechanism to track client activity and progress over time. The system should integrate clinical data with financial data and allow tracking of patients, services, supplies, and clinical information, including parameters of outcome. The ability to sort by age and diagnosis is self-evident. Mandated data collections such as the Outcome Assessment and Information Set (OASIS) will require integrated information systems.

Free flow of information is mandatory for a functioning QI/QA program. Departments must not be allowed to restrict the information available for QI activity.

▸ Director

The director of home care quality should have significant experience in pediatric home care. Direct access to the senior executive is critical to a successful QI program. Unrestricted access to providers allows for rapid collection and dissemination of data.

▸ Reporting Structure

Clear delineation of the responsibility for the oversight of QI activity is critical. Equally important is the delineation of the responsibility for tracking and implementing QI plans. Those responsible for QI must have the authority to ensure implementation. Some of that authority can be obtained through the reporting structure. Traditionally, QI activity has been a separate function, often reporting to a middle-level administrator. Added efficiency may be gained by direct reporting to the chief operating officer of the home care program.

▸ Committee Structure

Traditionally, QI activity has been committee based. This offers the advantage of inclusiveness and can offer planning and direction to the QI process. However, committees are labor intensive, periodic in activity, and consensual in style. These attributes can slow or actually impede the QI process. The QI infrastructure needs to have the ability to rapidly assess a process and implement changes. The director must have the ability to initiate quality processes independent of the committee. Membership should be limited to committed personnel with the ability to implement change. Too large a committee removes the sense of personal responsibility for the outcomes. Ad hoc members should be added to provide additional perspectives as needed.

▶ Issue Selection

Proper issue selection is critical to a successful QI program. The program must be able to perceive the important organizational issues. An intriguing study recently found that few home health agencies expect QA to find problems. One third or fewer felt QA would reveal a known problem. The most frequently cited methods of finding a problem were supervision/performance evaluation and formal feedback mechanisms. Formal QA strategies are perceived as relatively ineffective for problem identification. Most agencies rely on direct care staff and clients to alert the system to problems; therefore, direct contact with staff and clients should be integrated into the quality process.

Error analysis has been found to be another method of successful issue selection. Errors correlate with opportunities for system improvement.

Measuring Quality in Pediatric Home Care

The structure of QI is based on the theory that all health care consists of three fundamental components: structure, process, and outcome. Quality improvement/QA programs evaluate all three components. These components are evaluated through a theoretical cyclical process called Plan, Do, Study, Act (PDSA). Application of these theories results in four steps to all QA: delineation of standards, measurement, improvement, and remeasurement. Ideally, this is a seamless process that does not end and is called "continuous QI."

The first step in measuring home health care quality is for the organization to define its goals and desired outcomes. These are not the abstract goals of a mission statement, but concrete, discrete definitions of outcomes. Often they are client specific; QI in home health care frequently is described in terms of client satisfaction.

▶ Client Satisfaction

The measurement and application of client satisfaction in the improvement in home health care has been well studied. The use of client satisfaction reporting is an integral structure of quality measurement and improvement. There is, however, disagreement as to the methodology of measuring client satisfaction. Unresolved issues exist in the definition of client satisfaction, the lack of reliable and valid instruments to measure client satisfaction, and the lack of demonstrated translation to operational objectives and reality.

There are obstacles to accurately measuring satisfaction. Questions may have internal and social bias. Clients may fear reprisals resulting in loss of care. Guided interviews, open-ended questions, allowing clients to "tell their story," and responses to hypothetical scenarios have been found to overcome some of the obstacles. Unfortunately, the more accurate methods are more resource intensive. Information on commercial tools for measuring client satisfaction, such as internal consistency, discriminate validity, and convergent validity, allows the home health agency to evaluate a methodology of measuring client satisfaction. Unfortunately, few home health care tools for measuring satisfaction have been evaluated with such rigor.

The following two unique challenges of pediatric home care also influence the role of client satisfaction in quality improvement:

- Who is the client?
  - ~ Is the client of the home health care the child, parent, physician, or payer? At some time in home health care, all fill the role of the client. Whose satisfaction takes priority? Should all be measured simultaneously? Are there adverse institutional effects if only one client's satisfaction is measured? At this time, there are no readily available tools to measure the pediatric patient's or the parent's satisfaction. However, aspects of their satisfaction can be obtained through the application of tools designed for adult home care. These tools must be used with caution and should be adapted to pediatric use.

- What can be measured?
  - ~ There are multiple aspects to satisfaction. Some suggested components of client satisfaction include overall satisfaction, access, continuity, compliance, provider availability (physician and home health agency), communication, perceptions of provider competence, pain control, and family involvement. Despite these obstacles, regulatory agencies believe that formal satisfaction measurement is critical to quality care.

▶ Outcomes in Pediatric Home Care

Quality improvement activity is meaningless without quantitative improvement in outcome. Yet no specific data exist on pediatric home care outcomes. Significant work is being done in the adult home care environment to provide meaningful outcomes data with norms for comparing or benchmarking providers.

An example of a representative structured outcome measurement is OASIS. Now mandated by the CMS, it was developed by Peter Shaughnessy and associates at the University of Colorado from funding by the CMS and the Robert Wood Johnson Foundation. Initially the measurement system collected 79 items in 3 areas: patient identifiers, case mix, and outcomes. Recent concerns about health information confidentiality led the CMS to remove patient identifiers.

While its value to pediatric care has not been established, OASIS appears to offer value to pediatrics if age-specific adjustments to the reporting parameters are made. The system is specific for home care and is one of the first that offers outcomes-based quality improvement. Two stages of the system are delineated, data collection/patient assessment and benchmarking.

Data Collection

Data collection/patient assessment begins at the start of home health service and is repeated at an interval of 62 days or at discharge. Data that measure specific outcomes are collected. Interval, end-of-care, and utilization outcomes are measured. (These measures were developed for populations 21 years and older.) There are global measures for all patients and focused measures for specific patient conditions. These specific patient conditions have been named quality indicators groups. These measures provide quantitation of client improvement and stabilization.

The second stage of OASIS provides the ability to benchmark by comparing an individual home health agency's results internally over an interval or to outside standards.

Benchmarking

Knowing how an organization is doing compared to similar organizations is one of the most effective methods of improving care. A uniquely pediatric system could be valuable, but no such pediatric system exists. However, existing systems for home care such as OASIS may be able to be tailored to pediatric home care. Recent industry-wide initiatives may address this deficit.

ORYX

ORYX is the name of the JCAHO initiative to make performance measures part of the accreditation process. The JCAHO is attempting to make the accreditation process data driven and continuous. To accomplish this goal, the JCAHO has mandated that a home health agency measure quality through an approved measurement system.

The JCAHO has developed a list of available measurement systems to assist an organization in compiling and submitting the required data. This list is available at the JCAHO Web site, www.jcaho.org. The JCAHO reports that 68% of home care organizations found start-up costs for the project to be less than $10,000 and 62% estimated that one or less FTE was needed to fulfill the requirement.

Patient perception of care can include education, medication, pain management, communication of plans, preventive care, and improvement of health status.

Data collection will be monthly and submitted quarterly to the JCAHO. There are variations in the requirements if a home health agency has an annual volume of less than 120 patients.

Measures required by the JCAHO must be "clinical" or "patient perception of care." Clinical measures evaluate the delivery of clinical services and allow comparisons of health care organizations. The JCAHO states that for home health agencies with durable medical equipment, assessment of selection, delivery, setup, and maintenance are considered clinical measures.

Patient perception of care can include education, medication, pain management, communication of plans, preventive care, and improvement of health status. Organizations that provide multiple services such as home care, hospice, or pharmacy are required to select a specified number of measures as determined by the JCAHO.

As noted previously, one system for home health agency QI data collection and analysis has received significant attention. This system, OASIS, is the federally mandated data set for home care. It contains data that are part of the JCAHO listed measurement systems for ORYX. It is anticipated that OASIS will meet JCAHO requirements but this has not been clearly defined.

The JCAHO initiative offers promise for valid pediatric home health care quality data. If ORYX data are age specific and analyzed for validity in the pediatric age group, the data may become the first large-scale pediatric home care data.

Practice Guidelines

The federal Agency for Healthcare Research and Quality (AHRQ) has developed more than 19 practice guidelines. They are available along with many other guidelines through the National Guideline Clearinghouse on the Internet at www.guideline.gov. The clearinghouse is a public resource for evidence-based clinical practice guidelines. It is sponsored by the AHRQ in partnership with the American Medical Association and the American Association of Health Plans. A search of the site revealed 92 guidelines related directly to pediatrics.

The site contains thousands of evidence-based guidelines, many of which can be adapted to a home health agency's quality program.

▶ Sample Screens and Monitors

Tables 35-1, 35-2, and 35-3 list sample screens, monitors, and data collection sets that can be used for a home health agency's quality improvement process. These sample data sets should be modified to reflect an individual home health agency's patient population.

Summary

The following are pediatric home care QI structural guidelines:
- Clearly define desired outcomes.
- Structurally provide access to and impact on institutional resource allocation.
- Institutionally allocate sufficient resources and staff to QI process.
- Develop information system to support and enhance QI activity.
- Balance inclusion with effectiveness in determining QI committee membership.
- Seek input of providers when prioritizing issues for improvement.
- Errors and near errors have a high correlation with opportunities for improvement.

TABLE 35-1. Screens and Monitors for Pediatric Home Care

Clinical Parameter	Subset Screened
Screens	
Admissions to hospital	All
Transfer of care to another home care entity	All
Transfer of care from another entity	Selective
Satisfaction surveys	All; once per year
Central line infections	All
Central line loss	All
Decubiti	All
Malpractice cases	All
Monitors	
Medication compliance	Tailor to client
Pain management	Tailor to client
Mechanical ventilation	All
Hyperbilirubinemia	All
Acute gastroenteritis and fluid management	All

TABLE 35-2. Sample Data Collection: Medication

Clinical Scenario: Medication		
Structure		
Were orders received prior to initiation of therapy?	Y	N
Were orders comprehensive?		
Time of service	Y	N
Type of service	Y	N
Duration of service	Y	N
Were the desired outcomes of the medication clearly stated?	Y	N
Process		
Were the medications delivered on time to the family?	Y	N
Were instructions given to family and child?		
Verbal	Y	N
Written	Y	N
Were medications given by the family?	Y	N
At the proper time?	Y	N
Outcome		
Adverse reactions	Y	N

TABLE 35-3. Sample Data Collection: Hyperbilirubinemia

Clinical Scenario: Hyperbilirubinemia

Structure

Was diagnosis confirmed?	Y	N
Were intensity and wavelength of lights measured and calibrated?	Y	N
Were orders present before service was initiated?	Y	N
Was bilirubin level determined within 24 hours of initiation of therapy?	Y	N
Was child properly screened for sepsis?	Y	N

Process

Was family instructed in proper use, placement, and duration of therapy?	Y	N
Were follow-up bilirubin levels ordered?	Y	N
Was fluid status monitored?	Y	N

Outcome

Time to safe level of jaundice:		
Was subsequent hospitalization required?	Y	N

- Early successes in QI build support for the process. Address solvable problems first.
- Adapt adult models, develop pediatric data.

Bibliography

Forbes DA, Neufeld A. Strategies to address the methodological challenges of client-satisfaction research in home care. *Can J Nurs Res.* 1997;29:69-77

Kane RA, Frytak J, Eustis NN. Agency approaches to common quality problems in home care: a scenario study. *Home Health Care Serv Q.* 1997;16:21-40

Medicare and Medicaid programs: conditions of participation for home health agencies: proposed rule, 62 *Federal Register* 11005-11035 (1997)

Shaughnessy PW, Crisler KS, Schlenker RE, Arnold AG. Outcomes across the care continuum. Home health care. *Med Care.* 1997;35(11 suppl):NS115-123

Chapter 36

Wound Care, Catheter Care, and Infection Control in Home Care

Margaret C. Fisher, MD

Introduction

Infection control is important in every home care patient encounter. Understanding the routes of transmission of infectious agents is the first step in planning for infection control. By far the most frequent route of transmission involves the hands. Microbes are passed from person to person directly via the hands or indirectly on equipment and other objects. Organisms survive in the environment for variable periods of time. If a microbe is present on a doorknob, phone handle, or pencil, it can be transferred to a caregiver's hand and from there to a child's hands. Once on the child's hands, it rapidly gets to the nose and/ or mouth.

Some agents are transmitted via the air (eg, varicella-zoster virus, influenza, and tuberculosis). These agents stay suspended in small droplets and are truly airborne. Other agents are present in large droplets, which do not stay suspended. Large droplets are effective in transmitting agents during close face-to-face contact. Pathogens can be transmitted by contaminated water, food, or medications.

Hand Washing

Because hands are most important in the transmission of infectious agents, it follows that hand washing is the most important and effective way to decrease the spread of infection from person to person. Optimal hand washing requires running water with the hands rubbed together in the water. The type of soap used to clean the hands usually is not important; the goal is to wash off the agents, not to kill them. In some situations, such as performing surgery or rendering care to neonates, it is appropriate to wash hands with antibacterial soaps. Hand sanitizing agents are useful only as a supplement to routine hand washing, and not as a substitute. Organic debris should be removed with running water and soap by lathering for 10 seconds and then rinsing with running water, prior to the use of sanitizing agents. Antiseptic agents can be used in situations in which no clean water is available (eg, during patient transport). Skin emollients and lotions may be useful because they reduce dry, cracking skin that may harbor organisms. Liquid soap and skin lotions may become contaminated with bacteria, so containers of lotion and soap should not be refilled without careful cleaning and sterilization. Because artificial fingernails and hand jewelry may harbor a variety of infectious agents and have been implicated in several outbreaks, they should not be worn by home care providers.

Standard Precautions

Standard precautions have been recommended for patient encounters in the hospital. These precautions also are appropriate for care in the home or outpatient setting. The rationale for using standard precautions is that one cannot determine which child and which secretions are contagious; thus, all patient secretions are treated as if contagious. Gloves are used for contact with blood, body fluids, mucous membranes, non-intact skin, and items or surfaces contaminated with body fluids. Gloves need not be used for routine care of well children in the home, including wiping a nose and changing diapers. Gloves should be worn when performing venipuncture, during other vascular access procedures, and when changing dressings. Hands should be washed before donning gloves and after glove removal. Masks and protective eyewear or face shields should be used during procedures that are likely to generate droplets of blood or body fluids. Gowns or aprons are worn to protect clothing; gowns are appropriate whenever it is anticipated that there might be splashing of blood or body fluids. For example, a gown should be worn if irrigation is being performed. Needles and sharp instruments must be handled with great care. Needles should not be recapped, bent, broken, removed by hand from syringes, or manipulated by hand. Sharp instruments, including needles, should be placed in puncture-resistant containers for disposal. These disposal containers should be in easy reach of the care provider but out of reach of the child. Resuscitation equipment should be available so that mouth-to-mouth resuscitation is avoided.

All home care providers should receive training on infection control and blood-borne pathogens at the time of orientation and at least yearly. Such educational efforts increase compliance with hand washing. Home care providers should educate their patients about infection control.

Care of Equipment

Equipment must be cleaned properly before and after use. Stethoscopes should be wiped off between uses. Blood pressure cuffs should be placed on intact skin. Whenever feasible, disposable equipment should be used. Plastic shields are available for use with oral thermometers. If an electronic thermometer is used, it is important to remember to clean the box between patients. The box is easily contaminated with patients' secretions. If not wiped off, organisms can be transmitted to the next patient on the thermometer box.

Care of Intravenous Catheters

Many children require catheters for their care. These catheters increase the risk for infectious complications; care of the catheters must be meticulous. Vascular catheters provide direct access to the bloodstream. Organisms can enter the catheters via the hub, in the fluids being infused, or along the catheter as it enters the skin. Central catheters are designed to remain in the patient for prolonged periods of time. Usually a subcutaneous cuff anchors the catheter; as connective tissue invades the cuff, the catheter becomes secure and no longer moves in and out of the skin site. Peripheral catheters are not designed for prolonged use. In general, peripheral catheter sites should be changed every 3 days. Although there are some studies showing that longer times are safe, the longer a catheter is in place, the more likely it will become infected. Dressings usually are placed over the entry site of catheters. Transparent dressings are not necessary. Dressings should be changed whenever the dressing is wet, loosened, dirty, or when inspection of the entry site is necessary. Care should be taken to minimize the movement of the catheter during the dressing change. Topical agents, such as Betadine ointment, should not be applied to the entry site. The catheter should be manipulated as little as possible. When entering the system to

obtain blood samples or begin an infusion, an aseptic technique should
be used. The hub should be disinfected with tincture of iodine or povidone-
iodine. If povidone-iodine is used, it must be in contact for at least
30 seconds to allow for the release of the active agent. Fluid removed
to clear the line should be discarded, not reinfused. Policies for handling
catheters should be written and enforced. Part of the home care should
include educating the family about appropriate catheter care. There is no
consensus about bathing or showering when a central catheter is in place.
While some physicians instruct patients to keep the entrance site dry at all
times, others allow showers and even swimming. It is important that the
home care providers follow the instructions of the physician who is caring
for the child.

Care of Foley Catheters

Foley catheters are used to drain the bladder. In general, clean intermittent
catheterization is preferred to an indwelling catheter as there is a much
lower rate of bacteriuria. Indwelling catheters should be attached to a closed
drainage system. The drainage bag should be below the level of the bladder
to prevent reflux of urine into the catheter and back into the bladder.
Perineal care should be limited to maintaining hygiene. Studies comparing
frequent cleansing with no cleansing of the perineum showed an increased
infection rate in those who underwent cleansing. The foley catheter should
not be moved in and out of the bladder as this increases the risk for entry
of the perineal flora into the bladder. Symptoms of dysuria, fever, change in
the odor of the urine, or increase in urinary sediment should raise the possibility of a urinary tract infection. Urine should be collected using sterile
technique from the bladder, not from the drainage bag; urinalysis and culture
should be obtained. Bacteriuria is common and does not necessarily require
antibiotic therapy; symptomatic infection usually will respond to antibiotics.
Cultures must be obtained as the type of pathogen and susceptibilities are not
predictable. If the infection fails to clear, the catheter should be removed.

   Patients who are undergoing clean intermittent catheterization should
be educated in the clean technique. In this case, sterile catheters are not
used but cleaning of equipment with soap and water is required. Catheters
should be allowed to dry between uses. When urine is being obtained for

culture, sterile technique and a sterile catheter should be used. The perineum is cleansed with soap and a disinfectant; the catheter is introduced into the bladder. The first few milliliters of urine should be discarded as this represents urethral contamination.

Orogastric, Nasogastric, Jejunal, and Gastrostomy Tubes

Orogastric tubes may be used for feeding or for administering medications. The tube should be inserted with as little trauma as possible. In the older child, it is helpful to have the child swallow as the tube is passed. Correct placement is established by injecting air and listening to ensure that the end of the tube is in the stomach. This is done prior to infusion of fluids or medications. Orogastric tubes can be left in place but usually are withdrawn after use. Nasogastric tubes often are kept in place for longer periods of time. There are no studies about the optimal duration of catheterization; it is not clear whether it is safer to replace the catheter weekly or leave it in place for longer time periods. The tube often will occlude the eustachian tube and the ostia of the sinuses, thus increasing the risk for otitis and sinusitis. Jejunal tubes usually are left in place for longer periods of time. Any indwelling tube causes irritation to the local mucosa; the risk for perforation of the gastrointestinal tract is very low but must be remembered. Manipulation of the tube increases the trauma to the mucosa. Gastrostomy tubes often are used for long-term feeding; the stoma is on the abdominal wall. Complications include displacement of the tube and local inflammation or infection of the stoma site. Jejunostomy tubes sometimes are threaded through gastrostomies and placed percutaneously directly into the small bowel. The abdominal stoma often is preferable to an indwelling oral or nasal tube.

Care of Peritoneal Dialysis Catheters

Peritoneal dialysis catheters are tunneled from the peritoneum to the skin exit site. These catheters usually are dressed. Again there is not consensus as to whether the entrance site should be kept dry or whether bathing is permitted. Although topical agents usually are applied to the exit site, there are no controlled studies to suggest benefit. Signs of exit site inflammation often precede the development of peritonitis. Superficial exit site infection often responds to oral or systemic antibiotic therapy, while infection along the tunnel rarely improves without catheter removal. Signs of infection include erythema, heat, pain, and discharge. Signs of peritonitis include fever, abdominal pain, and cloudy dialysate. Methods to prevent infection in patients with peritoneal dialysis catheters include aseptic technique when changing bags of dialysate, careful care of the catheter exit site so that manipulation and maceration of the area are avoided, and placement of the catheter to ensure optimal drainage.

Wound Care

Wound care requires meticulous attention to aseptic technique. Most wounds are dressed to allow secondary healing from the base to the surface. The wounds frequently are packed open. Packing contains a variety of topical antimicrobials or disinfectants. Although povidone-iodine often is used for packing or irrigation, there is a risk of iodine intoxication and hyperthyroidism or hypothyroidism as a result of povidone-iodine irrigations. Thus, these should be avoided. It is important to remember that irrigation fluids may be absorbed across the wound surface. Dressing changes often are done daily or more depending on the type of wound and dressing. Hands should be washed and gloves should be donned prior to dressing change. The materials needed for the dressing change should be assembled and readied before gloves are donned. Skin and tissue should be handled with care and manipulation of the tissue should be minimized during dressing change. If debridement is undertaken, there is a risk for transient bacteremia during the procedure. Used dressings should be placed in impervious bags and disposed of carefully. Local, state, and federal standards for disposal of medical waste should be followed.

Ostomies and Stoma Care

Ostomies are surgically created openings of organs onto the skin surface. Examples include tracheostomies, vesicostomies, nephrostomies, gastrostomies, ileostomies, and colostomies. Stoma care varies depending on the age of the ostomy and the site. Tracheostomy tubes are secured with fabric tapes that go around the neck. Care must be taken to prevent damage to the skin of the neck with subsequent breakdown or infection. Suctioning of the trachea and/or lungs is performed as directed by the physician. Family members must be instructed in proper technique. Clean, rather than sterile, technique is used often in children in the home setting. Suction catheters are cleaned with soap and water between uses; the catheters should dry between uses. If the catheter is stored wet or in tap water, there will be colonization with pseudomonads and other water-loving organisms.

Ostomies drain body fluids that usually are not exposed to the skin. The skin around an ostomy site often becomes inflamed or macerated because of constant contact with body fluids. Drainage bags are used for colostomies, jejunostomies, and ileostomies. Vesicostomies are drained into a bag or diapers. There are a variety of appliances used to hold the bags in place. Topical agents are used to minimize skin exposure to irritating fluids. Stoma therapists are specially trained to deal with gut and urinary stomas. These caregivers are helpful in maintaining skin and preventing infection and inflammation.

Preventing Pressure Sores and Ulcers

Prevention of pressure sores and ulcers is essential and much preferred to treatment of sores and ulcers. Constant attention to areas of increased pressure is needed. The patient must be turned or moved frequently. As little as 60 mm Hg of pressure for 1 hour leads to tissue damage in animal models. Ongoing pressure will produce skin necrosis in time. Skin irritants such as stool or caustic fluids should be avoided because they can hasten the development of skin breakdown. Patient positioning and frequent repositioning are needed to minimize pressure.

Treatment of established sores is directed at prevention of extension of the injury and minimization of colonization and infection at the skin break. All skin is colonized by bacteria. Abnormal skin is colonized rapidly by a variety of pathogens including *Staphylococcus aureus* and groups A and B *streptococci*. If the area is exposed to tap water or bathwater, pseudomonads often colonize the macerated skin. As the sore progresses to ulceration and necrosis, the conditions become ideal for anaerobes. Thus, ulcers have mixed flora with gram-positive skin flora and pathogens, gram-negative enterics and pseudomonads, and gram-positive and gram-negative anaerobes. Transient bacteremia often follows debridement or manipulation of the ulcers and sores.

Antimicrobial Agent Resistance

Judicious use of antimicrobial agents is an important part of infection control and prevention of antimicrobial resistance. This is as important in home care as it is in the hospital. The American Academy of Pediatrics and the Centers for Disease Control and Prevention have published a compendium of articles dealing with the judicious use of antimicrobial agents.

Preventing Transmission of Infections Between Patient and Provider

Home care providers can transmit infections to their patients. Employee health services are essential to ensure the health of the home care staff. Staff with some contagious illnesses should be relieved of duties, especially if the patient is immunocompromised. The common cold may pose a significant risk to children with chronic lung disease; it may trigger bronchospasm in those with reactive airway disease. It is not practical to furlough staff with the common cold. It is not clear whether the use of masks is beneficial in preventing transmission of viruses from staff to patient. Hand washing is essential as nasal secretions frequently contaminate hands. Staff with some infectious diseases should not be caring for patients. Table 36-1 lists these conditions and suggestions for the type and duration of precautions.

Home care providers should be tested for tuberculosis at the time of employment. The frequency of subsequent testing will depend on the incidence of tuberculosis in the homes visited and state laws. There should be written policies about staff furlough.

Vaccination of home care staff is highly recommended; it should be a condition of employment (Table 36-2). All staff should be immune to hepatitis B, rubella, measles, and varicella. Yearly influenza vaccine should be provided free of charge; staff should be strongly encouraged to get vac-

TABLE 36-1. Work Restriction Policies for Employees

Infection	Restriction	Length of Restriction
Conjunctivitis	Restrict from direct patient care.	Until discharge resolved.
Gastroenteritis	Restrict from direct patient care and food preparation.	Until symptoms resolve or person is deemed noncontagious.
Hepatitis A	Restrict from direct patient care.	Until 1 week after onset of jaundice.
Hepatitis B	None unless performing procedures with a high risk of transmission of blood from provider to patient.	
Herpes simplex, orofacial	Cover lesions and avoid contact with lesions. Wash hands.	Until lesions dry.
Human immuno-deficiency virus	None unless performing procedures considered to be at risk for transmission of blood from provider to patient.	
Measles	Exclude from any patient contact.	Until 7 days after onset of rash.
Mumps	Exclude from any patient contact.	Until 9 days after onset of parotitis.
Pediculosis	Restrict from direct patient contact.	Until treated.
Pertussis	Exclude from any patient contact.	Until treated for 5 days.
Rubella	Exclude from any patient contact.	Until 5 days after onset of rash.
Scabies	Restrict from direct patient care.	Until treated.
Staphylococcal skin infection	Restrict from direct patient care.	Until treated for 24 hours.
Streptococcal infection, group A	Restrict from direct patient care.	Until treated for 24 hours.
Tuberculosis, active	Exclude from any patient contact.	Until proven noninfectious.
Varicella	Exclude from any patient contact.	Until lesions crusted.
Zoster	If covered, restrict from care of immunocompromised patients. If cannot be covered, restrict from patient care.	Until lesions crusted.

cinated. If a staff member refuses vaccination, this should be documented in employment records. Because no vaccination is currently available to protect against cytomegalovirus infection (CMV), home care agencies should have policies concerning pregnant employees who have contact with children infected with CMV.

Ideally there should be surveillance for infection in the home care setting. It is necessary to identify clusters of infections and investigate such outbreaks.

TABLE 36-2. Recommended Vaccines for Health Care Providers

Vaccine	Schedule	Comments	Contraindications
Hepatitis B	Three-dose series (initial, 1 month, 6 months)	All heath care providers Post-immunization titers recommended Boosters not needed	Anaphylaxis to prior dose or to baker's yeast
Measles, Mumps, and Rubella	Two doses at least 1 month apart	Not needed if proven immune	Pregnancy Immunocompromised Recent immune globulin
Varicella	Two doses at least 1 month apart	Not needed if history of varicella	Pregnancy Immunocompromised Recent immune globulin
Influenza	Yearly dose in October or November		History of anaphylaxis with egg products
Tetanus and diphtheria (Td)	Every 10 years	Recommended for all adults	History of anaphylaxis with previous dose
Inactivated polio vaccine	Three doses (initial, 1-2 months, booster 6-12 months later)	Not needed if immunized previously	Anaphylaxis after previous dose

Because various physicians are involved, surveillance must be conducted by the home care agency. Whenever possible, an infection control practitioner or a physician with expertise in infection control should be involved in surveillance for infection and in review and formulation of policies and procedures.

Control of Blood-Borne Infections

Home care providers are at risk for occupationally acquired illnesses. The best methods to avoid acquisition are hand washing, use of standard precautions, and vaccination. Identification and treatment of contagious patients also will decrease the risk to their caregivers. Home care providers should receive education and training on blood-borne infections. Precautions to prevent transmission of blood-borne agents include engineering controls, such as use of devices without needles or shielded needles; training on proper handling and disposal of needles and sharp instruments; common sense; and proper patient restraint when attempting to obtain blood samples. Policies should be in place to address procedures should a needle-stick injury occur. Immediate first aid is administered and the area is washed and rinsed. The injury should be reported to the health care agency and appropriate screening tests should be obtained. Screening for hepatitis B and C as well as for human immunodeficiency virus (HIV) should be obtained at baseline and after 1 and 6 months. Postexposure prophylaxis against hepatitis B should be considered if the employee is nonimmune and the patient is hepatitis B surface antigen (HBsAg) positive (Table 36-3). Postexposure prophylaxis for HIV should be considered for high-risk injuries with infected blood. Ideally, prophylaxis should be with multiple drugs and started within hours of injury;

TABLE 36-3. Postexposure Prophylaxis for Hepatitis B Virus

If exposed person is unvaccinated

Source hepatitis B surface antigen (HBsAg) positive: hepatitis B immunoglobulin (HBIG) intramuscularly and begin hepatitis B virus (HBV) vaccine series

Source HBsAg negative: begin HBV vaccine series

Source not tested or unknown: begin HBV vaccine series

If exposed person was vaccinated and responded

Source HBsAg positive: test exposed person for anti-hepatitis B surface antibodies (HBs) – if positive, no treatment; if negative, HBV booster dose

Source HBsAg negative: no treatment

Source not tested or unknown: no treatment

If exposed person was vaccinated and did not respond

Source HBsAg positive: HBIG immediately and in 1 month and a booster dose of HBV

Source HBsAg negative: no treatment

Source not tested or unknown: if high-risk source, consider HBIG as for positive source

If exposed person was vaccinated and not tested for a response

Source HBsAg positive: test exposed person for anti-HBs; if positive, no treatment; if negative, one dose of HBIG and a booster dose of HBV

Source HBsAg negative: no treatment

Source not tested or unknown: test exposed person for anti-HBs; if positive, no treatment; if negative, a booster dose of HBV recommendations for postexposure therapy are updated on a regular basis. The most current recommendations are given in Table 36-4.

TABLE 36-4. Postexposure Prophylaxis for Human Immunodeficiency Virus

---

Basic regimen: recommended when the degree of exposure is such that postexposure prophylaxis is appropriate but no increased risk for human immunodeficiency virus (HIV) transmission has been observed; examples include mucous membrane exposure or solid needle percutaneous exposure.

Four weeks (28 days) of both zidovudine and lamivudine.

Expanded regimen: recommended when the degree of exposure represents an increased HIV transmission risk; examples include percutaneous injury with large-bore hollow needle, deep puncture, or less severe injury but with blood from a patient known to have high titers of HIV.

Basic regimen plus either indinavir or nelfinavir.

Summary

To control infections in home care, be sure to heed the following recommendations:

- Hand washing is the most effective way to decrease the spread of infection from person to person.
- Standard precautions used in the hospital are appropriate for use in home care. All patient secretions should be treated as contagious and gloves should be used for contact with blood, body fluids, mucous membranes, non-intact skin, and items or surfaces contaminated by body fluids.
- Home care providers can transmit infections to their patients. Providers who have contagious illnesses should be relieved of their duties.
- Home care providers also can acquire illnesses from their patients. The best methods to avoid this are hand washing, using standard precautions, and vaccination.

Bibliography

Alvarado CJ, Farr BM, McCormick RD. *The Science of Hand Hygiene: Continuing Education Program for Healthcare Professionals.* University of Wisconsin Medical School: Sci-Health Communications. Available at: http://healthcare.gojo.com/programs.htm. Accessed August 30, 2001

American Academy of Pediatrics, Committee on Infectious Diseases and Committee on Practice and Ambulatory Medicine. Infection control in physicians' offices. *Pediatrics.* 2000;105:1361-1369

Avila-Aguero ML, Umana MA, Jimenez AL, Faingezicht I, Paris MM. Handwashing practices in a tertiary-care, pediatric hospital and the effect on an educational program. *Clin Perform Qual Health Care.* 1998;6:70-72

Bergstrom N, Allman RM, Alvarez OM, et al. *Treatment of Pressure Ulcers. Clinical Practice Guideline No. 15.* Rockville, MD: Agency for Health Care Policy and Research; December 1994. AHCPR publication 95-0652. Available at: http://www.ahrq.gov/clinic/cpgonline.htm. Accessed August 30, 2001

Bolyard EA, Tablan OC, Williams WW, Pearson ML, Shapiro CN, Deitchmann SD. Guideline for infection control in healthcare personnel, 1998. Hospital Infection Control Practices Advisory Committee. *Infect Control Hosp Epidemiol.* 1998;19:407-463

Bradley M, Pupiales M. Essential elements of ostomy care. *Am J Nurs.* 1997;97:38-46

Burke JP, Garibaldi RA, Britt MR, Jacobson JA, Conti M, Alling DW. Prevention of catheter-associated urinary tract infections. Efficacy of daily meatal care regimens. *Am J Med.* 1981; 70:655-658

Caplan ES, Hoyt NJ. Nosocomial sinusitis. *JAMA.* 1982;247:639-641

Centers for Disease Control and Prevention. Immunization of health-care workers: recommendations of the Advisory Committee on Immunization Practices (ACIP) and the Hospital Infection Control Practices Advisory Committee (HICPAC). *MMWR Morb Mortal Wkly Rep.* 1997;46:1-42

Centers for Disease Control and Prevention. Public health service guidelines for management of health-care worker exposures to HIV and recommendations for postexposure prophylaxis. *MMWR Morb Mortal Wkly Rep.* 1998;47:1-33

Diekema DJ, Doebbeling BN. Employee health and infection control. *Infect Control Hosp Epidemiol.* 1995;16:292-301

Do AN, Ray BJ, Banerjee SN, et al. Bloodstream infection associated with needleless device use and the importance of infection-control practices in the home health care setting. *J Infect Dis.* 1999;179:442-448

Doughty D. Role of the enterostomal therapy nurse in ostomy patient rehabilitation. *Cancer.* 1992;70:1390-1392

Dowell SF, Marcy SM, Phillips WR, Gerber MA, Schwartz B. Otitis media — principles of judicious use of antimicrobial agents. *Pediatrics*. 1998;101(suppl):165-171

Dowell SF, Marcy SM, Phillips WR, Gerber MA, Schwartz B. Principles of judicious use of antimicrobial agents for pediatric upper respiratory tract infections. *Pediatrics*. 1998;101(suppl):163-165

Dubbert PM, Dolce J, Richter W, Miller M, Chapman SW. Increasing ICU staff handwashing: effects of education and group feedback. *Infect Control Hosp Epidemiol*. 1990;11:191-193

Friedman C, Barnette M, Buck AS, et al. Requirements for infrastructure and essential activities of infection control and epidemiology in out-of-hospital settings: a consensus panel report. Association for Professionals in Infection Control and Epidemiology and Society for Healthcare Epidemiology of America. *Infect Control Hosp Epidemiol*. 1999;20:695-705

Garland JS, Dunne WM Jr, Havens P, et al. Peripheral intravenous catheter complications in critically ill children: a prospective study. *Pediatrics*. 1992;89:1145-1150

Garner JS, Hospital Infection Control Practices Advisory Committee. Guideline for isolation precautions in hospitals. *Infect Control Hosp Epidemiol*. 1996;17:53-80

Garvin G. Caring for children with ostomies. *Nurs Clin North Am*. 1994;29:645-654

George DL, Falk PS, Umberto Meduri G, et al. Nosocomial sinusitis in patients in the medical intensive care unit: a prospective epidemiological study. *Clin Infect Dis*. 1998;27:463-470

Glezen WP, Greenberg SB, Atmar RL, Piedra PA, Couch RB. Impact of respiratory virus infections on persons with chronic underlying conditions. *JAMA*. 2000;283:499-505

Herwaldt LA, Smith SD, Carter CD. Infection control in the outpatient setting. *Infect Control Hosp Epidemiol*. 1998;19:41-74

Hoffmann KK, Weber DJ, Samsa GP, Rutala WA. Transparent polyurethane film as an intravenous catheter dressing. A meta-analysis of the infection risks. *JAMA*. 1992;267:2072-2076

Hospital Infection Control Practices Advisory Committee. Recommendations for preventing the spread of vancomycin resistance. *Infect Control Hosp Epidemiol*. 1995;16:105-113

Keene JH. Regulated medical waste. In: Abrutyn E, ed. *Saunders Infection Control Reference Service*. Philadelphia, PA: WB Saunders Co; 1998:727-750

Krilov LR, Barone SR, Mandel FS, Cusack TM, Gaber DJ, Rubino JR. Impact of an infection control program in a specialized preschool. *Am J Infect Control*. 1996;24:167-173

Larson E. Skin hygiene and infection prevention: more of the same or different approaches? *Clin Infect Dis*. 1999;29:1287-1294

Larson EL. APIC guideline for handwashing and hand antisepsis in health care settings. *Am J Infect Control*. 1995;23:251-269

Lobato MN, Hannan J, Simonds RJ, Riske B, Evatt BL. Attitudes, practices, and infection risks of hemophilia treatment center nurses who teach infection control for the home. *Infect Control Hosp Epidemiol*. 1996;17:726-731

Mangram AJ, Horan TC, Pearson ML, Silver LC, Jarvis WR, Hospital Infection Control Practices Advisory Committee. Guideline for prevention of surgical site infection, 1999. *Infect Control Hosp Epidemiol.* 1999;20:250-280

Marinella MA, Pierson C, Chenoweth C. The stethoscope. A potential source of nosocomial infection? *Arch Intern Med.* 1997;157:786-790

Mermel LA. Prevention of intravascular catheter-related infections. *Ann Intern Med.* 2000;132: 391-402

Moolenaar RL, Crutcher JM, San Joaquin VH, et al. A prolonged outbreak of *Pseudomonas aeruginosa* in a neonatal intensive care unit: did staff fingernails play a role in disease transmission? *Infect Control Hosp Epidemiol.* 2000;21:80-85

O'Brien KL, Dowell SF, Schwartz B, Marcy SM, Phillips WR, Gerber MA. Acute sinusitis — principles of judicious use of antimicrobial agents. *Pediatrics.* 1998;101(suppl):174-177

O'Brien KL, Dowell SF, Schwartz B, Marcy SM, Phillips WR, Gerber MA. Cough illness/ bronchitis — principles of judicious use of antimicrobial agents. *Pediatrics.* 1998;101(suppl):178-181

Panel for the Prediction and Prevention of Pressure Ulcers in Adults. *Pressure Ulcers in Adults: Prediction and Prevention. Clinical Practice Guideline No 3.* Rockville, MD: Agency for Health Care Policy and Research; May 1992. AHCPR publication 92-0047. Available at: http://www.ahrq.gov/ clinic/cpgonline.htm. Accessed August 30, 2001

Pearson ML, Hospital Infection Control Practices Advisory Committee. Guideline for prevention of intravascular device-related infections. *Infect Control Hosp Epidemiol.* 1996;17:438-473

Raad II, Bodey GP. Infectious complications of indwelling vascular catheters. *Clin Infect Dis.* 1992;15:197-208

Reinhardt PA, Gordon JG, Alvarado CJ. Medical waste management. In: Mayhall CG, ed. *Hospital Epidemiology and Infection Control.* Baltimore, MD: Williams & Wilkins; 1996:1099-1108

Rosenstein N, Phillips WR, Gerber MA, Marcy SM, Schwartz B, Dowell SF. The common cold — principles of judicious use of antimicrobial agents. *Pediatrics.* 1998;101(suppl):181-184

Rutala WA. Disinfection and sterilization of patient-care items. *Infect Control Hosp Epidemiol.* 1996;17:377-384

Saint S, Lipsky BA. Preventing catheter-related bacteriuria: should we? Can we? How? *Arch Intern Med.* 1999;159:800-808

Schwartz B, Marcy SM, Phillips WR, Gerber MA, Dowell SF. Pharyngitis — principles of judicious use of antimicrobial agents. *Pediatrics.* 1998;101(suppl):171-174

Sepkowitz KA. Occupationally acquired infections in health care workers. Part I. *Ann Intern Med.* 1996;125:826-834

Sepkowitz KA. Occupationally acquired infections in health care workers. Part II. *Ann Intern Med.* 1996;125:917-928

Shlaes DM, Gerding DN, John JF Jr, et al. Society for Healthcare Epidemiology of America and Infectious Diseases Society of America Joint Committee on the Prevention of Antimicrobial Resistance: guidelines for the prevention of antimicrobial resistance in hospitals. *Infect Control Hosp Epidemiol.* 1997;18:275-291

Smith DM. Pressure ulcers in the nursing home. *Ann Intern Med.* 1995;123:433-442

Warady BA. Peritoneal dialysis catheter related infections in children. *Pediatr Infect Dis J.* 1998;17:1165-1166

Warren JW. Catheter-associated bacteriuria in long-term care facilities. *Infect Control Hosp Epidemiol.* 1994;15:557-562

Chapter 37

Out-of-Home Child Care and Medical Day Treatment Programs

Elizabeth Ruppert, MD; Nancy Host, MBA

Introduction

▶ The Need for Day Treatment Programs

Out-of-home medical day treatment is home care that is provided at the parents' request at a site other than the child's home. Some parents request this out-of-home day treatment for long periods of time, while others request it for weekends or regularly scheduled respite days. Parents want flexibility in scheduling and arrival and departure times and a quality staff.

Many of the following factors motivate parents to search for out-of-home medical day treatment:

- Parents tire from constant "traffic" of nurses, respiratory therapists, and durable medical equipment companies in their home.
- Parents and siblings want and need regularly scheduled time alone.
- Parents must return to work or school to improve the economic status of their family.
- Parents want their child to have some time away from home to participate in socialization experiences with children with and without disabilities.
- Parents want their child in an early childhood education and child care environment.
- Center-based care is a cost-effective alternative to in-home skilled nursing care and institutional care.

There are several exemplary programs nationwide that give parents access to a flexible and broad range of services. Some of these programs effectively integrate children in home care into the fabric of their communities.

▶ Models

In the late 1980s, the Prescribed Pediatric Extended Care Centers (PPEC) were established in Florida. This innovative day health care model is physician prescribed and qualifies for insurance reimbursement. The PPEC offers skilled nursing care in a group setting, respite, and parent education. This successful model strongly influenced the second-generation model established in 1993 by the Medical College of Ohio in Toledo. In this model, the Prescribed Pediatric Center (PPC) provides skilled nursing services, allied health services as prescribed, and developmentally appropriate education in a group setting for children from birth to 12 years. In addition, the PPC is located in an inclusive early childhood facility that provides supported opportunities for socialization with peers with and without disabilities and is the home base for early intervention activities in that county.

In the late 1990s, Respite House, Inc., became a reality in Illinois. A group of committed parents and professionals changed the way respite care was defined in the Illinois state statute by recognizing respite care as a medical necessity for children who are medically fragile. The term *medically fragile* was defined as a person who requires medical technology to sustain life and prevent death or further injury. Respite House, Inc., is a medical respite care facility for children up to 18 years old, based in a home-like environment. There is a maximum of 10 children at one time. Transitional training (ie, hospital-to-home training) is provided for families whose children are being discharged from the hospital and for foster families interested in fostering a child who is medically fragile. Child life services and education also are provided. Each of these programs provides year-round services with flexible scheduling for parents' convenience.

Program Design and Services

▶ Eligibility and Admissions

Referrals to Respite House, Inc., and other similar programs can be made by the family, school personnel, and the child's medical home. Parents should be made aware of this resource early in the course of the child's complex illness. If the child is dependent on a ventilator, has a tracheostomy, or has other complex health needs, the medical home or managing pediatric subspecialist should originate the referral. Referral during hospitalization facilitates collaborative planning and is appreciated by families.

▶ Assessment

A written individual health plan (IHP) for the child and family should be done prior to contracting for services. In some situations, the assessment is done by a hospital-based team and is shared and discussed with the facility staff. Pediatricians who personally communicate with the program staff help their patients get the best and most appropriate staff support. The following are key elements of the IHP:

- Brief health history and immunizations
- Special health care needs
- Medications
- Diet/nutrition
- Transportation
- Equipment
- Possible problems and interventions

The IHP should be written by the managing pediatric staff, be signed by one physician, and include a phone number, fax number, and mailing address. This initial assessment should indicate how often and by whom the identified services will be provided. If the facility generally does not provide the services, contracting or arranging with the appropriate professional should be detailed.

▶ Medical Role

Physicians have a major role in patient care, but a limited role in home care. Some pediatricians do remain involved in home care to monitor the quality of home care provided, coordinate the child's care and referrals that are made, ensure that the family and the medical home continue to work together, advocate for the child and family as problems arise, and confirm that the reordering of home care services continues to meet the needs of child and family.

▶ Nursing Care

Nursing care for children in a medical day treatment program is ordered
by each child's pediatrician or primary care physician. The following is general care for all children in the program:

- Temperature, pulse, respirations daily
- Pulse oximetry daily, if appropriate
- Weight weekly
- Cardiopulmonary assessment daily
- Gastrointestinal assessment daily
- Neurological assessment daily
- General assessment (skin color, temperature, turgor)
- Mouth care twice daily and as needed
- Skin care as needed
- Activities as appropriate

Universal precautions are practiced because of the vulnerable nature of
many of the children.

All food, medications, supplies, and equipment specific to each child are
provided by the child's family. Backup supplies are provided by the center,
as well as emergency equipment (eg, oxygen and suction). A variety of
general activity equipment is available, including standers, corner chairs,
slant pillows, sidelyers, and a water bed.

▶ Special Therapies

Important participants in a child's care team may include occupational
therapists, speech/language therapists, and physical therapists. Ideally, each
therapist will have excellent professional relationships with each home care
nurse. Such relationships will result in the therapist advising the nurse on
activities to reinforce, the nurse discussing with the therapist concerns
and questions about the patient, and a transdisciplinary relationship that
strengthens the quality and unique implementation of each child's care plan.

▶ Developmental Interventions

Safety and medical care are the primary concerns in caring for the child
with special health care needs. However, accepting the role of caregiver
includes attending to the developmental needs of the child and integrating
developmental services with the health care of the child. Staffing, consul-

tation with local early intervention and special education programs, and an overall philosophy of developmentally appropriate care are the basis for high-quality care.

▶ Family Support and Education

Public Law 105-17, the Individuals with Disabilities Education Act (IDEA) Amendments of 1997, established the early intervention program for infants and toddlers with disabilities, including free and appropriate public education for children with disabilities from age 3 to 21. Children who are medically fragile, and at risk for developmental delay, may be eligible for IDEA services. Early intervention services may include service coordination; transition planning; special instruction for the child; support and training for the child's family; therapies such as occupational, physical, and speech therapy; audiology; and assistive technology. Referrals are made through a state central resource directory or a local early intervention contact. Special education and related services (eg, speech therapy, occupational therapy, and assistive technology) are provided to eligible children from age 3. Referrals are made to the local education agency (ie, the public school) where the child resides. A Web site containing a complete listing of state early intervention and pre-school special education contacts can be found at www.nectas.unc.edu.

Every state and jurisdiction is responsible for providing early intervention or special educational services for eligible children with disabilities. Although IDEA provides statutory and regulatory guidance for these services, states have discretion in establishing some aspects of the services, including eligibility definitions. Service delivery mechanisms vary from state to state. Because many children served in medical day care may be eligible for IDEA services, staff should contact the state lead agency for early intervention and the local education agency (public school) to determine the policies and procedures within the community.

If the child qualifies for special education or early intervention services under the state's definition, all IDEA regulations apply. For example, a child younger than 3 years of age who is medically fragile would have all services described on an individual family service plan (IFSP); children from age 3 would have an individual education plan (IEP). These plans require that appropriate and individualized evaluations, assessments, and goals are established for enhancing the development of the child. Individual family service plans and IEPs are developed in conjunction with a multi-disciplinary team and with the active involvement and consent of the family. The family's concerns, priorities, and resources, as well as the fragility of the child's medical condition, should be taken into account in the writing of these plans.

Children from birth to 3 years of age with an IFSP are also entitled to a service coordinator, who serves as the primary contact for all intervention and care provided to the child and assists the family in obtaining needed services and supports. Although there are several public programs serving children with disabilities, it often is difficult for families to locate or access these programs, services may not be available or convenient, or the child's needs may not be completely met by the program. The service coordinator can help families determine which programs might be available. For children who are medically fragile, frequently it makes sense for the initial service coordinator to be the child's primary care nurse. The nurse then can ensure that developmental interventions are coordinated with nursing and medical care. The nurse serves as a liaison with the family, intervention team, and physician.

> *Children from birth to 3 years of age with an IFSP are also entitled to a service coordinator, who serves as the primary contact for all intervention and care provided to the child and assists the family in obtaining needed services and supports.*

For services to infants and toddlers, eligibility criteria and definitions vary from state to state. Under Part C of IDEA (Programs for Infants and Toddlers with Disabilities), states must provide services to children younger than 3 years of age who are experiencing developmental delays or who have a diagnosed physical or mental condition that has a high probability of resulting in developmental delay. States also may choose to provide early intervention services to children considered at risk of experiencing a substantial developmental delay if early intervention services were not provided.

Children age 3 to 21 who are medically fragile may qualify for special educational and related services. For the purposes of eligibility, a child with a disability is defined as a child with mental retardation, hearing impairment, speech and language impairments, visual impairments, severe emotional disturbances, orthopedic impairments, autism, traumatic brain injury, other health impairments, or specific learning disabilities *and* who, by reason thereof, needs special education and related services. For children ages 3 through

9, the term *child with a disability* may include a child experiencing a developmental delay (in cognitive, physical, adaptive, social, emotional, or communication areas) who needs special education and related services.

▶ Transition Planning

Children who are medically fragile will experience many changes in service setting, providers, routines, and procedures. Some of the most significant changes are those involving a change in location, including the transition from hospital (acute care) to home; transition from home care to a specialty child care center; and ultimately, transition into a natural environment (eg, typical child care, early childhood program, or school). All transitions must be planned, with attention given to the strengths and needs of the child and family, so the process allows the child's medical and developmental care to continue without interruption. The goal of transition planning is to ensure that the process of change is as smooth as possible; stress on the child and the family is kept to a minimum. The child's family, primary health care providers, and the local program or school staff should carefully plan transition from home care into community-based medical day treatment programs.

Identifying a transition team can help to identify appropriate community resources including family support, transportation, respite care, early intervention, and educational resources. A nurse who is familiar with the child should be present during the assessment and initial implementation of therapies to monitor for signs or symptoms of stress or intolerance of developmental interventions. Persons conducting the assessments should be familiar with children who are medically fragile. The rule of thumb for assessments and developmental therapies is to limit the number of people handling the child. Some intervention teams may be skilled in the transdisciplinary approach, where the team provides consultation to one or two direct service providers. Planning, observation, and flexibility should be guiding principles for the intervention team.

Personnel/Staffing

A medical day treatment program is staffed by experienced nurses with a pediatric background. At all times, a Pediatric Advanced Life Support (PALS)-certified registered nurse (RN) with pediatric ventilator experience is on site. Each child is assigned a primary nurse. The nurse-child ratio is determined by the acuity level of each child; average nurse-child ratio per experience is 1:3. An RN is on site while the center is open and licensed practical nurses (LPNs) serve as supplemental staff to maintain the nurse-child ratio. Licensed practical nurses also are used as transport nurses for children who require a medical professional while being transported from home to the day treatment program and back. The three acuity levels of care are listed in Table 37-1.

Program Management

▶ Licensure and Related Policies

Requirements for licensure of a medical day treatment program vary from state to state. State rules and regulations governing the particular owner type of the program (ie, acute care facility or health system, freestanding home health agency, extended care facility, school, etc) also may affect the need for and/or type of licensure required for the program. Classification or certification as a child care program, extension of the educational system, subacute

TABLE 37-1. Three Acuity Levels of Care

Level 1: Medically Complex
Ventilator dependent
Tracheostomy
Need for recurrent and/or frequent suctioning
Oxygen therapy in connection with apnea monitoring
Maintenance of intravenous therapy including indwelling catheters
Nutritional support – continuous nasogastric or gastrostomy tube feeding, central line

Level 2: Intermittent Skilled
Aerosol treatment with postural drainage
Nutritional support – intermittent nasogastric or gastrostomy tube feeding
Dressing changes
Daily injection therapy
Intravenous therapy – intermittent medication therapy
Oral medication therapy
Feeding program therapy
Monitored diet

Level 3: Continuous Skilled Monitoring
Apnea monitor without oxygenation
Seizures

center, or a combination thereof will dictate the need for and/or advantages of further certifications or accreditations, in addition to baseline requirements.

Each licensure type and certification or accreditation is accompanied by its own set of requirements for standards, outcome measures, reporting, record keeping, and periodic survey. The benefits of additional accreditations of the program should be weighed carefully against the cost, as well as the additional staff needed to maintain compliance with standards. Accreditations through organizations such as the Joint Commission on Accreditation of Healthcare Organizations, Community Health Accreditation Program, and other national accrediting bodies may carry significant financial obligations and possible imposition of sanctions, in addition to the outcome-based consumer and provider benefits.

▶ Medical Records/Record Keeping

Maintaining detailed individual medical record charts on a daily basis is critical to mapping the progress and measuring outcomes in accordance with stated, integrated clinical and developmental goals. Each chart should contain the following information:

- Signed physician orders for care
- A complete and thorough physical and developmental assessment updated at regular intervals
- Daily signed charting of the child's activity and performance of nursing tasks as related to the orders
- All collaborative intervention notes or reports that focus on the medical and/or developmental needs of the child
- Subsequent verbal physician orders
- Complete medication profile and subsequent updates
- Demographic, economic, environmental, and psychosocial data

Documentation in the child's chart must address performance of the physician's prescribed orders for medical care and the educational objectives identified by an early intervention specialist, early childhood teachers, and/ or a therapist. Typical pediatric-specific home health or acute care facility charting forms should be modified to include the developmental compo-nents typically found in the documentation used by an early intervention team or mental retardation/developmental disabilities (MR/DD) system.

Pertinent goals established within an IEP or IFSP also should be incorporated into the day treatment documentation. Embedding the developmental goals into the day treatment plan establishes a more complete, thorough picture of a child's total progress. The collaboration of the nursing and early intervention team to draft such documentation also fosters a closer team approach to delivery of family-focused care and the successful accomplishment of goals.

Each chart is a confidential record that contains sensitive information, including a child's medical condition, social and/or home environment concerns, and custody issues. Great care must be given to securing records to ensure limited, authorized access. Parental or guardian consent for publication of any child's information must be obtained and placed in the chart or other secure place.

▸ Physical and Learning Environment

Medical day treatment centers must provide opportunities for cognitive, language, social, emotional, adaptive, and physical development. Ideally, these learning opportunities include interaction with typically developing children, because children who are medically fragile have conditions that may stabilize or improve over time. Placement in a specialized child care setting with medical and nursing support should be considered transitional, not permanent. Developmental interventions and nursing care prepare the child for more natural, less restrictive settings in the future.

During the time that a child who is medically fragile is unstable, it is unlikely the child will be fully included in child care or other community programs. However, the ultimate goal of the IEP or IFSP should be to provide the child with as natural a learning experience as possible. For an infant, that might mean interaction with a small number of caring, consistent caregivers. For a young child, there might be opportunities for interaction with other children. For older children, there will be typical routines and activities. There may need to be modifications in toys, play equipment, play areas, and learning environments. Consultation with early childhood programs (eg, Head Start, Early Head Start, etc) and local school personnel will help to create a comprehensive program of health and educational services.

▶ Quality Assurance and Accountability

A quality or performance improvement plan that identifies mission, objectives, and performance of the program should be firmly established. Once developed, this plan should drive the collection of clinical and developmental data that support the day treatment role.

Clinical outcomes and developmental milestones should be measurable with the clinical chart documentation structured to capture and follow a child's progress. Standard clinical quality indicators include

- Efficacy of the procedures or treatments
- Appropriateness of the procedures or treatments
- Availability of needed procedures or treatments
- Timeliness with which needed procedures and treatments are provided
- Effectiveness with which procedures and treatments are provided
- Continuity of the services provided
- Safety of the client to whom the services are provided
- Efficiency with which the services are provided
- Respect and caring with which the services are provided

Additionally, measurement standards to benchmark a child's developmental progress against child-specific expected goals must be added. Professional tools such as the Hawaii Early Learning Profile, which measures the developmental progress from birth through 3 years of age, can assist in the periodic consistency with which data are captured.

Financing

▶ Medicaid Waivers

Each state's implementation of federal funding under a Medicaid medically fragile waiver or extended care reimbursement model program will vary. Most waiver programs are administered by the respective state's department of human services (health or similar division). While application needs to be made to the state, information about application for providership, eligibility criteria, and reimbursement and billing procedures should be available through each local county department of human services.

Waiver programs are designed to provide home- and community-based services to patients who have a chronic, unstable medical condition requiring the skills of an RN on a daily basis to detect and evaluate the need for possible treatment modification or for instituting other procedures. These patients otherwise would require long-term care, hospitalization, and potentially out-of-community placement at a residential facility designed to accommodate such cases. A cap rate for expenditures per participant per month or annually usually is established by each state. This cap rate may include all authorized medical/health-related expenses incurred by the child. Reimbursement to providers normally is set at one statewide maximum rate per service type. State waiver programs may cover services to include private duty (hourly) nursing, respite care, home medical equipment and supplies, adaptive/assistive devices, therapy services, and social work/counseling. Patients who have been authorized to receive services under a state waiver program normally require the highest level or combination of services. Each child has an assigned RN or social work case manager who is responsible for the coordination of collective services each child receives and awards hours of nursing services in the day treatment and/or home setting.

▶ Public and Private Health Insurance

Alternative public funding sources, in addition to the Medicaid and Medicaid waiver programs, will vary from state to state. Providers should investigate eligibility for providership under all programs administered through the health and human services state department, as well as the MR/DD and state educational system. A provider of medical day treatment may be successful in obtaining financial support for school-aged children who cannot attend a typical classroom. Contact with the local county board of MR/DD should assist in accessing alternative funding streams under the Medicaid system.

Because of the high cost and long-term nature of many of these cases, the private insurance industry has been a reluctant payer source. A strong case can be made for private insurance case management and authorization of payment for services rendered at a medical day treatment program. The delivery option provides a safe environment, is cost-effective compared to the institutional inpatient setting or seclusion of home care, and has evidence of marked decreased use of emergency rooms and subsequent hospitalization. The collaborative efforts of all providers of care under one roof also increases the continuity of care and case coordination, thereby decreasing the numerous interruptions, invasions of family privacy, or interferences in the family home.

▶ Title V and Children With Special Health Care Needs

Title V programs of the Maternal and Child Health Bureau and programs for children with special health care needs have federal and/or state resources. States have choices as to how these funds are allocated. Some states fund care coordination for children with special health care needs. However, few state Title V programs provide/fund home care services. Grant funding often is available for innovative activities but does not support ongoing reimbursement for home care services.

▶ Contracts With Public Agencies

Financial support on a contracted basis for services rendered in the medical day treatment setting to like clients is available by establishing working relationships with area school systems, county boards for MD/DD, county boards for children's services, and other collaborative agency network support programs that provide services to families and children with special needs. Often, pooled community funding support programs are available and can be found by contacting the local United Way. Because of the stringent fiscal funding cycles of many county agencies, budget submission deadlines and application dates must be adhered to.

▶ Private Philanthropy

The financial viability, growth, and expansion of a medical day treatment program and the services it provides will be related directly to the volume of philanthropic dollars generated to support it on an ongoing basis. Because of the cap rates, lifetime benefit maximums, and the intensive/extensive nature of skilled and social interventions needed for these children and their families, cost for services often exceeds reimbursement, leaving a gap to be filled by charitable dollars. In addition to funding support for direct care, grants for new program development and research, tuition assistance, private endowment, and deferred giving options will provide longevity to the financial integrity of the program and increase the options available to all families regardless of their ability to pay. Funding available through locally based foundations, local branches of national foundations, hospital systems and corporate foundations, and the local United Way are excellent options to pursue.

Partnerships

▶ Role of the Advisory Board

Development of a diverse, well-rounded advisory board or committee serves several key purposes for successful development of a medical day treatment program. An integrated team of medical professionals, educators, parents of children with special needs, third-party payer representatives, and community/county/state representatives of programs that serve or coordinate services for special needs population can be invaluable in establishing a firm strategic base of knowledge and information sharing. The advisory board may serve in various capacities depending on the structure of the program owner, business operation, and established board or committee goals. Goals of the advisory board include but may not be limited to the following:

- Identifying families of children with special needs who may be appropriate for the day treatment program
- Creating a nonthreatening mechanism for the services of the day treatment program to be introduced to those families
- Serving as a means for dissemination of information on legislative-related activities and a forum for ongoing and acquiring support, as needed
- Identifying and communicating with possible funding sources that may support payment for or expansion of medical day treatment services or enable research opportunities
- Working in conjunction with appropriate resources to provide a uniform and consistent message that will increase the knowledge level of the general public about how children with special needs and their families are similar to all other children and families, yet also face unique challenges and demands
- Educating health insurance companies to acknowledge and meet the needs of the family and child with special needs

The following community agency members are recommended for inclusion on an advisory board:

- Local pediatricians serving children who are medically complex
- County early intervention representatives
- County MR/DD board
- County children's services board representatives

- Physical, occupational, speech therapists
- Area hospital pediatric unit representation
- Local special education school board representation
- Special education teachers
- Area philanthropy specialists
- Any other agency representation whose focus of service is on the population of children with special needs
- Local organization of parents of children with special health care needs — with at least one parent who currently uses the program, if possible

▶ Early Intervention, Early Care, and Education Programs

Forming relationships with organizations that provide early care and education promotes community-wide awareness and commitment to serve children with complex health problems. Head Start and public preschools can be helpful as a curriculum resource and as a resource for care when transition is appropriate, and may be of help financially with some children.

▶ Hospitals, Other Health Care Providers, Colleges, and Universities

Strong relationships with the major providers for acute pediatric care promote timely referrals, cooperation between hospital nursing staff and center-based home health staff, and open lines of communication for all future needs. Out-of-home medical day treatment centers are excellent sites for supervised clinical training of medical students, pediatric and rehabilitation residents, nurses, allied health students, and early childhood educators. Because children attend the program over a long period of time, the experience also provides excellent opportunities to teach best practices for pediatricians who are the medical home for patients with high-tech needs or chronic complex health issues.

Summary

Out-of-home medical day treatment programs provide respite for the family. The central role of the family in the ongoing care of the child is supported when center-based medical day treatment programs are accessible and operated by a quality nursing staff in a natural environment (home or school) that promotes socialization with peers with and without disabilities and developmentally appropriate education. Because the number of children with chronic diseases that may be appropriate for home care is increasing, this specialized medical day treatment should be of interest to all pediatricians and be considered when developing the continuance of care options for children who are medically fragile. This is a cost-effective alternative to pediatric home care delivered exclusively in the home.

Bibliography

American Public Health Association, American Academy of Pediatrics. *Caring for Our Children: National Health and Safety Performance Standards: Guidelines for Out-of-Home Child Care Programs.* 2nd ed. Washington, DC: American Public Health Association. In press

Government Accounting Office. *SSI Children: Multiple Factors Affect Families' Costs for Disability-Related Services.* Washington, DC: GAO/HEHS-99-99; June 1999

The Individuals with Disabilities Education Act Amendments of 1997, 20USC §1400-1485 (1997)

Lally R. *Caring for Infants and Toddlers in Groups: Developmentally Appropriate Practice.* Washington, DC: Zero to Three: National Center for Clinical Infant Programs; 1995

O'Brien M. *Inclusive Child Care for Infants and Toddlers: Meeting Individual and Special Needs.* Baltimore, MD: Paul H. Brooks Publishing Co; 1997:25-77

Perrin JM, Shayne MH, Bloom SR. *Home and Community Care for Chronically Ill Children.* New York, NY: Oxford University Press; 1993:118-135

Pierce PM, Lester DG, Fraze DE. Prescribed pediatric extended care, the family centered health care alternative for medically and technology-dependent children. In: Hochstad NJ, Yost DM, eds. *The Medically Complex Child: The Transition to Home Care.* Chur, Switzerland: Harwood Academic Publishers; 1991:177-190

Porter S, Hayrie M, Bierle T, Caldwell TH, Palfrey JS. *Children and Youth Assisted by Medical Technology in Educational Settings.* Baltimore, MD: Paul H. Brooks Publishing Co; 1997:41-55

Shackelford J. State and jurisdictional eligibility definitions for infants and toddlers with disabilities under IDEA. *NECTAS Notes.* April 2000:1-14

Storgion SA. From hospital to home: transitioning children from acute care facilities. A special report. Available at: http://pedsccm.wustl.edu/file-cabinet/special/special_needs_kids.html. Accessed July 31, 2001

Resources

Illinois Department of Public Health Office of Health Care Regulations
525 W Jefferson
Springfield, IL 62761
William Bell
217/782-2913
www.idph.state.il.us/home.htm

Respite House, Inc.
3510 Hobson Rd
Suite 104 C
Woodbridge, IL 60517
Denise Callerman — Founder
www.respitehouse.org

PART FIVE

Appendices

Home Care Curriculum

Sonia O. Imaizumi, MD; Jay Perman, MD; Mary Elaine Patrinos, MD; Mark Magnusson, MD; Claire Cowen, MA

Home Health Care Curriculum for Residents in Pediatrics

The training of pediatric residents is evolving from a primarily inpatient, acute or critical care/specialty model toward an ambulatory/primary care/preventive medicine community-based model. The Residency Review Committee (RRC) now asks for "Community Medicine" to be an integral part of approved Pediatric Residency Programs. Home care education needs to be a part of that experience and is an area that is currently absent from most pediatric training programs.

The lack of adequate training in this area has contributed to pediatricians largely remaining on the periphery of this reemerging area of pediatric health care. Our vision for the future is to integrate the home setting into pediatric practices and to foster physician participation in home care, service delivery, program planning, and evaluation.

▶ Goals

- Provide pediatric residents experiential learning that will equip them with the knowledge and skills to deliver and supervise health care in the home, through direct "hands-on" learning with increasing levels of responsibility throughout the 3 years of training.
- Upon the completion of the home health care curriculum, residents will understand the value, nature, culture, and philosophy of home care.
- Upon the completion of the home health care curriculum, residents will understand the physician's role and responsibilities, the scope of services available, how to access and utilize those services, and how to coordinate home care services with ambulatory and hospital care.
- Upon the completion of the home health care curriculum, residents will consider the home setting and physician case management an intrinsic part of their practice, and be able to work as a partner with his or her patients and families.

▶ **Objectives**

1. The resident/physician will correctly identify patients eligible for home care.
2. The resident/physician will demonstrate an understanding of the importance of discharge planning, process of referral, and responsibility of care plan oversight.
3. The resident/physician will be aware of required community resources and how to access those resources.
4. The resident/physician will become familiar with current home care cost reimbursement issues along with the impact of managed care on home care.
5. The resident/physician will demonstrate awareness of the types of technology and range of services that can be provided in the home.
6. The resident/physician will understand the physician's role as an active home care team member.
7. The resident/physician will understand the importance of the physician's role in integrating and planning for care across the continuum, including home care.
8. The resident/physician will independently coordinate and perform home care visits for selected patients.
9. The resident/physician will demonstrate awareness of cultural health beliefs and stress factors when deciding the level of support each family requires.
10. The resident/physician will evaluate the adequacy of family and other care providers to provide care in the home.
11. The resident/physician will understand the importance of the primary care physician's or the specialist's role in coordinating and overseeing home care services.

▶ **I. PL-1**

A. Understand the integration of ambulatory and hospital care through participation in
   1. Discharge planning.
   2. Parent teaching.
   3. Coordination of appropriate home care referrals.

B. Develop awareness of available home care technology.

C. Identify, access, and utilize community resources.

D. Effectively employ and evaluate services that can be provided in the home.

E. Effectively recognize the role of the home care nurse.

F. Understand the organizational structure and function of a home care agency, including the role of the medical director.

G. Understand the role of the primary care physician in home care and as a member of an integrated team.

H. Understand core services required for successful home health care.
   1. Intermittent visits
   2. Continuous care
   3. Respite care
   4. Hospice care
   5. Psychological support
   6. Self-help strategies
   7. Infusion/enteral
   8. Nutrition
   9. Durable medical equipment (DME)
   10. Other professionals: respiratory therapists (RTs), occupational therapists (OTs), physical therapists (PTs), etc

▶ II. PL-2

A. Practice appropriate home care assessment skills.
   1. Physical assessments; general assessment, vital signs, nutritional status, etc
   2. Infants: physiological and behavioral competencies
   3. Family readiness from a strengths model rather than deficit model
   4. Psychosocial screening/evaluation
   5. Knowledge of available validated assessment tools (eg, Home Scale, etc)

B. Develop an appropriate plan of care for individual patients, and write the appropriate orders consistent with that plan.

C. Modify a home care plan as necessary after the initial care plan is implemented.

D. Recognize home care issues relative to specific diseases that include but are not limited to the following:
1. IV antibiotics.
2. Home care of infants and children with apnea.
3. Home care of infants and children dependent on a ventilator, including tracheostomy care guidelines.
4. Home care of the child with short bowel syndrome.
5. Home care of the child with bronchopulmonary dysplasia (BPD).
6. Home care of the child with hydrocephalus.
7. Home care of the child with total parenteral nutrition (TPN) and/or enteral feeds.
8. Home care of the child with oncology-related disorders.
9. Home care of the child with human immunodeficiency virus (HIV).
E. Access and/or prescribe other supplemental services (eg, rehabilitative, developmental, occupational, physical and speech therapy, nutrition, home infusion, education, transportation, etc).

▶ III. PL-3

A. Actively coordinate discharge planning and home care plans.
B. Assume the role of case manager.
C. Enhance awareness of financial issues.
1. Reimbursement
2. Insurance/managed care issues
3. Supplemental Security Income (SSI); Women, Infants, and Children (WIC) program; and other local systems
4. Family financial resources

Methodology

▶ I. PL-1

Those who are involved in the planning and provision of home care need to be involved in teaching. Families of children receiving home care must also be involved in educating the residents. The individual institution needs to construct as inclusive a team of teachers as its individual circumstances permit.

The topics outlined in the units of study for a home care curriculum offer a comprehensive outline of the content that needs to be covered. Each institution will need to integrate that content into the recommended methodology described for PL-1s, PL-2s, and PL-3s, as described below.

Suggestions for integration are in italics.

A. Introduction to home care: *Unit I, II, III, IV, V, VI, VII, IX.*
    1. Sufficient lectures and/or panel discussions by those physicians, therapists, nurses, parents, and social workers to provide a basic working knowledge of home care
    2. One case discussed in depth
B. Discharge planning conferences (may vary per institution) — active participation during their regular rotations: *Unit X.*
C. One home visit required. Accompany nurse, physician, therapist, or whoever is responsible for home visits.
D. Case discussions with discharging physicians and write up on patient's chart.

▶ II. PL-2

A. Home visits: *Minimum* of one home visit during the appropriate pediatrics rotation.
B. Specific cases.
    • Standard cases need to be developed that are relevant to each institution.
    • Nursing team meeting.
    • Supervision of these left to each individual institution (advanced practice nurse [APN], MD, etc).
C. Summary evaluation should be in a form of a seminar lead by supervising physician, and possibly other professionals and parents, with each resident presenting the history of the patient and family whose home visit in which the resident participated.

▶ III. PL-3

A. Supervisory role of PL-1 and PL-2, with active teaching role
B. Home visit
C. Agency visit
D. Case management/Discharge planning: *Unit X*

E. QI: *Unit XI*

F. Reimbursement: *Unit VIII*

Concerns

1. Articulated curriculum: undergraduate — graduate — postgraduate medical education.

2. An evaluative component.

  a. Summary evaluation: as in (C) above.

  b. National standards to be developed with an objective evaluation tool (sample attached).

3. Safety concern issues should be addressed by individual institution.

4. Residents must have one-to-one supervision.

Suggested Units

Units may be grouped for lectures and during PL-1 year may occur during regular didactic lectures.

I. **Unit I Overview**

  History of home care

  Organization

  Mission

  Program development

II. **Unit II Nursing Overview**

  Field staff

  Types of patients

  Clinical management philosophy

  Communications

  On-call roles and responsibilities

  Geography

III. **Nursing Intake Functions**

  Flow of intake

  Physician role/responsibility

  Documentation/medical records

  Vendor resources

IV.   **Unit IV Pharmacy**
        Physician orders
        Clinical monitoring
        Maintaining pharmacy orders

V.   **Unit V DME/RT**
        Flow of intake
        Coordination of services
        Documentation/medical record
        Vendor resources

VI.   **Unit VI Patient Services**
        Review patient census
        Patient supply management
        Patient communication
        Physician communication
        Nutritional monitoring program

VII. **Unit VII Warehouse and Delivery**
        Review home care equipment purchasing, maintenance,
            and biomed
        Shipping

VIII. **Unit VIII Reimbursement**
        Team overview
        Role on intake
        Contracts
        Physician orders

IX.   **Unit IX Social Work**
        Overview of staff
        Support groups
        Bereavement
        Referral

X.   **Unit X Case Management**
        Community resources
        Utilization

XI. Unit XI CQI

Rounds

Nursing team meeting

Care team meeting

Case management

Visits

Home visit with nursing x 2

Supportive care visit x 1

Homeless health visit x 1

Home visit with respiratory therapist

Home delivery x 1

The Children's Regional Hospital at the Cooper Health System
Department of Pediatrics

INTERN/RESIDENT EVALUATION FOR HOME HEALTH CARE EXPERIENCE

Name: _____ Date: _____

Site(s): _____

Preceptor: _____

Goal: Engage in an interactive experience outside the clinical setting in preparation for assuming the role of advocate for the health and well-being of the children and families within the community.

Objectives:
1. The resident will develop an appreciation of the complex social, emotional, and physical needs of the child and family.
2. The resident will understand the role of this preceptor in the life of the child and family.

1. Was the resident on time? _____

2. Did the resident evidence interest and willingness? _____

3. Was the resident able to acquire appropriate information while taking history? _____

4. Did the resident interact appropriately?   ☐ yes ☐ no
   Please elaborate. _____

5. Please write a brief description of the resident's activities during the time he or she was with you. _____

HOME CARE EDUCATION
GENERAL EVALUATION

Describe two or three of the most significant learning experiences.

1.

2.

3.

Describe two or three of the least valuable learning experiences.

1.

2.

3.

List suggestions for improvement.

1.

2.

3.

Please provide an overall evaluation of your experience with
Home Care Education:

Evaluation Form
Home Care
Field Experience

LOW				HIGH
1	2	3	4	5

Date: _____

Location: _____

Family/Facilitator at Site: _____

Complete the following questions by circling the one number that describes your rating.

The rating scale ranges from 1-5; 1=not at all and 5=very much so.

Did your introductory lectures prepare you appropriately for your field experience?   1 2 3 4 5

Did you feel supported and well guided during the experience?   1 2 3 4 5

Did your facilitator guide you in understanding the goal of the experience in the context of the individual child and family needs?   1 2 3 4 5

Did your facilitator guide you in understanding of your role in supporting the child, parent, family, and/or caregiver through the experience?   1 2 3 4 5

Were your expectations of the session met?   1 2 3 4 5

Was the session motivating and energizing toward your own work?   1 2 3 4 5

What prepared you the most for this experience?

What did you find most valuable of this experience toward your work with children and families in your work?

Comments and Recommendations:

Year of Pediatric Resident: Yr. 1   Yr. 2   Yr. 3

Name: _____ Age:_____(Optional)
Years Experience in Pediatrics: _____

Emergency Information Form

Emergency Information Form for Children With Special Needs

American College of Emergency Physicians®	American Academy of Pediatrics DEDICATED TO THE HEALTH OF ALL CHILDREN™	Date Form Completed By Whom	Revised Revised	Initials Initials

Name:	Birth Date: Nickname:
Home Address:	Home/Work Phone:
Parent/Guardian:	Emergency Contact Names and Relationship:
Signature/Consent*:	
Primary Language:	Phone Number(s):

Physicians:

Primary Care Physician:	Emergency Phone:
	Fax:
Current Specialty Physician: Specialty:	Emergency Phone: Fax:
Current Specialty Physician: Specialty:	Emergency Phone: Fax:
Anticipated Primary ED:	Pharmacy:
Anticipated Tertiary Care Center:	

Diagnoses/Past Procedures/Physical Exam:

1. _____   Baseline Physical Findings: _____

2. _____   _____

3. _____   Baseline Vital Signs: _____

4. _____   _____

Synopsis: _____   Baseline Neurological Status: _____

*Consent for release of this form to health care providers

521

Last name:

Diagnoses/Past Procedures/Physical Exam continued:

Medications:

1.

2.

3.

4.

5.

6.

Significant Baseline Ancillary Findings (lab, x-ray, ECG):

Prostheses/Appliances/Advanced Technology Devices:

Management Data:

Allergies: Medications/Foods to Be Avoided   **and why:**

1.

2.

3.

Procedures to Be Avoided   **and why:**

1.

2.

3.

Immunizations

Dates						Dates					
DPT						Hep B					
OPV						Varicella					
MMR						TB status					
HIB						Other					

Antibiotic Prophylaxis: Indication: Medication and Dose:

Common Presenting Problems/Findings With Specific Suggested Managements

Problem   Suggested Diagnostic Studies   Treatment Considerations

---

Comments on Child, Family, or Other Specific Medical Issues:

Physician/Provider Signature: **Print Name:**

Self-Assessment Inventory for Family-Centered Pediatric Home Care

Institute for Family-Centered Care

7900 Wisconsin Ave, Suite 405, Bethesda, MD 20814, Phone: 301/652-0281, Fax: 301/652-0186

MOVING TOWARD FAMILY-CENTERED PEDIATRIC HOME CARE

A Self-Assessment Inventory

Instructions: This tool will help you think about family-centered care in relation to pediatric home care policies, programs, practices, and environments. This tool can help prioritize the next steps for moving forward with family-centered care and creating a process of change. It is designed for use with a multidisciplinary, multiperspective team that includes families who have experienced pediatric home care.

The checklist is divided into the following nine sections:

- Philosophy of Care
- Patterns of Care
- Family Participation in Caregiving
- Information Sharing
- Child and Family Support
- Documentation
- Environment and Design
- Families as Advisors
- Personnel Practices

Your team can choose to work on selected sections, or to complete the entire checklist. The team should discuss each item and decide on one team response. Some users have found it helpful to have individuals complete the tool and then meet as a group, discuss responses, and formulate a group response. We recommend setting aside several hours for the team to complete this checklist.

The first task is to rate each item as 0, 1, or 2 according to how well you think your home care program is applying the concepts of family-centered care. Rate each statement 0=we are not doing well, 1=we are doing okay, or 2=we are doing very well. This 3-point scale is not an attempt to get a precise numerical rating, but rather is a way to begin thinking as a team about the degree to which family-centered concepts are reflected in home care policies and programs, in facility design, and in staff interactions. Be aware that if you complete this tool more than once, you may find that your scores go *down* before they go up. As your awareness of family-centered care increases, you will rate the home care program more critically.

After rating an item, describe one or more specific examples that illustrate how family-centered care is or is not happening in your home care program in relation to that item. The examples provided in this section are the most important and most useful part of your response, so we recommend that you spend the most time in your team discussion on developing specific examples.

When you have completed all of the items in the entire checklist, answer the open-ended questions at the end of this inventory and discuss next steps to further implement family-centered concepts in your program or practice.

Philosophy of Care

0=not well, 1=okay, or 2=very well

	0	1	2	Specific Examples (positive or negative)
Does the home care program or agency have a written philosophy statement that				
• Recognizes the importance of conveying respect and preserving the dignity of each individual and family?				
• Acknowledges the individuality, strengths, and culture of each family?				
• Acknowledges the importance of families and other support persons to the care and comfort of the child or adolescent?				
• Promotes information sharing with each family and supports their participation in decision-making about their child's care?				

Philosophy of Care (continued)

0=not well, 1=okay, or 2=very well

	0	1	2	**Specific Examples (positive or negative)**
• Respects and supports the choices of each family for how they participate in caregiving and care planning?				
• Recognizes the importance of continuity of care between hospital and home?				
• Recognizes emotional, spiritual, and practical support as essential components of care?				
• Affirms the importance of having meaningful opportunities for families who have experienced pediatric home care to collaborate in policy formulation and in program planning, implementation, and evaluation?				
Is there a process in place to review, and if necessary, revise your home care agency's philosophy of care statement?				
Is the philosophy of care reflected in				
• Home care policies?				
• Operating procedure?				
• Staff selection, evaluation, and promotion?				
• Staffing patterns?				
• Strategic planning?				
Is the philosophy of care statement communicated to the families who are served by the home care program or agency?				
Were families who have experienced home care involved in developing the philosophy of care statement?				

Additional notes:

Patterns of Care

0=not well, 1=okay, or 2=very well

	0	1	2	Specific Examples (positive or negative)
Do home care staff interact respectfully with all children, youth, and families?				
Do home care staff introduce themselves to children, youth, and family members in all interactions?				
Are the roles of all team members clear to the family and, when developmentally appropriate, the child?				
Do pediatric home care staff collaborate/interact respectfully with each other?				
Are contributions from different disciplines coordinated and integrated into the care plan?				
Is there one individual designated to work with the family as the care coordinator or case manager?				
Do staffing patterns promote continuity and predictability for infants, children, youth, and their families?				
Are back-up plans in place for providing services when regular providers are not available?				
Is there continuity in equipment and approaches to care between the hospital and home setting?				
Is there a commitment to collaborative decision making?				

Patterns of Care (continued)

0=not well, 1=okay, or 2=very well

	0	1	2	**Specific Examples (positive or negative)**
Do pediatric home care staff respect and support decisions made by families, even when there is disagreement?				
Are there supportive procedures for resolving disputes between families and pediatric home care staff?				
Is there an ethics committee available to families and pediatric home care staff?				

Additional notes:

Family Participation in Caregiving

0=not well, 1=okay, or 2=very well

	0	1	2	Specific Examples (positive or negative)
Are families recognized as integral members of the child's health care team?				
• Is a child or adolescent recognized as an integral member of his or her health care team?				
Do families participate from the beginning in hospital discharge planning and other transition planning for home care?				
Are families provided with criteria or short-term goals specific for determining their child's discharge from the hospital?				
Are families, and when developmentally appropriate, children and youth, encouraged to participate in the development of home care plans?				
Are policies and practices flexible in order to meet individual preferences and needs?				
Are cultural beliefs and practices of each family respected and followed whenever possible?				
Do pediatric home care staff support family members in their nurturing and caregiving roles?				
Do staff support families in helping their children cope with stress?				
Do home care staff work in ways that enhance families' self-sufficiency?				

Additional notes:

Information Sharing

0=not well, 1=okay, or 2=very well

	0	1	2	Specific Examples (positive or negative)
Do families receive complete, unbiased information about the care plan and various approaches to treatment?				
Do families receive written information about their rights and responsibilities in home care?				
Are families and home care staff provided with guidelines for setting appropriate boundaries in therapeutic relationships?				
Do families have information about • Specific services? • Equipment/supplies? • Medications? • Laboratory specimens? • Personnel? • Frequency and duration of home care visits covered by their health plan or insurance? • Alternative sources of equipment, supplies, services?				
Are meetings, conference calls, and e-mail used regularly with families and other care providers to facilitate communication, coordination of care, and reassessment of the care plan?				
Do families, and when developmentally appropriate, children and youth, have the opportunity to identify their priorities for health information, education, and training?				

Information Sharing (continued)

0=not well, 1=okay, or 2=very well

	0	1	2	Specific Examples (positive or negative)
Do families receive education and the opportunity to practice new caregiving skills and procedures to *their* level of satisfaction?				
In hospital or clinic settings, do families have the opportunity to practice using equipment that is the same as what they will use at home?				
Are there varied ways in which information is shared with families? With children and youth? • Do home care providers bring to the home setting information (eg, brochures, videos, Web site information) to the family and, when developmentally appropriate, to the child?				
Is there a family resource center available to families? • Are pediatric home care providers knowledgeable about family resource libraries and how to access their services?				
Are information and educational materials for children, youth, and families developed in a collaborative manner that involves these consumers in planning the content, design, and dissemination of materials?				
Are information materials for children, youth, and families available in a range of reading levels (eg, 5th grade to more advanced reading levels)?				

Information Sharing (continued)

0=not well, 1=okay, or 2=very well

	0	1	2	Specific Examples (positive or negative)
Is written information provided in the primary languages of the families served by the home care agency? • Are translators and interpreters available for families who do not speak English or who use sign language?				
Are information materials available in audio/visual formats?				
Are pediatric home care staff able to communicate with families who are deaf or hearing impaired? • Is a TTY or relay system available for people who are deaf or hearing impaired?				

Additional notes:

Child and Family Support

0=not well, 1=okay, or 2=very well

	0	1	2	**Specific Examples** (positive or negative)
Are pediatric home care services coordinated with, and specific referrals made to, services and programs that families may want or need				
• Community-based primary care providers?				
• Specialists and other hospital-based health care team members?				
• Classes in CPR and emergency care planning?				
• Family-to-family support programs?				
• Peer support programs for children and youth?				
• Organizations for children with special needs?				
• Respite care?				
• Mental health services?				
• Social services?				
• Financial support services?				
• Domestic violence prevention programs?				
• Substance abuse prevention and treatment programs?				
• Child abuse prevention and treatment programs?				
• Early childhood development services?				
• School programs and tutoring?				
• Child care agencies?				

Child and Family Support (continued)

0=not well, 1=okay, or 2=very well

	0	1	2	Specific Examples (positive or negative)
Are pediatric home care services coordinated with, and specific referrals made to, services and programs that families may want or need (continued) • Parenting education? • Hospice services? • Bereavement groups? • Other services identified by families?				
Do pediatric home care staff help families connect with other families who are having or have had similar experiences?				

Documentation

0=not well, 1=okay, or 2=very well

	0	1	2	Specific Examples (positive or negative)
Are pediatric home care documentation procedures and forms developed in consultation with families who have experienced home care?				
Do methods of documentation obtain and convey information in ways that protect the privacy and respect the choices of families?				
Do documentation procedures and charting forms encourage • The family, and when possible the child, to identify their strengths and needs? • The recording of the child's and family's goals, priorities, and preferences as identified by family and child, when possible?				

Documentation (continued)

0=not well, 1=okay, or 2=very well

	0	1	2	Specific Examples (positive or negative)
Is the documentation system used as a tool to facilitate communication among • Family and all other members of the interdisciplinary health care team? • Providers across shifts and the family? • In-home providers, primary care providers, and specialists involved in the child's health care? • Family, home care staff, and other community agencies, such as schools and child care and recreation programs?				
Do families have access to their child's chart?				
Can families write comments, observations, or questions in their child's chart?				

Additional notes:

Environment and Design

0=not well, 1=okay, or 2=very well

	0	1	2	Specific Examples (positive or negative)
Do home care providers work with the family to arrange the physical environment for care in the home to				
• Honor the privacy of the child? Privacy of the family?				
• Promote normalcy and natural routines for the child and family?				
• Enable the child, as much as possible to ~ Actively participate in care?				
~ Carry out developmentally appropriate tasks?				
~ Have fun?				
~ Be as independent as possible (in what may be a very dependent situation)?				
• Minimize intrusiveness in family living spaces?				
• Facilitate ease and convenience of caregiving?				
• As appropriate, ensure that phone and electric companies are aware of the need for priority service?				
• Adapt equipment to the family's home?				
• Allow for adequate storage of supplies and equipment?				
• Ensure the safety of the child and other family members?				

Additional notes:

Families as Advisors

0=not well, 1=okay, or 2=very well

	0	1	2	Specific Examples (positive or negative)
Are families who received pediatric home care, and their family members, involved in advisory activities such as • A family advisory council? • Formal committees and task forces? • Informal workgroups and discussions?				
Are there formal or informal opportunities for families to share good ideas, insights, strategies, and resources with staff and other families?				
Do families served by the pediatric home care program participate in designing, evaluating, and interpreting quality improvement initiatives?				
Are there systematic procedures for gathering information about families' perceptions of care and satisfaction with home care policies, programs, and practices?				
Are families served by the home care program involved in the collection and analysis of information about experiences and perceptions of care?				
Are families involved in responding to and finding solutions to the ideas, suggestions, and concerns expressed by other consumers of the pediatric home care program or agency?				
In academic medical centers, are patients and families involved in teaching students and professionals-in-training about pediatric home care and the family experience of this type of care?				

Personnel Practices

0=not well, 1=okay, or 2=very well

	0	1	2	Specific Examples (positive or negative)
Do home care staff have the training and technical competence to provide care in the home to infants, children, and youth?				
Do home care staff have the training and expertise to work in a collaborative manner with families from diverse backgrounds?				
Do pediatric home care staff ask families about their preferences, priorities, concerns, and goals for home care?				
Are policies and practices in place that encourage the recruiting and hiring of individuals with age-appropriate pediatric experience, and family-centered skills and attitudes?				
Do the individuals providing pediatric home care reflect the cultural and ethnic diversity of families served?				
Do all pediatric home care staff, both direct service providers and others, such as receptionists, secretaries, supervisors, and administrators, view every encounter with a family receiving home care services as an opportunity to contribute to the family's competence and confidence?				
Do position descriptions and performance appraisals clearly state that all home care employees demonstrate the knowledge, skills, and attitudes consistent with philosophy of care (described on pages 524–525)?				

Personnel Practices (continued)   0=not well, 1=okay, or 2=very well

	0	1	2	**Specific Examples** (positive or negative)
Do position descriptions and performance appraisals clearly articulate the importance of working in respectful, supportive, and collaborative ways with children, youth, and families?				
Do supervisors of staff providing home care services check in with families about employee performance on a regular basis?				
Are families asked to participate in search committees or interviews for leadership staff for pediatric home care?				
Are orientation and in-service programs provided to support all home care staff in acquiring family-centered, culturally competent knowledge, skills, and attitudes?				
Are there supervised opportunities for hospital-based staff and home care staff to learn about home care and family perspectives in families' homes? • Are families trained and supported in serving as faculty for these educational home visits?				
Does in-service programming include discussions about • Family-centered principles? • Effective interpersonal communication? • Cultural competence? • Child development?				

Personnel Practices (continued)

0=not well, 1=okay, or 2=very well

	0	1	2	Specific Examples (positive or negative)
Does in-service programming include discussions about (continued)				
• Identifying and building on child and family strengths?				
• Providing care in a developmentally supportive manner?				
• Supporting families in appropriate ways?				
• Sharing medical and other information with children, youth, and families?				
• Adapting care to individual home situations?				
• Collaborating with consumers?				
Are strategies in place to support staff and address issues of social isolation and other challenging aspects of working alone in a home setting?				
Do families who have been consumers of pediatric home care services participate as faculty for staff orientation and in-service programs?				
Are there rewards for staff who demonstrate excellence in providing family-centered pediatric home care?				

Additional notes:

Questions for Discussion:

Are there other ways that your pediatric home care program demonstrates a commitment
to family-centered care?

What are the biggest challenges your home care program faces in implementing family-centered
care (eg, identifying family members to serve on committees, attitudes of administrative staff, cut-
backs in personnel)?

What are the opportunities for family-centered change in your home care program at this time (eg, new staff recently hired, a continuous quality improvement team with energy and creativity)?

What are the 3-5 top priorities for family-centered change in your home care program?

Name of home care program: _____

Team members who completed this checklist:

Name	Professional Discipline/Patient/Family Members

Web Sites for Home Care-Related Organizations

Organization		URL
AAHCP	American Academy of Home Care Physicians	http://www.aahcp.org/
AAHomecare	American Association for Homecare	http://www.aahomecare.org/
AAHP	American Association of Health Plans	http://www.aahp.org/
AAP	American Academy of Pediatrics	http://www.aap.org/
AARC	American Association for Respiratory Care	http://www.aarc.org/
AFHHA	American Federation of Home Health Agencies	http://www.his.com/~afhha/usa.html/
CHAP	Community Health Accreditation Program	http://www.chapinc.org/
CHCA	Child Health Corporation of America	http://www.chca.com/
CMS	Centers for Medicare and Medicaid Services (formerly Health Care Financing Administration [HCFA])	http://cms.hhs.gov/
HIAA	Health Insurance Association of America	http://www.hiaa.org/
INS	Infusion Nurses Society	http://www.ins1.org/
JCAHO	Joint Commission on Accreditation of Healthcare Organizations	http://www.jcaho.org/
NACHRI	National Association of Children's Hospitals and Related Institutions	http://www.childrenshospitals.net/index.htm/
NAHC	National Association for Home Care	http://www.nahc.org/

Organization		URL
NAPHAC[2]	National Association of Pediatric Home and Community Care	http://www.gnofn.org/~naphacc/whatis.html/
NAPNAP	National Association of Pediatric Nurse Practitioners	http://www.napnap.org/
NCQA	National Committee for Quality Assurance	http://www.ncqa.org/
NHIA	National Home Infusion Association	http://www.nhianet.org/

Index